W9-ARF-034

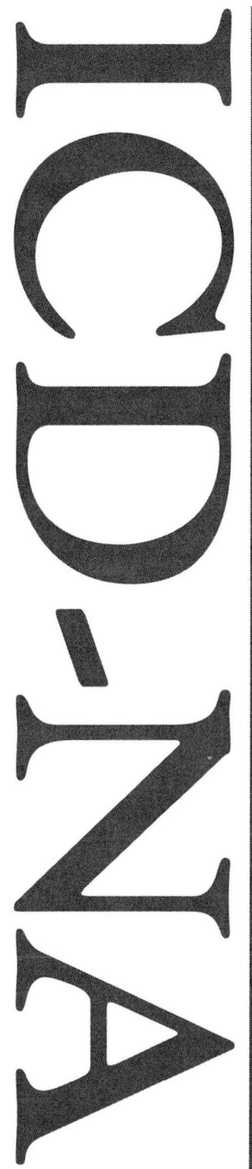

Application of the International Classification of Diseases to Neurology

Second Edition

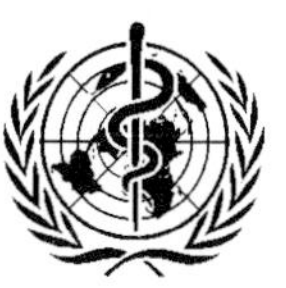

World Health Organization
Geneva
1997

First edition 1987
Second edition 1997

Application of the international classification of diseases to neurology: ICD-NA – 2nd ed.

1. Neurology — classification 2. Nervous system diseases — classification I. Title: ICD-NA

ISBN 92 4 154502 X (NLM Classification: WL 15)

Typeset in Hong Kong
Printed in Canada
95/10663–Best-set/Tri-Graphics–8000

Contents

Preface

The Application of the International Classification of Diseases to Neurology (ICD-NA) is one of several adaptations of the Tenth Revision of the International Statistical Classification of Diseases and Related Health Problems (ICD-10) being produced by the World Health Organization to respond to the needs of specialist disciplines such as neurology. A previous edition of ICD-NA was developed in 1984–85 with the help of a group of experts convened by Dr L. Bolis (International Foundation Fatebenefratelli, Milan, Italy), then in charge of activities dealing with the prevention and control of neurological disorders in WHO's Division of Mental Health (MNH). Taking into account the recommendations of this expert group and advice received from the Neuroepidemiology Group of the World Federation of Neurology, chaired by the late Professor B.S. Schoenberg (National Institutes of Health, Bethesda, MD) and from other nongovernmental organizations, Professor J.-M. Orgogozo and Professor J.F. Dartigues (University of Bordeaux, France) drafted the text of the first edition in English and French. That edition provided an extensive selection, but a limited expansion, of the neurologically relevant codes of ICD-9. The present edition has been developed with the broader aim of providing an individual code for almost every neurological condition, so that a uniform classification is available for epidemiological and clinical research as well as for routine statistical reporting.

The synopsis of the second edition of ICD-NA was produced by Professor W.G. Bradley (University of Miami, Miami, FL), Professor J.-M. Orgogozo, Dr N. Sartorius (then Director of WHO's Division of Mental Health) and Dr J. van Drimmelen (WHO, Geneva, Switzerland). It was discussed with representatives of nongovernmental organizations active in the field of neurology and with experts in WHO and from various Member countries and then used as a framework for the development of the ICD-NA.

The initial draft of ICD-NA was produced by Professors Bradley and Orgogozo with the help of Dr van Drimmelen on the basis of the first edition and of detailed suggestions from the Ad Hoc Committee on Disease Classification of the American Neurological Association, chaired by Professor Bradley; in the Acknowledgements section (pages ix–xii), the names of the members of the committee are marked with an asterisk. The draft was examined by nongovernmental organizations active in the field of neurology (listed on page xi) and by numerous advisers. Their valuable comments contributed to the production of the penultimate version of ICD-NA, which was again reviewed by the participating nongovernmental organizations.

The final version reflects the best resolution of many, often competing, needs. It should be kept in mind that ICD-NA had to be based upon the structure of ICD-10. This has prevented the introduction of some changes that were recommended, but has ensured that all of the 5-, 6- and 7-character codes of the ICD-NA can be contracted back into the original 3- or 4-character codes of ICD-10; compatibility with the official classification can therefore be maintained, whatever the purpose or level of utilization.

The ICD-NA index was produced by Mr M. Catan and Dr van Drimmelen of WHO, using a preliminary partial draft produced by Drs H.J. Freyberger and C. Kessler (Lübeck, Germany), with extensive help from Mr A. L'Hours of WHO's Division of Health Situation and Trend Assessment. Guidance from Mr l'Hours also helped to ensure the congruence of ICD-NA with the parent ICD-10.

An outline of the history of the International Classification of Diseases, information on the structure of ICD-NA and instructions on its use are given in Sections I and II of this publication.

Dr N.P. Napalkov
Assistant Director-General
World Health Organization

Acknowledgements

The following organizations provided invaluable support to the development of this publication:

American Academy of Neurology
American Neurological Association
American Sleep Disorders Association
European Federation of Neurological Societies
European Stroke Council
International Brain Research Organization
International Bureau for Epilepsy
International Cerebral Palsy Society
International Child Neurology Association
International Federation of Multiple Sclerosis Societies
International Headache Society
International League Against Epilepsy
International Movement Disorder Society
International Society of Neuropathology
International Stroke Society
World Federation for Mental Health
World Federation of Neurology
World Federation of Neurosurgical Societies

Special thanks are due to Lord Walton of Detchant, whose continuing and strong support greatly facilitated the work on this publication, and to Professor Armand Lowenthal, of the World Federation of Neurology (WFN), who was particularly helpful in obtaining comments from Committees and Research Groups of the World Federation of Neurology.

Administrative support for this work was provided by Ms J. Gilmore, Mrs J. Joseph and Mrs T. Drouillet.

The work done by the following individuals, whose comments were particularly helpful and thoughtful, is gratefully acknowledged. Members of the Ad Hoc Committee on Neurological Classification of the American Neurological Association are indicated with an asterisk (*).

*Dr R. Ackerman, Boston, MA, USA
*Dr H. Adams, Glasgow, Scotland

Dr Y. Agid, Paris, France
Dr A. Ahmed, Karachi, Pakistan
Dr L. Amaducci, Florence, Italy
Dr S. Araki, Kumamoto, Japan
*Dr B. Arnason, Chicago, IL, USA
*Dr J. Bale, Iowa City, IA, USA
*Dr B. Banker, Hanover, Germany
Sir Roger Bannister, Oxford, England
Dr B. Barac, Zagreb, Croatia
Dr H. Barnett, London, Ontario, Canada
*Dr R.W. Beck, Tampa, FL, USA
*Dr W. Bell, Iowa City, IA, USA
*Dr D.F. Benson, Los Angeles, CA, USA
Dr A. Beraldelli, Rome, Italy
*Dr J. Berger, Miami, FL, USA
Dr N.E. Bharucha, Bombay, India
Dr K.L. Bick, Washington, DC, USA
Dr C.D. Binnie, London, England
*Dr P. Black, Boston, MA, USA
Dr J.P. Blass, New York, NY, USA
*Dr J. Blavis, New York, NY, USA
Dr J. Bogousslavsky, Lausanne, Switzerland
*Dr W.G. Bradley, Miami, FL, USA
*Dr B. Brookes, Madison, WI, USA
*Dr J. Bruni, Mississauga, Ontario, Canada
*Dr L. Caplan, Boston, MA, USA
Dr P. Casaer, Louvain, Belgium
Dr J.-P. Castel, Bordeaux, France
*Dr M. Cohen, Buffalo, NY, USA
*Dr M. Cole, Mayfield Heights, OH, USA
*Dr P. Cooper, London, Ontario, Canada
Dr R. Currier, Jackson, MS, USA
*Dr D. Dalessio, La Jolla, CA, USA
*Dr A. Damasio, Iowa City, IA, USA
Dr J.P. Dartigues, Bordeaux, France
*Dr J. Daube, Rochester, MN, USA
Dr D.E. Deisenhammer, Vienna, Austria
*Dr R. DeLorenzo, Richmond, VA, USA
*Dr S. Diamond, Chicago, IL, USA
*Dr R. Dorwart, Burlington, VT, USA
*Dr D. Drachman, Worcester, MA, USA
Dr C. Dravet, Marseilles, France
*Dr F.E. Dreifuss, Charlottesville, VA, USA
*Dr R. Duvoisin, New Brunswick, NJ, USA

*Dr P. Dyck, Rochester, MN, USA
*Dr A.G. Engel, Rochester, MN, USA
*Dr O.B. Evans, Jackson, MS, USA
*Dr S. Fahn, New York, NY, USA
Dr N. Fejerman, Buenos Aires, Argentina
*Dr R. Feldman, Boston, MA, USA
*Dr G. Fenichel, Nashville, TN, USA
*Dr P. Finelli, Providence, RI, USA
*Dr R.A. Fishman, San Francisco, CA, USA
Dr S. Flache, Geneva, Switzerland
Dr D. Gardner-Medwin, Newcastle-upon-Tyne, England
Dr C. Goetz, Chicago, IL, USA
*Dr M. Gomez, Rochester, MN, USA
*Dr B. Griggs, Rochester, MN, USA
*Dr C. Gross, Burlington, VT, USA
*Dr A. Harding, London, England
Dr O. Henriksen, Sandvika, Norway
Dr P. Henry, Bordeaux, France
Dr A. Huber, Zurich, Switzerland
*Dr J.T. Hughes, Oxford, England
*Dr C. Jablecki, San Diego, CA, USA
Dr P. Jallon, Geneva, Switzerland
Dr J. Jancovic, Houston, TX, USA
*Dr P.J. Janetta, Pittsburgh, PA, USA
Dr F.R. Jeri, Lima, Peru
*Dr R.T. Johnson, Baltimore, MD, USA
*Dr B. Katzman, La Jolla, CA, USA
Dr J. Kesselring, Bad Ragaz, Switzerland
*Dr A. Khachaturian, Bethesda, MD, USA
*Dr J. Kimura, Kyoto, Japan
*Dr E. Kolodny, Waltham, MA, USA
Dr K. Kondo, Sapporo, Japan
*Dr A.E. Lang, Toronto, Canada
*Dr P. Lavin, Nashville, TN, USA
Dr H. Lechner, Graz, Austria
Dr M. Leonardi, Geneva, Switzerland
*Dr P. Lequesne, London, England
Dr I. Lesny, Prague, Czech Republic
*Dr J. Lieberman, Sacramento, CA, USA
*Dr A. Lockwood, Houston, TX, USA
Dr C. Loeb, Genoa, Italy
Dr J.N. Loeber, Heemstede, Netherlands
Dr P. Loiseau, Bordeaux, France
*Dr P.A. Low, Rochester, MN, USA

Dr A. Lowenthal, Antwerp, Belgium
Dr S.K. Ludwin, Toronto, Ontario, Canada
Dr C.D. Marsden, London, England
*Dr J. Martin, Boston, MA, USA
Dr J.M. Martinez-Lage, Pamplona, Spain
*Dr C.J. Mathias, London, England
Dr W.I. McDonald, London, England
*Dr D. McFarlin, Bethesda, MD, USA
Dr H. Meinardi, Heemstede, Netherlands
*Dr M. Mendez, Cleveland, OH, USA
*Dr M. Mesulam, Boston, MA, USA
*Dr R. Miller, San Francisco, CA, USA
Dr G.R.W. Moore, Vancouver, Canada
*Dr H. Moser, Baltimore, MD, USA
Dr C. Munari, Grenoble, France
Dr N.J.M. Mwang'Ombe, Nairobi, Kenya
Dr G. Nappi, Pavia, Italy
*Dr F. Norris Jr, San Francisco, CA, USA
Dr J. Olesen, Hellerup, Denmark
Dr A.T. Ordinario, Manila, Philippines
*Dr D. Parks, London, England
Dr D.W. Paty, Vancouver, Canada
*Dr W. Pendlebury, Burlington, VT, USA
*Dr D. Perl, New York, NY, USA
Mr T. Petzal, London, England
Dr K. Poeck, Aachen, Germany
*Dr R. Polinsky, Bethesda, MD, USA
Dr R.J. Porter, Bethesda, MD, USA
*Dr J. Posner, New York, NY, USA
Dr S.B. Prusiner, San Francisco, CA, USA
Dr N.P. Quinn, London, England
Dr F. Regli, Lausanne, Switzerland
*Dr S. Reichlin, Boston, MA, USA
Dr Rhong-Chi Chen, Taiwan, China
*Dr K. Ricker, Wurzburg, Germany
*Dr J. Riggs, Morgantown, WV, USA
Dr P. Rodgers-Johnson, Bethesda, MD, USA
Dr J. Roger, Marseilles, France
*Dr L.P. Rowland, New York, NY, USA
*Dr D. Rushton, London, England
*Dr D.B. Sanders, Durham, NC, USA
Dr J.R. Santoni M., Santo Domingo, Dominican Republic
*Dr H. Schaumburg, New York, NY, USA
*Dr J. Schmidley, Cleveland, OH, USA

Dr M. Seino, Shizuoka, Japan
Dr S. Sen, Calcutta, India
Dr D. Simpson, Adelaide, Australia
Dr V. Smirnov, Moscow, Russian Federation
*Dr B. Snyder, St Paul, MN, USA
Dr A. Spina-Franca, São Paulo, Brazil
*Dr R. Sriram, Nashville, TN, USA
Dr H. Stefan, Erlangen, Germany
*Dr D. Stumpf, Chicago, IL, USA
Dr L. Symon, London, England
*Dr R. Tandan, Burlington, VT, USA
*Dr G. Teasdale, Glasgow, Scotland
*Dr R. Terry, La Jolla, CA, USA
Dr F. Tison, Bordeaux, France
Dr E. Tolosa, Barcelona, Spain
*Dr R. Tomsak, Cleveland, OH, USA
*Dr B.T. Troost, Winston-Salem, NC, USA
Dr N. Vereschagin, Moscow, Russian Federation
*Dr S. Wald, Burlington, VT, USA
Dr S. Walker III, La Jolla, CA, USA
Lord Walton of Detchant, Oxford, England
Dr P. Wolf, Bielefeld, Germany
*Dr J. Wolinsky, Houston, TX, USA
*Dr S. Wolpert, Boston, MA, USA
Dr M.D. Yahr, New York, NY, USA
Dr N. Yanagisawa, Matsumoto, Japan
*Dr F. Yatsu, Houston, TX, USA
Dr Zhi Ping Qu, Shanghai, China

SECTION I

Introduction

1. What is the International Classification of Diseases (ICD)?

1.1 The history of ICD

Classification is fundamental to science and a standard classification of diseases and injury is essential for systematic, statistical studies of illness and death. This was recognized as early as the seventeenth century when such studies started. In 1853, Dr William Farr of London and Dr Marc d'Espine of Geneva were entrusted by the first International Statistical Congress (ISC), held in Brussels, with the task of preparing "a uniform nomenclature of causes of death applicable to all countries". They submitted two separate lists, based on very different principles. The classification of Dr William Farr was arranged under five groups: epidemic diseases, constitutional (general) diseases, local diseases arranged by anatomical site, developmental diseases, and diseases that are the direct result of violence. Dr Marc d'Espine had classified diseases according to their nature (gouty, herpetic, haematic, etc.). The Congress adopted a compromise list of 139 rubrics.

Although there was never any universal acceptance of this classification, the general arrangement, including the principle of classifying diseases by anatomical site proposed by Farr, has survived as the basis of the *International List of Causes of Death.* At its meeting in Vienna in 1891, the International Statistical Institute, successor to the ISC, charged a committee, under the chairmanship of Jacques Bertillon (Paris), with the preparation of a classification of causes of death. In 1893, at the meeting in Chicago, the Institute adopted Bertillon's proposal. His classification was based on the principle of distinguishing between general diseases and those localized to a particular organ or anatomical site. It represented a synthesis of French, English, German, and Swiss classifications. Bertillon included three versions: the first an abridged classification of 44 titles, the second a classification of 99 titles, and the third a classification of 161 titles.

The Bertillon Classification of Causes of Death, as it was initially called, received general approval and was adopted by several countries, as well as by many individual cities, and was revised about every 10 years. In 1948, the newly created World Health Organization was asked to undertake the regular review and revision of the classification. Thus WHO took responsibility for the Sixth Revision, which for the first time provided a single list applicable to both morbidity and mortality. This list was renamed "The International Statistical Classification of Diseases, Injuries and Causes of Death (ICD)".

Since that time, ICD — in addition to its traditional application to epidemiology — has been increasingly used for the indexing and retrieval of medical records and for statistics concerning the planning, monitoring, and evaluation of health services. The Eighth Revision Conference met in Geneva in 1965; the resulting ICD-8 was of a more radical nature than the Seventh Revision but left unchanged the basic structure of the Classification and the general philosophy of classifying diseases according to their etiology rather than a particular manifestation. A major innovation was the development of descriptions for the Mental Disorder Chapter, which was published separately with a view to overcoming the particular difficulties in a field where international terminology had not been standardized.

The Ninth Revision was adopted in 1976. Although it was considered that this ought to have been a limited revision, a much more radical revision was being demanded by specialists in many fields of medicine. The structure of several of the ICD chapters appeared to be out of touch with modern clinical concepts. Nevertheless it was felt that the Ninth Revision, compared with its predecessors, presented many new features in its content and quality, making it more flexible and up-to-date and also more adaptable to various purpose-oriented uses. One of its innovations was to make it possible to code diseases according to important manifestations, e.g. to classify mumps encephalitis to a category for encephalitis. The new codes for manifestation were marked with an asterisk (*), while the corresponding etiology codes were marked with a dagger (†). However, it became apparent that much of the subject matter being suggested for incorporation into the new revision did not belong in the main ICD classification itself but would be more appropriately placed in a series, or "family", of related classifications developed from and around the "core" classification. Preparation of the Tenth Revision of ICD started even before the work on ICD-9 was completed, and the final draft of ICD-10 was adopted in 1990 under a slightly different title — *International Statistical Classification of Diseases and Related Health Problems* — which better reflected its content.[1]

A new code structure was designed to facilitate the function of ICD-10 and to allow future changes to be made without the need for major changes to the basic structure. Numeric codes (001-999) were used in ICD-9, but for ICD-10 an alphanumeric coding scheme was adopted, based on a single letter followed by two numbers at the three-character level (A00-Z99). This has significantly enlarged the number of categories available for the classification. Further detail is provided at the four-character level by means of decimal numeric subdivisions. Specialty-based adaptations of ICD then provide extension

[1] *International Statistical Classification of Diseases and Related Health Problems. Tenth Revision.* Geneva, World Health Organization.
Vol. 1. Tabular list, 1992
Vol. 2. Instruction manual, 1993
Vol. 3. Index, 1994

of detail at the fifth character and beyond, without changing the "core" classification.

The need for the ICD to be internationally acceptable makes an extensive and continuing process of consultation with WHO's Member States and their professional organizations essential, to ensure that as many viewpoints as are practicable and compatible are represented. Every effort has been made to achieve clear presentation, plus adequate description and explanation, so that the final version of ICD-10 is potentially of unrivalled importance as an instrument of international communication, education, and research.

1.2 The structure of ICD-10

The Tenth Revision of ICD came into effect on 1 January 1993 and consists of three volumes. Volume 1 includes a tabular (alphanumeric) presentation of the classification, Volume 2 provides instructions for use of the classification, including rules and guidance for the single cause coding of mortality and the single condition coding of morbidity; definitions, recommendations, and reporting requirements for fetal, perinatal, neonatal, infant, and maternal mortality; and a brief history of the development of the ICD. Volume 3 is the index, listing all items of the classification alphabetically, as well as a large number of additional terms and synonyms that cannot be found in the tabular list.

The taxonomic philosophy of ICD is somewhat eclectic: no strictly systematic classification is entirely practicable, because of different national views on disease classification and terminology. The main emphasis, however, is on etiology, since etiology codes are to be given priority for the statistics of mortality. In principle, codes for manifestation are secondary, except when the cause of the manifestation is unknown or unspecified, in which case the non-asterisk code for the manifestation (e.g. meningitis, G03.9) is used as the primary code. A coded nomenclature of the morphology of neoplasms is also provided in ICD-10, an extract of which is included in this edition of ICD-NA (pages 459–476).

Not every condition is assigned an individual rubric, but there is always a category to which any condition or disease can be referred. This has been achieved by the method of selective grouping. The principles used to determine the conditions that should be specified as definite categories are based on frequency, cost, public health importance, research interest, and clarity of characterization of the condition.

In the alphanumeric system of numbering that has been adopted, each general category in the classification is designated by a letter. For instance, "G" is the letter corresponding to diseases of the nervous system. In most instances, the first digit after the letter (i.e. the second character) designates important or summary groups of diseases that are related by topography or by physiopathology. The second digit (i.e. the third character) divides each group into categories that represent specific disease entities, or classes of diseases or conditions that are related according to some significant axis such as etiology, symptomatology, anatomical site, or pathology. This is the reason that the three-character categories have not all been numbered consecutively: some numbers have been omitted so that the summary character of the first two characters is preserved wherever it is meaningful. Because the three-character codes are the legal base for reporting and classifying causes of death in all countries that submit data to the WHO mortality data bank, no additional three-character categories may be introduced in the classification, except when the list is revised by international agreement.

For the majority of codes, ICD-10 also contains a fourth character level of subdivision, designed for more comprehensive description of the types and causes of illness and injury. According to the guidelines established for the development of specialty-based applications of the ICD, four-character categories cannot be created except during the official process of the periodic revisions of the ICD. At both three- and four-character levels, an attempt has been made to include most of the diagnostic terms given in the standard or official nomenclatures, as well as terms most commonly used in different countries. These terms, synonyms, or eponyms, have been called "inclusion terms", of which a more extensive list is to be found in the Index (Volume 3) of ICD-10.

Where there is an appreciable risk that a condition will be wrongly classified, cross-reference to relevant categories is achieved by "exclusion terms". The numbers .8 and .9 in the fourth-character position frequently carry the connotation "other" and "unspecified", respectively; "NOS" is an abbreviation for "not otherwise specified" and is virtually the equivalent of "unspecified" or "unqualified".

2. The ICD family of classifications

ICD-10 provides a central or "core" classification, from which a "family" of classifications is being derived (see figure opposite), with each "member" of the family being adapted to a particular medical specialty or type of user and each reaching a different degree of specificity. For certain purposes, e.g. in oncology, dentistry, neurology, and psychiatry, the ICD classification is substantially expanded; for other purposes however, categories have been condensed and emphasis given to some less precise diagnostic terminology (such as would be suitable for general medical practice).

Family of disease and health-related classifications

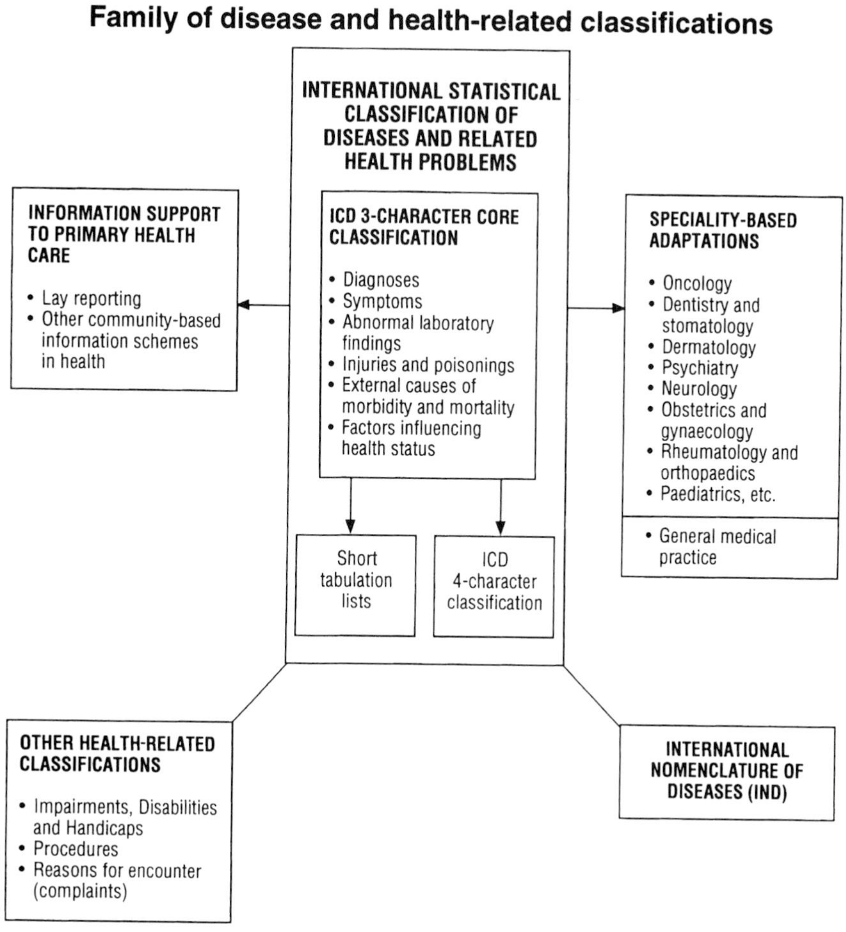

The speciality-based adaptations of ICD-10 do not amend the classification at the four-character level but provide extension of detail at and beyond the fifth character. A further group of classifications covers information that is not presented in the main ICD but that has important medical or health implications, such as classifications of impairments, disabilities, and handicaps, and procedures in medicine and reasons for encounters.

The ICD is complemented by the International Nomenclature of Diseases (IND). Whereas the ICD is a list of "categories", grouping diagnoses in a way convenient for the collection, recording, and analysis of statistical data, the IND is a comprehensive listing of recommended names of all specific, identified morbid entities. Its purpose is to improve communication and to facilitate the retrieval of information from different sources.

3. What is ICD-NA?

3.1 History of ICD-NA

In response to numerous requests for a more detailed classification of neurological disorders — for use in morbidity statistics, hospital record indexing, and research — the Neuroscience programme of WHO's Division of Mental Health convened a consultation in 1984 to consider the development of an adaptation of ICD-9 to neurology, under the responsibility of Dr C.L. Bolis. With the help of consultants and a group of experts, supported by research groups of several nongovernmental organizations, such as the World Federation of Neurology, an Application of ICD-9 to Neurology was prepared by Professors J.M. Orgogozo and J.F. Dartigues (University of Bordeaux, France) and published for trial purposes in 1987 in English[1], followed by French[2], German[3], and Italian[4]. It was received with interest by the scientific community and other users. The classification and coding systems of ICD-9 were retained to ensure compatibility but further subdivisions were introduced at the fifth-character level and beyond, to provide codes for each recognized neurological disorder. WHO has since prepared this second edition of ICD-NA, as explained in the Preface.

3.2 The role of ICD-NA

The aims of ICD-NA are as follows:

- To provide specialists in the clinical neurosciences with a classification that provides a unique code for each recognized neurological disease or injury.
- To focus the attention of specialists in the clinical neurosciences on the desirability of a detailed diagnosis for each patient, using a comprehensive and consistent classification of neurological diseases and of neurological manifestations of other diseases.
- To provide an improved standard recording system for neurological diseases and conditions, available in several languages and prepared under the auspices of WHO.
- To make possible the collection of epidemiological data, comparisons of the prevalence of individual neurological diseases, and identification of the risk

---

[1] *Application of the International Classification of Diseases to Neurology*. Geneva, World Health Organization, 1987.

[2] *Application à la neurologie de la classification internationale des maladies*. Geneva, World Health Organization, 1989.

[3] *Neurologisches Diagnosenschlüssel den internationalen Klassifikation der Krankeheiten den WHO*. Berlin, Springer-Verlag, 1987.

[4] *Applicazione alla Neurologia della Classificazione Internazionale delle Mallattie*. Padua, Fidia S.p.A. Edizione, 1989.

factors for these diseases at both national and international levels. It is hoped that the system will also facilitate the collection of epidemiological data on the rarer neurological diseases, which are urgently needed to support national programmes of prevention and control.

ICD-NA thus aims to be of value to a great variety of users, from government and other health agencies concerned with the collection of statistical data under relatively few main headings, to individual physicians or researchers requiring a convenient tool for indexing their clinical and teaching material in sufficient detail. The classification may be contracted to a few broad categories or further expanded in areas in which the user may have a special interest. Through its direct compatibility with the "parent" ICD-10, ICD-NA provides a method of classification that should facilitate international collaboration and exchange of information.

ICD-NA is intended to remain "open", to allow its adaptation to future advances in the neurological sciences, particularly in the domains of diagnosis, etiopathogenesis, nosology, and classification. For this reason premature use of still questionable classifications has been avoided, and as few individual codes as possible have been allocated to entities whose status remains uncertain. Unavoidable changes in concepts, technology, and even the diseases themselves will occur, and revisions of ICD-NA will be essential. New codes will be added and obsolete codes deleted, in such a way that each new revision will remain compatible with the previous one(s). The hope is that the users of ICD-NA will contribute to this evolution by sending their suggestions and comments to WHO. In addition, users who encounter problems or difficulties in the application of this classification are asked to communicate with the Programme Manager, Mental Health, Division of Mental Health and Prevention of Substance Abuse, World Health Organization, 1211 Geneva 27, Switzerland.

It should be noted that this edition of ICD-NA was constructed at the beginning of the era of genetic and biochemical definition of diseases. As this era advances, an ever-increasing number of diseases in ICD-NA will become genetically and biochemically defined and the number of allelic forms recognized will rise similarly. These advances will probably require a total reclassification of many diseases. In the meantime, the classifications in ICD-NA are based on the best currently available evidence concerning etiology.

3.3 The structure of ICD-NA

Like ICD-10, ICD-NA has a tabular (alphanumeric) section and a comprehensive alphabetical index. In the tabular section, liberal use has been made of inclusion and exclusion terms; the latter are provided with the relevant codes, so that the user will have as much assistance as possible in finding the correct category for any condition diagnosed. In addition, certain notes and cross-references (given in round brackets) have been added to facilitate use. When necessary, synonyms and eponyms are given in square brackets.

The classification and coding systems of ICD-10 have been strictly retained in ICD-NA for the sake of compatibility. In some instances, this may have resulted in a degree of awkwardness or even in an apparent lack of logic. It may seem that certain diseases would be better classified in other categories than those in which they appear, but the alternative would have meant a loss of compatibility with ICD-10. On the whole, ICD-10 was easier to adapt to neurology and neurosurgery than ICD-9.

Each main alphanumeric heading in ICD-NA is an ICD-10 code at the three- or four-character level. Titles for each of these rubrics and for groups of codes and main sections remain exactly the same as those given in ICD-10. However, the originality and potential usefulness of ICD-NA is based on the five-, six- and seven-character codes. Thus the first three or four characters of any ICD-NA code, and the corresponding terms, are those of ICD-10, but most of the fifth and all of the sixth and seventh characters are exclusive to ICD-NA. These subdivisions allow for increased specificity within the broader three- and four-character categories. For instance, mutually exclusive inclusion terms listed under a single ICD-10 code are given individual codes in ICD-NA where it is felt that this separate classification could be of interest for neurological practice, teaching, or research. In other cases, subdivisions used or recommended by experts, committees, or international organizations have been introduced within the broader categories of ICD-10. When it was not possible to subdivide under a defined four-character code, for example because of inappropriateness, the subcategories to classify are listed whenever possible under the "other" category (.8). In the rare cases where there is no four-character category in ICD-10, the subdivisions are made directly at the five-character level, after a dash that symbolizes the unused fourth character (.–). It should be noted, however, that in ICD-10 the convention .– is used to indicate that the three-character category has been subdivided. This numbering system enables the relationship between the ICD-NA category and the parent ICD-10 category to be established from the code itself, and should facilitate comparisons between statistics compiled according to ICD-NA and, for instance, national morbidity or mortality statistics compiled according to ICD-10.

Section IV of ICD-NA includes an excerpt from Chapter XX of ICD-10 for the classification of external causes of morbidity and mortality. Only those codes thought to be pertinent to neurology are included. In Section V a complete list of the morphology of neoplasms is to be found, which can be used in addition to the codes provided in Chapter II (Neoplasms). (See also Section II, 1.7, and Section IV, introduction to Chapter II.)

SECTION II

Instructions and recommendations for the use of ICD-NA

1. Instructions for use of the tabular list

The basic principles of classification and coding that apply to ICD-10 are retained in ICD-NA, so that users familiar with the one will encounter no difficulty with the other. For less experienced users, the recommendations that follow may be helpful.

1.1 Until thoroughly familiar with ICD-NA, the user should consult the index, main headings, and inclusion/exclusion terms before recording a diagnosis.

1.2 The fourth characters .8 and .9 have usually been reserved for "other" and "unspecified" categories, respectively. The category "unspecified" is used where there has been an omission in diagnosis, or where it is impossible to be specific, and — in most cases — is not used beyond the four-character level. With the much higher degree of specification achieved by ICD-NA, it should seldom be necessary to use this code.

1.3 If an uncertain diagnosis is to be classified, the appropriate category for the maximal level of certainty, for instance the general nature or site of the lesion, must be used. Many examples of such general categories of symptoms or signs are to be found in Chapter XVIII, Symptoms, signs and abnormal clinical and laboratory findings, not elsewhere classified (particularly under R25–R29 and R40–R49).

1.4 Provision is made for recording neurological manifestations of a general disease or condition. Such manifestations are indicated by an asterisk (*) code and have a corresponding dagger (†) code to indicate etiology. For example, tuberculous meningitis has its dagger code (A17.0†) in Chapter I, for infectious and parasitic diseases, and its asterisk code (G01*) in Chapter VI, for diseases of the nervous system. Another example would be: Lyme disease (A69.2†) and meningitis in bacterial diseases classified elsewhere (G01*). Use of the asterisk/dagger system provides for the recording of neurological manifestations of a general disease or condition classified elsewhere. All asterisk and dagger code pairs are cross-referenced to each other. It is a principle of the ICD that the dagger code is the primary one for coding purposes and must always be used. The use of the additional asterisk coding is entirely optional. *The asterisk code must never be used alone.* It should never be employed in coding the underlying cause of death (only dagger coding should be used for this purpose), but it may be used in morbidity coding and in multiple-condition coding in relation to either morbidity or mortality. Asterisk and dagger codes can, in fact, be used even if there is no dagger associated with a particular etiology in the tabular list, provided that the manifestation is an unquestionable consequence of that etiology.

1.5 *Multiple coding.* Even when asterisk and dagger coding is not applicable, the use of additional codes (i.e. multiple coding) is encouraged in all cases where the different aspects of a disease need to be described more extensively. In the absence of explicit rules for multiple coding in ICD-NA at present (except for the asterisk/dagger codes), it is suggested that multiple codes be used in the following rank order for each principal disease or condition diagnosed in an individual patient:

- Etiology
- Manifestation
- Other relevant code(s).

An example would be: Manganese poisoning (T57.2) leading to secondary parkinsonism (G21.2). When the etiology is not known or is unspecified, the rank order will be:

- Manifestation (e.g. meningitis NOS (G03.9) or tremor, unspecified (R25.1))
- Other relevant code(s).

Other relevant codes are used to describe associated diseases, conditions, or external factors that are part of, or contribute to, the principal diagnosis.

Concomitant diseases and diagnoses in the same patient, which in the opinion of the user are unrelated to the principal diagnosis, should be given additional codes and listed separately, e.g. in separate data fields.

Coding of late effects. ICD-10 provides a number of categories entitled "Sequelae of . . ." (B90–B94, E64.–, G09, I69.–, T90–T98), which may be used to indicate conditions no longer present as the cause of a current problem under treatment or investigation. The preferred code for the "main condition" is, however, the code for the nature of the sequela itself, to which the code for "Sequelae of . . ." may be added as an optional additional code. Where a number of different, very specific sequelae are present and no one of them predominates in severity and use of resources for treatment, it is permissible for the description "Sequelae of . . ." to be recorded as the main condition. *Example*: main condition: motor aphasia (R47.00), Sequelae of cerebral infarction (I69.3).

1.6 Synonyms and eponyms are provided in square brackets or listed under the title of the category, but the official ICD-10 title is preferred. It is hoped that a concerted attempt will be made in the near future to standardize nomenclature, thus obviating the need for such synonyms.

1.7 In the coding of neoplasms, those desiring more histological specificity should use, in addition, the morphology codes relevant to neurology and neurosurgery, given on pages 459–476. These morphology codes are the same as those used in the special adaptation of the ICD for oncology (ICD-O).[1] Care should be taken that these morphology codes, which begin with M, are not confused with the ICD codes in Chapter XIII (M00–M99).

1.8 Only terms relating in some way to the nervous system and its diseases are included in ICD-NA. If a diagnosed disease is missing from ICD-NA, ICD-10 should be used. Every effort has been made to ensure that such instances will occur infrequently.

1.9 As mentioned earlier, use of a dash (–) in ICD-NA indicates a space within a code that cannot contain any number. For example, the code for chronic progressive multiple sclerosis is G35.–1; the dash indicates that the first position to the right of the decimal point has no digit in ICD-10. However, in instances where ICD-NA provides no five-character subdivision, the dash indicates that ICD-10 contains four-character subdivisions that are not reproduced in ICD-NA. A typical example is A00.– Cholera.

An "*x*" indicates a space within a code that is supposed to contain a number. The actual number to be substituted is dictated by the specific set of instructions pertaining to that code. For example, the code for cerebral infarction due to embolism of a precerebral artery by atrial fibrillation is I63.1*x*2. The number that replaces the "*x*" designates the particular artery involved.

2. Instructions for use of the index

The index to ICD-NA is an alphabetical list of all key items in the classification, as well as a large number of synonyms and eponyms, together with the corresponding code. Items are generally listed by noun, followed by adjective. Thus, "tuberculous meningitis" would appear in the index as "meningitis, tuberculous". Eponymous syndromes and diseases are listed alphabetically both under the corresponding eponym and under "syndrome" or "disease" as appropriate. For example, Guillain–Barré syndrome will be found in the index under "Guillain–Barré" and under "syndrome".

[1] *International Classification of Diseases for Oncology*, 2nd ed. Geneva, World Health Organization, 1990.

The reader is cautioned against using only the index for purposes of coding. The index is simply intended as a guide, indicating the appropriate place in the ICD-NA classification to consult for the proper code. The classification often contains explanatory notes regarding the condition and special rules of inclusion and exclusion that must be considered in choosing the correct code.

The abbreviation "NEC" ("not elsewhere classified") is added after terms classified to residual or unspecified categories and to terms in themselves ill-defined, as a warning that specified forms of the condition are classified differently. In these cases, the defined category should be sought.

SECTION III

List of block titles[1]

[1] The chapters of ICD-10 are divided into homogeneous "blocks" of three-character categories. The listing of a block title in Section III does not imply that all three-character categories from the block can be found in ICD-NA; it is intended only as an indication that at least one of those categories is represented.

Chapter I
Certain infectious and parasitic diseases (A00–B99)

A00–A09 Intestinal infectious diseases
A15–A19 Tuberculosis
A20–A28 Certain zoonotic bacterial diseases
A30–A49 Other bacterial diseases
A50–A64 Infections with a predominantly sexual mode of transmission
A65–A69 Other spirochaetal diseases
A70–A74 Other diseases caused by chlamydiae
A75–A79 Rickettsioses
A80–A89 Viral infections of the central nervous system
A90–A99 Arthropod-borne viral fevers and viral haemorrhagic fevers
B00–B09 Viral infections characterized by skin and mucous membrane lesions
B15–B19 Viral hepatitis
B20–B24 Human immunodeficiency virus [HIV] disease
B25–B34 Other viral diseases
B35–B49 Mycoses
B50–B64 Protozoal diseases
B65–B83 Helminthiases
B90–B94 Sequelae of infectious and parasitic diseases
B95–B97 Bacterial, viral and other infectious agents

Chapter II
Neoplasms (C00–D48)

C00–C75 Malignant neoplasms
C76–C80 Malignant neoplasms of ill-defined, secondary and unspecified sites
C81–C96 Malignant neoplasms of lymphoid, haematopoietic and related tissue
C97 Malignant neoplasms of independent (primary) multiple sites.
D10–D36 Benign neoplasms
D37–D48 Neoplasms of uncertain or unknown behaviour

Chapter III
Diseases of the blood and blood-forming organs and certain disorders involving the immune mechanism (D50–D89)

D50–D53 Nutritional anaemias
D55–D59 Haemolytic anaemias

D65–D69 Coagulation defects, purpura and other haemorrhagic conditions
D70–D77 Other diseases of blood and blood-forming organs
D80–D89 Certain disorders involving the immune mechanism

Chapter IV
Endocrine, nutritional and metabolic diseases (E00–E90)

E00–E07 Disorders of thyroid gland
E10–E14 Diabetes mellitus
E15–E16 Other disorders of glucose regulation and pancreatic internal secretion
E20–E35 Disorders of other endocrine glands
E40–E46 Malnutrition
E50–E64 Other nutritional deficiencies
E65–E68 Obesity and other hyperalimentation
E70–E90 Metabolic disorders

Asterisk categories for this chapter are provided as follows:
E35* Endocrine disorders in diseases classified elsewhere
E90* Nutritional and metabolic disorders in diseases classified elsewhere

Chapter V
Mental and behavioural disorders (F00–F99)

F00–F09 Organic, including symptomatic, mental disorders
F10–F19 Mental and behavioural disorders due to psychoactive substance use
F30–F39 Mood [affective] disorders
F40–F48 Neurotic, stress-related and somatoform disorders
F50–F59 Behavioural syndromes associated with physiological disturbances and physical factors
F60–F69 Disorders of adult personality and behaviour
F70–F79 Mental retardation
F80–F89 Disorders of psychological development
F90–F98 Behavioural and emotional disorders with onset usually occurring in childhood and adolescence

Asterisk categories for this chapter are provided as follows:
F00* Dementia in Alzheimer's disease
F02* Dementia in other diseases classified elsewhere

Chapter VI
Diseases of the nervous system (G00–G99)

G00–G09 Inflammatory diseases of the central nervous system
G10–G13 Systemic atrophies primarily affecting the central nervous system
G20–G26 Extrapyramidal and movement disorders
G30–G32 Other degenerative diseases of the nervous system
G35–G37 Demyelinating diseases of the central nervous system
G40–G47 Episodic and paroxysmal disorders
G50–G59 Nerve, nerve root and plexus disorders
G60–G64 Polyneuropathies and other disorders of the peripheral nervous system
G70–G73 Diseases of myoneural junction and muscle
G80–G83 Cerebral palsy and other paralytic syndromes
G90–G99 Other disorders of the nervous system

Asterisk categories for this chapter are provided as follows:

G01* Meningitis in bacterial diseases classified elsewhere
G02* Meningitis in other infectious and parasitic diseases classified elsewhere
G05* Encephalitis, myelitis and encephalomyelitis in diseases classified elsewhere
G07* Intracranial and intraspinal abscess and granuloma in diseases classified elsewhere
G13* Systemic atrophies primarily affecting the central nervous system in diseases classified elsewhere
G22* Parkinsonism in diseases classified elsewhere
G26* Extrapyramidal and movement disorders in diseases classified elsewhere
G32* Other degenerative disorders of nervous system in diseases classified elsewhere
G46* Vascular syndromes of brain in cerebrovascular diseases
G53* Cranial nerve disorders in diseases classified elsewhere
G55* Nerve root and plexus compressions in diseases classified elsewhere
G59* Mononeuropathy in diseases classified elsewhere
G63* Polyneuropathy in diseases classified elsewhere
G73* Disorders of myoneural junction and muscle in diseases classified elsewhere
G94* Other disorders of brain in diseases classified elsewhere
G99* Other disorders of nervous system in diseases classified elsewhere

Chapter VII
Diseases of the eye and adnexa
(H00–H59)

H00–H06 Disorders of eyelid, lacrimal system and orbit
H15–H22 Disorders of sclera, cornea, iris and ciliary body
H25–H28 Disorders of lens
H30–H36 Disorders of choroid and retina
H40–H42 Glaucoma
H46–H48 Disorders of optic nerve and visual pathways
H49–H52 Disorders of ocular muscles, binocular movement, accommodation and refraction
H53–H54 Visual disturbances and blindness
H55–H59 Other disorders of eye and adnexa

Asterisk categories for this chapter are provided as follows:

H28* Cataract and other disorders of lens in diseases classified elsewhere
H32* Chorioretinal disorders in diseases classified elsewhere
H36* Retinal disorders in diseases classified elsewhere
H42* Glaucoma in diseases classified elsewhere
H48* Disorders of optic [2nd] nerve and visual pathways in diseases classified elsewhere
H58* Other disorders of eye and adnexa in diseases classified elsewhere

Chapter VIII
Diseases of the ear and mastoid process
(H60–H95)

H65–H75 Diseases of middle ear and mastoid
H80–H83 Diseases of inner ear
H90–H95 Other disorders of ear

Asterisk categories for this chapter are provided as follows:

H82* Vertiginous syndromes in diseases classified elsewhere
H94* Other disorders of ear in diseases classified elsewhere

Chapter IX
Diseases of the circulatory system
(I00–I99)

I00–I02 Acute rheumatic fever
I05–I09 Chronic rheumatic heart diseases
I10–I15 Hypertensive diseases
I20–I25 Ischaemic heart diseases

I30–I52 Other forms of heart disease
I60–I69 Cerebrovascular diseases
I70–I79 Diseases of arteries, arterioles and capillaries
I80–I89 Diseases of veins, lymphatic vessels and lymph nodes, not elsewhere classified
I95–I99 Other and unspecified disorders of the circulatory system

Asterisk categories for this chapter are provided as follows:
I39* Endocarditis and heart valve disorders in diseases classified elsewhere
I41* Myocarditis in diseases classified elsewhere
I43* Cardiomyopathy in diseases classified elsewhere
I68* Cerebrovascular disorders in diseases classified elsewhere
I79* Disorders of arteries, arterioles and capillaries in diseases classified elsewhere
I98* Other disorders of the circulatory system in diseases classified elsewhere

Chapter X
Diseases of the respiratory system
(J00–J99)

J00–J06 Acute upper respiratory infections
J10–J18 Influenza and pneumonia
J30–J39 Other diseases of upper respiratory tract
J40–J47 Chronic lower respiratory diseases
J60–J70 Lung diseases due to external agents
J80–J84 Other respiratory diseases principally affecting the interstitium
J85–J86 Suppurative and necrotic conditions of lower respiratory tract
J90–J94 Other diseases of pleura
J95–J99 Other diseases of the respiratory system

An asterisk category for this chapter is provided as follows:
J17* Pneumonia in diseases classified elsewhere

Chapter XI
Diseases of the digestive system
(K00–K99)

K00–K14 Diseases of oral cavity, salivary glands and jaws
K20–K31 Diseases of oesophagus, stomach and duodenum
K50–K52 Noninfective enteritis and colitis
K55–K63 Other diseases of intestines
K65–K67 Diseases of peritoneum
K70–K77 Diseases of liver

K80–K87 Disorders of gallbladder, biliary tract and pancreas
K90–K93 Other diseases of the digestive system

Chapter XII
Diseases of the skin and subcutaneous tissue (L00–L99)

L50–L54 Urticaria and erythema
L80–L99 Other disorders of the skin and subcutaneous tissue

An asterisk category for this chapter is provided as follows:
L99* Other disorders of skin and subcutaneous tissue in diseases classified elsewhere

Chapter XIII
Diseases of the musculoskeletal system and connective tissue (M00–M99)

M00–M25 Arthropathies
M30–M36 Systemic connective tissue disorders
M40–M54 Dorsopathies
M60–M79 Soft tissue disorders
M80–M94 Osteopathies and chondropathies
M95–M99 Other disorders of the musculoskeletal system and connective tissue

Asterisk categories for this chapter are provided as follows:
M03* Postinfective and reactive arthropathies in diseases classified elsewhere
M14* Arthropathies in other diseases classified elsewhere
M36* Systemic disorders of connective tissues in diseases classified elsewhere

Chapter XIV
Diseases of the genitourinary system (N00–N99)

N00–N08 Glomerular diseases
N17–N19 Renal failure
N25–N29 Other disorders of kidney and ureter
N30–N39 Other diseases of the urinary system
N40–N51 Diseases of male genital organs
N60–N64 Disorders of breast
N80–N98 Noninflammatory disorders of female genital tract

Chapter XV
Pregnancy, childbirth and the puerperium (O00–O99)

O00–O08 Pregnancy with abortive outcome
O10–O16 Oedema, proteinuria and hypertensive disorders in pregnancy, childbirth and the puerperium
O20–O29 Other maternal disorders predominantly related to pregnancy
O30–O48 Maternal care related to the fetus and amniotic cavity and possible delivery problems
O60–O75 Complications of labour and delivery
O85–O92 Complications predominantly related to the puerperium
O95–O99 Other obstetric conditions, not elsewhere classified

Chapter XVI
Certain conditions originating in the perinatal period (P00–P99)

P00–P04 Fetus and newborn affected by maternal factors and by complications of pregnancy, labour and delivery
P05–P08 Disorders related to length of gestation and fetal growth
P10–P15 Birth trauma
P20–P29 Respiratory and cardiovascular disorders specific to the perinatal period
P35–P39 Infections specific to the perinatal period
P50–P61 Haemorrhagic and haematological disorders of fetus and newborn
P70–P74 Transitory endocrine and metabolic disorders specific to fetus and newborn
P90–P96 Other disorders originating in the perinatal period

Chapter XVII
Congenital malformations, deformations and chromosomal abnormalities (Q00–Q99)

Q00–Q07 Congenital malformations of the nervous system
Q10–Q18 Congenital malformations of eye, ear, face and neck
Q20–Q28 Congenital malformations of the circulatory system
Q65–Q79 Congenital malformations and deformations of the musculoskeletal system
Q80–Q89 Other congenital malformations
Q90–Q99 Chromosomal abnormalities, not elsewhere classified

Chapter XVIII
Symptoms, signs and abnormal clinical and laboratory findings not elsewhere classified
(R00–R99)

R00–R09	Symptoms and signs involving the circulatory and respiratory systems
R10–R19	Symptoms and signs involving the digestive system and abdomen
R20–R23	Symptoms and signs involving the skin and subcutaneous tissue
R25–R29	Symptoms and signs involving the nervous and musculoskeletal systems
R30–R39	Symptoms and signs involving the urinary system
R40–R46	Symptoms and signs involving cognition, perception, emotional state and behaviour
R47–R49	Symptoms and signs involving speech and voice
R50–R69	General symptoms and signs
R70–R79	Abnormal findings on examination of blood, without diagnosis
R83–R89	Abnormal findings on examination of other body fluids, substances and tissues, without diagnosis
R90–R94	Abnormal findings on diagnostic imaging and in function studies, without diagnosis
R95–R99	Ill-defined and unknown causes of mortality

Chapter XIX
Injury, poisoning and certain other consequences of external causes
(S00–T98)

S00–S09	Injuries to the head
S10–S19	Injuries to the neck
S20–S29	Injuries to the thorax
S30–S39	Injuries to the abdomen, lower back, lumbar spine and pelvis
S40–S49	Injuries to the shoulder and upper arm
S50–S59	Injuries to the elbow and forearm
S60–S69	Injuries to the wrist and hand
S70–S79	Injuries to the hip and thigh
S80–S89	Injuries to the knee and lower leg
S90–S99	Injuries to the ankle and foot
T00–T07	Injuries involving multiple body regions
T08–T14	Injuries to unspecified part of trunk, limb or body region
T15–T19	Effects of foreign body entering through natural orifice
T36–T50	Poisoning by drugs, medicaments and biological substances
T51–T65	Toxic effects of substances chiefly nonmedicinal as to source
T66–T78	Other and unspecified effects of external causes

T79 Certain early complications of trauma
T80–T89 Complications of surgical and medical care, not elsewhere classified
T90–T98 Sequelae of injuries, of poisoning and of other consequences of external causes

Chapter XX
External causes of morbidity and mortality (V00–Y98)

X40–X49 Accidental poisoning by and exposure to noxious substances
Y40–Y84 Complications of medical and surgical care
Y90–Y98 Supplementary factors related to causes of morbidity and mortality classified elsewhere

Chapter XXI
Factors influencing health status and contact with health services (Z00–Z99)

Z00–Z13 Persons encountering health services for examination and investigation
Z20–Z29 Persons with potential health hazards related to communicable diseases
Z30–Z39 Persons encountering health services in circumstances related to reproduction
Z40–Z54 Persons encountering health services for specific procedures and health care
Z70–Z76 Persons encountering health services in other circumstances
Z80–Z99 Persons with potential health hazards related to family and personal history and certain conditions influencing health status

SECTION IV

Tabular list of neurological and related disorders

Certain infectious and parasitic diseases (A00–B99)

Intestinal infectious diseases (A00–A09)

A00.– Cholera

A01 Typhoid and paratyphoid fevers

A01.0 Typhoid fever
Meningitis in typhoid fever† (G01*)

A02 Other salmonella infections

A02.2† Localized salmonella infections
Salmonella:
- meningitis (G01*)
- intracranial and intraspinal abscess (G07*)

A03.– Shigellosis

A04 Other bacterial intestinal infections

A04.5 Campylobacter enteritis

A05 Other bacterial foodborne intoxications

A05.1 Botulism

A06 Amoebiasis

A06.6† Amoebic brain abscess (G07*)

Tuberculosis (A15–A19)

A17† Tuberculosis of nervous system

A17.0† **Tuberculous meningitis (G01*)**
Tuberculous (lepto)meningitis (cerebral)(spinal)

A17.1† **Meningeal tuberculoma (G07*)**

A17.8† **Other tuberculosis of nervous system**
Tuberculoma } of { brain (G07*)
Tuberculosis } of { spinal cord (G07*)
Tuberculous:
- abscess of brain (G07*)
- meningoencephalitis (G05.0*)
- myelitis (G05.0*)
- polyneuropathy (G63.0*)

A17.9† **Tuberculosis of nervous system, unspecified (G99.8*)**

A18 Tuberculosis of other organs

A18.0† **Tuberculosis of bones and joints**
Tuberculosis of vertebral column [Pott] (M49.0*)

A18.8† **Tuberculosis of other specified organs**
Tuberculosis of thyroid gland (E35.0*)
Tuberculous cerebral arteritis (I68.1*)

Certain zoonotic bacterial diseases (A20–A28)

A20 Plague

A20.3 **Plague meningitis**

A20.7 **Septicaemic plague**

A21.– Tularaemia

A22 Anthrax

A22.7 **Anthrax septicaemia**

A22.8 **Other forms of anthrax**
Anthrax meningitis† (G01*)

A23 Brucellosis

Includes: fever:
- Malta

- Mediterranean
- undulant

A23.0 Brucellosis due to *Brucella melitensis*

A23.1 Brucellosis due to *Brucella abortus*

A23.2 Brucellosis due to *Brucella suis*

A23.9 Brucellosis, unspecified

A27.– Leptospirosis

Other bacterial diseases (A30–A49)

A30 Leprosy [Hansen's disease]

Includes: infection due to *Mycobacterium leprae*
mononeuropathy in leprosy† (G59.8*)
polyneuropathy in leprosy† (G63.0*)

Excludes: sequelae of leprosy (B92)

A30.0 Indeterminate leprosy
I leprosy

A30.1 Tuberculoid leprosy
TT leprosy

A30.2 Borderline tuberculoid leprosy
BT leprosy

A30.3 Borderline leprosy
BB leprosy

A30.4 Borderline lepromatous leprosy
BL leprosy

A30.5 Lepromatous leprosy
LL leprosy

A30.8 Other forms of leprosy

A30.9 Leprosy, unspecified

A32 Listeriosis

Includes: listerial food-borne infection

Excludes: neonatal (disseminated) listeriosis (P37.2)

A32.1† **Listerial meningitis and meningoencephalitis**
Listerial:
- meningitis (G01*)
- meningoencephalitis (G05.0*)

A32.8 **Other forms of listeriosis**
Listerial cerebral arteritis† (I68.1*)

A33 Tetanus neonatorum

A34 Obstetrical tetanus

A35 Other tetanus
Tetanus NOS

A36 Diphtheria

A36.8 **Other diphtheria**
Diphtheritic polyneuritis† (G63.0*)

A37.– Whooping cough

A38 Scarlet fever
Scarlatina

A39 Meningococcal infection

A39.0† **Meningococcal meningitis (G01*)**

A39.1† **Waterhouse–Friderichsen syndrome (E35.1*)**
Meningococcic adrenal syndrome

A39.2 **Acute meningococcaemia**

A39.3 **Chronic meningococcaemia**

A39.4 **Meningococcaemia, unspecified**

A39.5 **Meningococcal heart disease**

A39.8 **Other meningococcal infections**
Meningococcal:
- encephalitis† (G05.0*)
- retrobulbar neuritis† (H48.1*)

A40 Streptococcal septicaemia

A40.0 **Septicaemia due to streptococcus, group A**

A40.1 **Septicaemia due to streptococcus, group B**

A40.2 **Septicaemia due to streptococcus, group D**

A40.3 **Septicaemia due to *Streptococcus pneumoniae***
Pneumococcal septicaemia

A40.8 **Other streptococcal septicaemia**

A40.9 **Streptococcal septicaemia, unspecified**

A41 Other septicaemia

A41.0 **Septicaemia due to *Staphylococcus aureus***

A41.1 **Septicaemia due to other specified staphylococcus**
Septicaemia due to coagulase-negative staphylococcus

A41.2 **Septicaemia due to unspecified staphylococcus**

A41.3 **Septicaemia due to *Haemophilus influenzae***

A41.4 **Septicaemia due to anaerobes**

A41.5 **Septicaemia due to other Gram-negative organisms**
Gram-negative septicaemia NOS

A41.8 **Other specified septicaemia**

A41.9 **Septicaemia, unspecified**
Septic shock

A42.– Actinomycosis

A43.– Nocardiosis

A44 Bartonellosis

A44.8 **Other forms of bartonellosis**
Neurological manifestations of bartonellosis

A48 Other bacterial diseases, not elsewhere classified

A48.3 **Toxic shock syndrome**

Infections with a predominantly sexual mode of transmission (A50–A64)

Excludes: human immunodeficiency virus [HIV] disease (B20–B24)

A50 Congenital syphilis

A50.0 Early congenital syphilis, symptomatic

Any congenital syphilitic condition specified as early or manifest less than two years after birth.

A50.1 Early congenital syphilis, latent

Congenital syphilis without clinical manifestations, with positive serological reaction and negative spinal fluid test, less than two years after birth.

A50.2 Early congenital syphilis, unspecified

Congenital syphilis NOS less than two years after birth.

A50.3 Late congenital syphilitic oculopathy

A50.4 Late congenital neurosyphilis [juvenile neurosyphilis]

Includes: late congenital syphilitic:
- encephalitis† (G05.0*)
- meningitis† (G01*)
- polyneuropathy† (G63.0*)

Use additional code, if desired, to identify any associated mental disorder.

A50.40 Juvenile general paresis
Dementia paralytica juvenilis
A50.41 Juvenile tabes dorsalis
A50.42 Juvenile taboparetic neurosyphilis

A50.5 Other late congenital syphilis, symptomatic

Clutton's joints

A51 Early syphilis

A51.0 Primary genital syphilis

A51.1 Primary anal syphilis

A51.2 Primary syphilis of other sites

A51.3 Secondary syphilis of skin and mucous membranes

Condyloma latum
Syphilitic:
- alopecia† (L99.8*)
- leukoderma† (L99.8*)
- mucous patch

A51.4 Other secondary syphilis

Secondary syphilitic:
- meningitis† (G01*)

- myositis† (M63.0*)
- oculopathy NEC† (H58.8*)

A51.5 Early syphilis, latent

Syphilis (acquired) without clinical manifestations, with positive serological reaction and negative spinal fluid test, less than two years after infection.

A51.9 Early syphilis, unspecified

A52 Late syphilis

A52.0† Cardiovascular syphilis

Cardiovascular syphilis NOS (I98.0*)
Syphilitic:
- aneurysm of aorta (I79.0*)
- endocarditis (I39.–*)

A52.1 Symptomatic neurosyphilis

Charcot's arthropathy† (M14.6*)
Late syphilitic:
- encephalitis† (G05.0*)
- general paresis† (G05.0*)
- meningitis† (G01*)
- optic atrophy† (H48.0*)
- polyneuropathy† (G63.0*)
- retrobulbar neuritis† (H48.1*)

Syphilitic:
- Argyll Robertson pupil† (H58.0*)
- parkinsonism† (G22.–2*)

Tabes dorsalis† (G05.01*)

A52.2 Asymptomatic neurosyphilis

A52.3 Neurosyphilis, unspecified

Gumma (syphilitic) } of central nervous system NOS
Syphilis (late) } of central nervous system NOS
Syphiloma } of central nervous system NOS

A52.7 Other symptomatic late syphilis

Syphilis [stage unspecified] of muscle† (M63.0*)

A52.8 Late syphilis, latent

Syphilis (acquired) without clinical manifestations, with positive serological reaction and negative spinal fluid test, two years or more after infection.

A52.9 Late syphilis, unspecified

A53 Other and unspecified syphilis

A53.0 Latent syphilis, unspecified as early or late

A53.9 Syphilis, unspecified

A54 Gonococcal infection

A54.8 Other gonococcal infections
Gonococcal:
- brain abscess† (G07*)
- meningitis† (G01*)

Other spirochaetal diseases (A65–A69)

Excludes: leptospirosis (A27.–)
syphilis (A50–A53)

A68.– Relapsing fevers

Includes: recurrent fever

A69 Other spirochaetal infections

A69.2 Lyme disease
Erythema chronicum migrans due to *Borrelia burgdorferi*

Other diseases caused by chlamydiae (A70–A74)

A71.– Trachoma

Excludes: sequelae of trachoma (B94.0)

Rickettsioses (A75–A79)

A75 Typhus fever

A75.0 Epidemic louse-borne typhus fever due to *Rickettsia prowazekii*

A77.– Spotted fever [tick-borne rickettsioses]

A79.– Other rickettsioses

Viral infections of the central nervous system (A80–A89)

Excludes: sequelae of:
- poliomyelitis (B91)
- viral encephalitis (B94.1)

A80 Acute poliomyelitis

A80.0 Acute paralytic poliomyelitis, vaccine-associated

A80.1 Acute paralytic poliomyelitis, wild virus, imported

A80.2 Acute paralytic poliomyelitis, wild virus, indigenous

A80.3 Acute paralytic poliomyelitis, other and unspecified

A80.4 Acute nonparalytic poliomyelitis

A80.9 Acute poliomyelitis, unspecified

A81 Slow virus infections of central nervous system

Includes: prion diseases of the central nervous system
Excludes: HIV-associated encephalopathy (B22.0)
HIV vacuolar myelopathy (B23.8)
HTLV-1-associated myelopathy (G04.1)

A81.0 Creutzfeldt–Jakob disease
Subacute spongiform encephalopathy

A81.1 Subacute sclerosing panencephalitis
Dawson's inclusion body encephalitis
Van Bogaert's sclerosing leukoencephalopathy

A81.2 Progressive multifocal leukoencephalopathy
Multifocal leukoencephalopathy NOS

A81.8 Other slow virus infections of central nervous system
Excludes: rubella:
- encephalitis (acute) (B06.00)
- meningitis (B06.01)
- meningoencephalitis (B06.02)
- subacute panencephalitis (B06.03)

A81.80 Kuru
A81.81 Gerstmann–Straüssler–Scheinker disease or syndrome

A81.9 **Slow virus infection of central nervous system, unspecified**

A82 Rabies

A82.0 **Sylvatic rabies**

A82.1 **Urban rabies**

A82.9 **Rabies, unspecified**

A83 Mosquito-borne viral encephalitis

Includes: mosquito-borne viral meningoencephalitis
Excludes: Venezuelan equine encephalitis (A92.2)

A83.0 **Japanese encephalitis**

A83.1 **Western equine encephalitis**

A83.2 **Eastern equine encephalitis**

A83.3 **St Louis encephalitis**

A83.4 **Australian encephalitis**
Kunjin virus disease

A83.5 **California encephalitis**
California meningoencephalitis
La Crosse encephalitis

A83.6 **Rocio virus disease**

A83.8 **Other mosquito-borne viral encephalitis**

A83.9 **Mosquito-borne viral encephalitis, unspecified**

A84 Tick-borne viral encephalitis

Includes: tick-borne viral meningoencephalitis

A84.0 **Far Eastern tick-borne encephalitis [Russian spring–summer encephalitis]**

A84.1 **Central European tick-borne encephalitis**

A84.8 **Other tick-borne viral encephalitis**
Louping ill
Powassan virus disease

A84.9 **Tick-borne viral encephalitis, unspecified**

A85 Other viral encephalitis, not elsewhere classified

Includes: specified viral:
- encephalomyelitis NEC
- meningoencephalitis NEC

Excludes: benign myalgic encephalomyelitis (G93.3)
encephalitis due to:
- herpesvirus [herpes simplex] (B00.4)
- measles virus (B05.0)
- mumps virus (B26.2)
- poliomyelitis virus (A80.–)
- zoster (B02.0)

lymphocytic choriomeningitis (A87.2)

A85.0† Enteroviral encephalitis (G05.1*)
Enteroviral encephalomyelitis

A85.1† Adenoviral encephalitis (G05.1*)
Adenoviral meningoencephalitis

A85.2 Arthropod-borne viral encephalitis, unspecified

A85.8 Other specified viral encephalitis
Encephalitis lethargica
Von Economo–Cruchet disease

A86 Unspecified viral encephalitis

Viral:
- encephalomyelitis NOS
- meningoencephalitis NOS

A87 Viral meningitis

Excludes: meningitis due to:
- herpesvirus [herpes simplex] (B00.3)
- measles virus (B05.1)
- mumps virus (B26.1)
- poliomyelitis virus (A80.–)
- zoster (B02.1)

A87.0† Enteroviral meningitis (G02.0*)
Coxsackievirus meningitis
Echovirus meningitis

A87.1† Adenoviral meningitis (G02.0*)

A87.2 Lymphocytic choriomeningitis
Lymphocytic meningoencephalitis

A87.8 Other viral meningitis

A87.9 Viral meningitis, unspecified

A88 Other viral infections of central nervous system, not elsewhere classified

Excludes: viral:
- encephalitis NOS (A86)
- meningitis NOS (A87.9)

A88.0 **Enteroviral exanthematous fever [Boston exanthem]**

A88.1 **Epidemic vertigo**

A88.8 **Other specified viral infections of central nervous system**

A89 Unspecified viral infection of central nervous system

Arthropod-borne viral fevers and viral haemorrhagic fevers (A90–A99)

A90 Dengue fever [classical dengue]

Excludes: dengue haemorrhagic fever (A91)

A91 Dengue haemorrhagic fever

A92 Other mosquito-borne viral fevers

A92.2 **Venezuelan equine fever**

Venezuelan equine:
- encephalitis
- encephalomyelitis virus disease

A95.– Yellow fever

A96 Arenaviral haemorrhagic fever

Includes: arenaviral meningitis† (G02.0*)

A96.2 **Lassa fever**

A98 Other viral haemorrhagic fevers, not elsewhere classified

A98.2 **Kyasanur Forest disease**

A98.3 **Marburg virus disease**

A98.4 **Ebola virus disease**

Viral infections characterized by skin and mucous membrane lesions (B00–B09)

B00 Herpesviral [herpes simplex] infections

Excludes: congenital herpesviral infection (P35.2)

B00.3† Herpesviral meningitis (G02.0*)

B00.4† Herpesviral encephalitis (G05.1*)
Herpesviral meningoencephalitis
Simian B disease

B00.7 Disseminated herpesviral disease
Herpesviral septicaemia

B01 Varicella [chickenpox]

B01.0† Varicella meningitis (G02.0*)

B01.1† Varicella encephalitis (G05.1*)
Postchickenpox encephalitis
Varicella encephalomyelitis

B02 Zoster [herpes zoster]

B02.0† Zoster encephalitis (G05.1*)
Zoster meningoencephalitis

B02.1† Zoster meningitis (G02.0*)

B02.2† Zoster with other nervous system involvement
Acute herpetic geniculate ganglionitis (G53.04*)
Acute trigeminal herpes zoster neuropathy (G53.00*)
Postherpetic:
- geniculate ganglionitis (G53.05*)
- ocular nerve palsy (G53.06*)
- polyneuropathy (G63.0*)

Postzoster:
- glossopharyngeal neuralgia (G53.03*)
- trigeminal neuralgia (G53.01*)

B03 Smallpox[1]

[1] In 1980 the 33rd World Health Assembly declared that smallpox had been eradicated. The classification is retained for surveillance purposes.

B05 Measles

Includes: morbilli
Excludes: subacute sclerosing panencephalitis (A81.1)

B05.0† Measles complicated by encephalitis (G05.1*)
Postmeasles encephalitis

B05.1† Measles complicated by meningitis (G02.0*)
Postmeasles meningitis

B06 Rubella [German measles]

Excludes: congenital rubella (P35.0)

B06.0† Rubella with neurological complications

B06.00† Rubella encephalitis (acute) (G05.1*)
B06.01† Rubella meningitis (G02.0*)
B06.02† Rubella meningoencephalitis (G05.1*)
B06.03† Rubella subacute panencephalitis (G05.1*)

Viral hepatitis (B15–B19)

B15 Acute hepatitis A

B15.0 Hepatitis A with hepatic coma

B16 Acute hepatitis B

B16.0 Acute hepatitis B with delta-agent (coinfection) with hepatic coma

B16.2 Acute hepatitis B without delta-agent with hepatic coma

B17.– Other acute viral hepatitis

B18.– Chronic viral hepatitis

Chronic hepatitis B

B19 Unspecified viral hepatitis

B19.0 Unspecified viral hepatitis with coma

Human immunodeficiency virus [HIV] disease (B20–B24)

Note: The fourth-character subcategories of B20–B23 are provided for optional use where it is not possible or not desired to use multiple coding to identify the specific conditions.

Excludes: asymptomatic human immunodeficiency virus [HIV] infection status (Z21)

B20 Human immunodeficiency virus [HIV] disease resulting in infectious and parasitic diseases

Excludes: acute HIV infection syndrome (B23.0)

B20.0 HIV disease resulting in mycobacterial infection
HIV disease resulting in tuberculosis

B20.1 HIV disease resulting in other bacterial infections

B20.2 HIV disease resulting in cytomegaloviral disease

B20.3 HIV disease resulting in other viral infections

B20.4 HIV disease resulting in candidiasis

B20.5 HIV disease resulting in other mycoses

B20.6 HIV disease resulting in *Pneumocystis carinii* pneumonia

B20.7 HIV disease resulting in multiple infections

B20.8 HIV disease resulting in other infectious and parasitic diseases

B20.9 HIV disease resulting in unspecified infectious or parasitic disease
HIV disease resulting in infection NOS

B21 Human immunodeficiency virus [HIV] disease resulting in malignant neoplasms

B21.0 HIV disease resulting in Kaposi's sarcoma

B21.1 HIV disease resulting in Burkitt's lymphoma

B21.2 HIV disease resulting in other types of non-Hodgkin's lymphoma

B21.3 HIV disease resulting in other malignant neoplasms of lymphoid, haematopoietic and related tissue

B21.7 **HIV disease resulting in multiple malignant neoplasms**

B21.8 **HIV disease resulting in other malignant neoplasms**

B21.9 **HIV disease resulting in unspecified malignant neoplasm**

B22 Human immunodeficiency virus [HIV] disease resulting in other specified diseases

B22.0 **HIV disease resulting in encephalopathy**
HIV dementia
HIV leukoencephalopathy

B22.1 **HIV disease resulting in lymphoid interstitial pneumonitis**

B22.2 **HIV disease resulting in wasting syndrome**
HIV disease resulting in failure to thrive
Slim disease

B23 Human immunodeficiency virus [HIV] disease resulting in other conditions

B23.0 **Acute HIV infection syndrome**

B23.1 **HIV disease resulting in (persistent) generalized lymphadenopathy**

B23.2 **HIV disease resulting in haematological and immunological abnormalities, not elsewhere classified**

B23.8 **HIV disease resulting in other specified conditions**
HIV peripheral neuropathy† (G63.0*)
Vacuolar myelopathy† (G99.2*)

B24 Unspecified human immunodeficiency virus [HIV] disease
Acquired immunodeficiency syndrome [AIDS] NOS
AIDS-related complex [ARC] NOS

Other viral diseases (B25–B34)

B25 Cytomegaloviral disease
Excludes: congenital cytomegalovirus infection (P35.1)
cytomegaloviral mononucleosis (B27.1)

B25.8 **Other cytomegaloviral diseases**

B26 Mumps

B26.1† Mumps meningitis (G02.0*)

B26.2† Mumps encephalitis (G05.1*)

B26.8 Mumps with other complications
Mumps polyneuropathy† (G63.0*)

B27 Infectious mononucleosis

B27.0 Gammaherpesviral mononucleosis
Mononucleosis due to Epstein–Barr virus

B27.1 Cytomegaloviral mononucleosis

B33 Other viral diseases, not elsewhere classified

B33.0 Epidemic myalgia
Bornholm disease

B33.1 Ross River disease

Mycoses (B35–B49)

B37 Candidiasis

Includes: candidosis
moniliasis

Excludes: neonatal candidiasis (P37.5)

B37.5† Candidal meningitis (G02.1*)

B38 Coccidioidomycosis

B38.4† Coccidioidomycosis meningitis (G02.1*)

B39.– Histoplasmosis

B40 Blastomycosis

B40.7 Disseminated blastomycosis
Generalized blastomycosis

B40.8 Other forms of blastomycosis

B41 Paracoccidioidomycosis

Includes: Brazilian blastomycosis
Lutz' disease

B41.7 Disseminated paracoccidioidomycosis
Generalized paracoccidioidomycosis

B41.8 Other forms of paracoccidioidomycosis

B43 Chromomycosis and phaeomycotic abscess

B43.1 Phaeomycotic brain abscess
Cerebral chromomycosis

B44 Aspergillosis

Includes: aspergilloma

B44.7 Disseminated aspergillosis
Generalized aspergillosis

B44.8 Other forms of aspergillosis

B45 Cryptococcosis

B45.1 Cerebral cryptococcosis
Cryptococcal:
- brain abscess† (G07*)
- meningitis† (G02.1*)

Cryptococcoma of brain† (G07*)
Cryptococcosis meningocerebralis

B45.7 Disseminated cryptococcosis
Generalized cryptococcosis

B46 Zygomycosis

B46.1 Rhinocerebral mucormycosis

B48 Other mycoses, not elsewhere classified

B48.7 Opportunistic mycoses
Mycoses caused by fungi of low virulence that can establish an infection only as a consequence of factors such as the presence of debilitating disease or the administration of immunosuppressive and other therapeutic agents or radiation therapy. Most of the causal fungi are normally saprophytic in soil and decaying vegetation.

Protozoal diseases (B50–B64)

B50 *Plasmodium falciparum* malaria

Includes: mixed infections of *Plasmodium falciparum* with any other *Plasmodium* species

B50.0 *Plasmodium falciparum* malaria with cerebral complications
Cerebral malaria NOS

B51 *Plasmodium vivax* malaria

Includes: mixed infections of *Plasmodium vivax* with other *Plasmodium* species, except *Plasmodium falciparum*
Excludes: when mixed with *Plasmodium falciparum* (B50.–)

B51.8 *Plasmodium vivax* malaria with other complications

B52 *Plasmodium malariae* malaria

Includes: mixed infections of *Plasmodium malariae* with other *Plasmodium* species, except *Plasmodium falciparum* and *Plasmodium vivax*
Excludes: when mixed with *Plasmodium*:
- *falciparum* (B50.–)
- *vivax* (B51.–)

B52.8 *Plasmodium malariae* malaria with other complications

B53.– Other parasitologically confirmed malaria

B54 Unspecified malaria

Clinically diagnosed malaria without parasitological confirmation.

B56 African trypanosomiasis

B56.0 Gambiense trypanosomiasis
Infection due to *Trypanosoma brucei gambiense*
West African sleeping sickness

B56.1 Rhodesiense trypanosomiasis
East African sleeping sickness
Infection due to *Trypanosoma brucei rhodesiense*

B56.9 African trypanosomiasis, unspecified
Sleeping sickness NOS
Trypanosomiasis NOS, in places where African trypanosomiasis is prevalent

B57 Chagas' disease

Includes: American trypanosomiasis
infection due to *Trypanosoma cruzi*

B57.0† Acute Chagas' disease with heart involvement (I41.2*, I98.1*)

B57.2† Chagas' disease (chronic) with heart involvement (I41.2*, I98.1*)
American trypanosomiasis NOS
Chagas' disease NOS
Trypanosomiasis NOS, in places where Chagas' disease is prevalent

B57.4 Chagas' disease (chronic) with nervous system involvement

B58 Toxoplasmosis

Includes: infection due to *Toxoplasma gondii*
Excludes: congenital toxoplasmosis (P37.1)

B58.0† Toxoplasma oculopathy
Toxoplasma chorioretinitis (H32.0*)

B58.2† Toxoplasma meningoencephalitis (G05.2*)

B58.3† Pulmonary toxoplasmosis (J17.3*)

B60 Other protozoal diseases, not elsewhere classified

B60.2 Naegleriasis
Primary amoebic meningoencephalitis† (G05.2*)

Helminthiases (B65–B83)

B65.– Schistosomiasis [bilharziasis]

Includes: snail fever

B66 Other fluke infections

B66.4 Paragonimiasis
Infection due to *Paragonimus* species

B67 Echinococcosis

Includes: hydatidosis

B67.3 *Echinococcus granulosus* infection, other and multiple sites

B67.6 *Echinococcus multilocularis* infection, other and multiple sites

B67.7 *Echinococcus multilocularis* infection, unspecified

B67.9 Echinococcosis, other and unspecified
Echinococcosis NOS

B69 Cysticercosis

Includes: cysticerciasis infection due to larval form of *Taenia solium*

B69.0 Cysticercosis of central nervous system

B69.1 Cysticercosis of eye

B69.8 Cysticercosis of other sites

B69.9 Cysticercosis, unspecified

B70 Diphyllobothriasis and sparganosis

B70.0 Diphyllobothriasis
Diphyllobothrium (adult) (*latum*) (*pacificum*) infection
Fish tapeworm (infection)

B73 Onchocerciasis

Onchocerca volvulus infection
Onchocercosis
River blindness

B74.– Filariasis

Excludes: onchocerciasis (B73)

B75 Trichinellosis

Infection due to *Trichinella* species
Trichiniasis

B77 Ascariasis

Includes: ascaridiasis
roundworm infection

B77.8 Ascariasis with other complications

B83 Other helminthiases

B83.2 Angiostrongyliasis due to *Parastrongylus cantonensis*
Eosinophilic meningoencephalitis† (G05.2*)

Sequelae of infectious and parasitic diseases (B90–B94)

Note: These categories are to be used to indicate conditions in categories A00–B89 as the cause of sequelae, which are themselves classified elsewhere. The "sequelae" include conditions specified as such; they also include late effects of diseases classifiable to the above categories if there is evidence that the disease itself is no longer present. (See also Section II, note 1.5, coding of late effects.)

B90 Sequelae of tuberculosis

B90.0 Sequelae of central nervous system tuberculosis

B91 Sequelae of poliomyelitis

B91.–0 Progressive postpolio muscular atrophy
B91.–1 Postpolio pain syndrome due to joint deformity
B91.–2 Postpolio pain syndrome, idiopathic

B92 Sequelae of leprosy

B94 Sequelae of other and unspecified infectious and parasitic diseases

B94.0 Sequelae of trachoma

B94.1 Sequelae of viral encephalitis

B94.8 Sequelae of other specified infectious and parasitic diseases

B94.9 Sequelae of unspecified infectious or parasitic disease

Bacterial, viral and other infectious agents (B95–B97)

Note: These categories should never be used in primary coding. They are provided for use as supplementary or additional codes when it is desired to identify the infectious agent(s) in diseases classified elsewhere.

B95 Streptococcus and staphylococcus as the cause of diseases classified to other chapters

B95.0 **Streptococcus, group A, as the cause of diseases classified to other chapters**

B95.1 **Streptococcus, group B, as the cause of diseases classified to other chapters**

B95.2 **Streptococcus, group D, as the cause of diseases classified to other chapters**

B95.3 ***Streptococcus pneumoniae*** **as the cause of diseases classified to other chapters**

B95.4 **Other streptococcus as the cause of diseases classified to other chapters**

B95.5 **Unspecified streptococcus as the cause of diseases classified to other chapters**

B95.6 ***Staphyloccus aureus*** **as the cause of diseases classified to other chapters**

B95.7 **Other staphylococcus as the cause of diseases classified to other chapters**

B95.8 **Unspecified staphyloccus as the cause of diseases classified to other chapters**

B96 Other bacterial agents as the cause of diseases classified to other chapters

B96.0 ***Mycoplasma pneumoniae*** **[*M. pneumoniae*] as the cause of diseases classified to other chapters**
Pleuro-pneumonia-like-organism [PPLO]

B96.1 ***Klebsiella pneumoniae*** **[*K. pneumoniae*] as the cause of diseases classified to other chapters**

B96.2 ***Escherichia coli*** **[*E. coli*] as the cause of diseases classified to other chapters**

B96.3 ***Haemophilus influenzae*** **[*H. influenzae*] as the cause of diseases classified to other chapters**

B96.4 ***Proteus*** **(*mirabilis*)(*morganii*) as the cause of diseases classified to other chapters**

B96.5 ***Pseudomonas*** **(*aeruginosa*)(*mallei*)(*pseudomallei*) as the cause of diseases classified to other chapters**

B96.6 ***Bacillus fragilis*** **[*B. fragilis*] as the cause of diseases classified to other chapters**

B96.7 ***Clostridium perfringens* [*C. perfringens*] as the cause of diseases classified to other chapters**

B96.8 **Other specified bacterial agents as the cause of diseases classified to other chapters**

B97 Viral agents as the cause of diseases classified to other chapters

B97.0 **Adenovirus as the cause of diseases classified to other chapters**

B97.1 **Enterovirus as the cause of diseases classified to other chapters**
Coxsackievirus
Echovirus

B97.2 **Coronavirus as the cause of diseases classified to other chapters**

B97.3 **Retrovirus as the cause of diseases classified to other chapters**
Lentivirus
Oncovirus

B97.4 **Respiratory syncytial virus as the cause of diseases classified to other chapters**

B97.5 **Reovirus as the cause of diseases classified to other chapters**

B97.6 **Parvovirus as the cause of diseases classified to other chapters**

B97.7 **Papillomavirus as the cause of diseases classified to other chapters**

B97.8 **Other viral agents as the cause of diseases classified to other chapters**

CHAPTER II

Neoplasms (C00–D48)

Notes

1. Primary, ill-defined, secondary and unspecified sites of malignant neoplasms

Categories C76–C80 include malignant neoplasms where there is no clear indication of the original site of the cancer or the cancer is stated to be "disseminated", "scattered" or "spread" without mention of the primary site. In both cases the primary site is considered to be unknown.

2. Functional activity

All neoplasms are classified in this chapter, whether they are functionally active or not. An additional code from Chapter IV may be used, if desired, to identify functional activity associated with any neoplasm. For example, catecholamine-producing malignant phaeochromocytoma of adrenal gland should be coded to C74 with additional code E27.5; basophil adenoma of pituitary gland with Cushing's syndrome should be coded to D35.2 with additional code E24.0.

3. Morphology

There are a number of major morphological (histological) groups of malignant neoplasms: carcinomas including squamous (cell) and adenocarcinomas; sarcomas; other soft tissue tumours including mesotheliomas; lymphomas (Hodgkin's and non-Hodgkin's); leukaemia; other specified and site-specific types; and unspecified cancers. Cancer is a generic term and may be used for any of the above groups, although it is rarely applied to the malignant neoplasms of lymphatic, haematopoietic and related tissue. "Carcinoma" is sometimes used incorrectly as a synonym for "cancer".

In Chapter II neoplasms are classified predominantly by site within broad groupings for behaviour. In a few exceptional cases morphology is indicated in the category and subcategory titles.

For those wishing to identify the histological type of neoplasm, comprehensive separate morphology codes are provided on pages 459–476. These morphology codes are derived from the second edition of International Classification of Diseases for Oncology (ICD-O), which is a dual-axis classification providing independent coding systems for topography and morphology. Morphology codes have six digits: the first four digits identify the histological type; the fifth digit is the behaviour code (malignant primary, malignant secondary (metastatic), in situ, benign, uncertain whether malignant or benign); and the sixth digit is a grading code (differentiation) for solid tumours, and is also used as a special code for lymphomas and leukaemias.

4. Use of subcategories in Chapter II

Attention is drawn to the special use of subcategory .8 in this chapter [see note 5]. Where it has been necessary to provide subcategories for "other", these have generally been designated as subcategory .7.

5. Malignant neoplasms overlapping site boundaries and the use of subcategory .8 (overlapping lesion)

Categories C00–C75 classify primary malignant neoplasms according to their point of origin. Many three-character categories are further divided into named parts or subcategories of the organ in question. A neoplasm that overlaps two or more contiguous sites within a three-character category and whose point of origin cannot be determined should be classified to the subcategory .8 ("overlapping lesion"), unless the combination is specifically indexed elsewhere. "Overlapping" implies that the sites involved are contiguous (next to each other). Numerically consecutive subcategories are frequently anatomically contiguous, but this is not invariably so (e.g. bladder C67.–) and the coder may wish to consult anatomical texts to determine the topographical relationships.

Sometimes a neoplasm overlaps the boundaries of three-character categories within certain systems. To take care of this, subcategories have been designated for overlapping lesions, e.g. carcinoma of the stomach and small intestine, which should be coded to C26.8 (Overlapping lesion of digestive system).

C02.8 Overlapping lesion of tongue
C14.8 Overlapping lesion of lip, oral cavity and pharynx
C21.8 Overlapping lesion of rectum, anus and anal canal
C24.8 Overlapping lesion of biliary tract
C26.8 Overlapping lesion of digestive system
C39.8 Overlapping lesion of respiratory and intrathoracic organs
C41.8 Overlapping lesion of bone and articular cartilage
C49.8 Overlapping lesion of connective and soft tissue
C57.8 Overlapping lesion of female genital organs
C63.8 Overlapping lesion of male genital organs
C68.8 Overlapping lesion of urinary organs

C72.8 Overlapping lesion of brain and other parts of central nervous system

6. Malignant neoplasms of ectopic tissue

Malignant neoplasms of ectopic tissue are to be coded to the site mentioned, e.g. malignant neoplasms of ectopic testis are coded to C62.0.

7. Use of the Alphabetical Index in coding neoplasms

In addition to site, morphology and behaviour must also be taken into consideration when coding neoplasms. However, the index of this book provides only the alphanumeric codes used in the tabular lists. The morphology codes for neoplasms are not indexed, and must be looked for, if desired, in the numerical list of Section V.

8. Use of the second edition of International Classification of Diseases for Oncology (ICD-O)

For certain morphological types, Chapter II provides a rather restricted topographical classification, or none at all. The topography codes of ICD-O use for all neoplasms essentially the same three- and four-character categories that Chapter II uses for malignant neoplasms (C00–C77, C80), thus providing increased specificity of site for other neoplasms (malignant secondary (metastatic), benign, in situ and uncertain or unknown).

It is therefore recommended that those interested in identifying both the site and morphology of tumours, e.g. cancer registries, cancer hospitals, pathology departments and other agencies specializing in cancer, use ICD-O.

Malignant neoplasms (C00–C97)

Malignant neoplasms of lip, oral cavity and pharynx (C00–C14)

C02 Malignant neoplasm of other and unspecified parts of tongue

C02.8 Overlapping lesion of tongue

C07 Malignant neoplasm of parotid gland

C10.– **Malignant neoplasm of oropharynx**

C11.– **Malignant neoplasm of nasopharynx**

C14 **Malignant neoplasm of other and ill-defined sites in the lip, oral cavity and pharynx**

C14.0 **Pharynx, unspecified**

C14.8 **Overlapping lesion of lip, oral cavity and pharynx**

Malignant neoplasms of digestive organs (C15–C26)

C15.– **Malignant neoplasm of oesophagus**

C16.– **Malignant neoplasm of stomach**

C17.– **Malignant neoplasm of small intestine**

C18.– **Malignant neoplasm of colon**

C19 **Malignant neoplasm of rectosigmoid junction**
Colon with rectum
Rectosigmoid (colon)

C20 **Malignant neoplasm of rectum**
Rectal ampulla

C21 **Malignant neoplasm of anus and anal canal**

C21.8 **Overlapping lesion of rectum, anus and anal canal**

C22.– **Malignant neoplasm of liver and intrahepatic bile ducts**
Excludes: secondary malignant neoplasm of liver (C78.–)

C23 **Malignant neoplasm of gallbladder**

C24 **Malignant neoplasm of other and unspecified parts of biliary tract**

C24.8 **Overlapping lesion of biliary tract**

C25.– Malignant neoplasm of pancreas

C26 Malignant neoplasm of other and ill-defined digestive organs

Excludes: peritoneum and retroperitoneum (C48.–)

C26.8 Overlapping lesion of digestive system

Malignant neoplasms of respiratory and intrathoracic organs (C30–C39)

C30 Malignant neoplasm of nasal cavity and middle ear

C30.0 Nasal cavity

C30.1 Middle ear

C31 Malignant neoplasm of accessory sinuses

C31.0 Maxillary sinus
Antrum (Highmore)(maxillary)

C31.1 Ethmoidal sinus

C31.2 Frontal sinus

C31.3 Sphenoidal sinus

C31.8 Overlapping lesion of accessory sinuses

C32 Malignant neoplasm of larynx

C32.0 Glottis

C32.1 Supraglottis

C32.2 Subglottis

C32.3 Laryngeal cartilage

C32.8 Overlapping lesion of larynx

C33 Malignant neoplasm of trachea

C34.– Malignant neoplasm of bronchus and lung

C37 Malignant neoplasm of thymus

C38 Malignant neoplasm of heart, mediastinum and pleura

Excludes: mesothelioma (C45.–)

C38.1 **Anterior mediastinum**

C38.2 **Posterior mediastinum**

C38.3 **Mediastinum, part unspecified**

C38.8 **Overlapping lesion of heart, mediastinum and pleura**

C39 Malignant neoplasm of other and ill-defined sites in the respiratory system and intrathoracic organs

C39.8 **Overlapping lesion of respiratory and intrathoracic organs**

Malignant neoplasms of bone and articular cartilage (C40–C41)

C40.– Malignant neoplasm of bone and articular cartilage of limbs

C41 Malignant neoplasm of bone and articular cartilage of other and unspecified sites

Excludes: bones of limbs (C40.–)
cartilage of larynx (C32.3)

C41.0 **Bones of skull and face**
Maxilla (superior)
Orbital bone
Excludes: carcinoma, any type except intraosseous or odontogenic, of maxillary sinus (C31.0)
jaw bone (lower) (C41.1)

C41.1 **Mandible**
Lower jaw bone

C41.2 **Vertebral column**
Excludes: sacrum and coccyx (C41.4)

C41.3 **Ribs, sternum and clavicle**

C41.4 **Pelvic bones, sacrum and coccyx**

C41.8 **Overlapping lesion of bone and articular cartilage**

Melanoma and other malignant neoplasms of skin (C43–C44)

C43.– Malignant melanoma of skin

C44.– Other malignant neoplasms of skin

Includes: malignant neoplasm of:
- sebaceous glands
- sweat glands

Excludes: Kaposi's sarcoma (C46.–)
malignant melanoma of skin (C43.–)
skin of genital organs (C51–C52, C60.–, C63.–)

Malignant neoplasms of mesothelial and soft tissue (C45–C49)

C45 Mesothelioma

C45.1 Mesothelioma of peritoneum

C46 Kaposi's sarcoma

C46.1 Kaposi's sarcoma of soft tissue

C46.7 Kaposi's sarcoma of other sites

C46.8 Kaposi's sarcoma of multiple organs

C47 Malignant neoplasm of peripheral nerves and autonomic nervous system

C47.0 Peripheral nerves of head, face and neck

C47.00 Cervical nerve roots
C47.01 Cervical nerves
C47.02 Cervical sympathetic chain and plexus
C47.07 Other peripheral nerves of head, face and neck

C47.1 Peripheral nerves of upper limb, including shoulder

C47.10 Brachial plexus
C47.11 Radial nerve and branches
C47.12 Median nerve and branches
C47.13 Ulnar nerve and branches
C47.17 Other peripheral nerves of upper limb

C47.2 Peripheral nerves of lower limb, including hip

C47.20 Sciatic nerve
C47.21 Gluteal nerve
C47.22 Peroneal nerve and branches
C47.23 Tibial nerve and branches
C47.27 Other peripheral nerves of lower limb

C47.3 Peripheral nerves of thorax

C47.30 Thoracic nerve roots
C47.31 Thoracic nerve
C47.32 Thoracic sympathetic chain and plexus
C47.37 Other peripheral nerves of thorax

C47.4 Peripheral nerves of abdomen

C47.40 Lumbar nerve roots
C47.41 Lumbar nerve
C47.42 Lumbar plexus
C47.47 Other peripheral nerves of abdomen

C47.5 Peripheral nerves of pelvis

C47.50 Sacral nerve roots
C47.51 Sacral nerve
C47.52 Pudendal nerve
C47.53 Obturator nerve
C47.57 Other peripheral nerves of pelvis

C47.6 Peripheral nerves of trunk, unspecified

C47.8 Overlapping lesion of peripheral nerves and autonomic nervous system

C47.9 Peripheral nerves and autonomic nervous system, unspecified

C48.– Malignant neoplasm of retroperitoneum and peritoneum

Excludes: Kaposi's sarcoma (C46.1)
mesothelioma (C45.–)

C49 Malignant neoplasm of other connective and soft tissue

Includes: muscle
tendon (sheath)

Excludes: cartilage (of):
- articular (C40–C41)
- larynx (C32.3)

Kaposi's sarcoma (C46.–)
mesothelioma (C45.–)
peripheral nerves and autonomic nervous system (C.47.–)

C49.0 Connective and soft tissue of head, face and neck

C49.1 Connective and soft tissue of upper limb, including shoulder

C49.2 Connective and soft tissue of lower limb, including hip

C49.3 Connective and soft tissue of thorax

C49.4 Connective and soft tissue of abdomen

C49.5 Connective and soft tissue of pelvis

C49.6 Connective and soft tissue of trunk, unspecified

C49.8 Overlapping lesion of connective and soft tissue

C49.9 Connective and soft tissue, unspecified

Malignant neoplasm of breast (C50)

C50.– Malignant neoplasm of breast

Malignant neoplasms of female genital organs (C51–C58)

C51.– Malignant neoplasm of vulva

C52 Malignant neoplasm of vagina

C53.– Malignant neoplasm of cervix uteri

C54.– Malignant neoplasm of corpus uteri

C55 Malignant neoplasm of uterus, part unspecified

C56 Malignant neoplasm of ovary

C57 Malignant neoplasm of other and unspecified female genital organs

C57.8 Overlapping lesion of female genital organs

C58 Malignant neoplasm of placenta

Choriocarcinoma NOS
Chorionepithelioma NOS

Malignant neoplasms of male genital organs (C60–C63)

C60.– Malignant neoplasm of penis

C61 Malignant neoplasm of prostate

C62 Malignant neoplasm of testis

C62.0 Undescended testis

Ectopic testis [site of neoplasm]
Retained testis [site of neoplasm]

C63 Malignant neoplasm of other and unspecified male genital organs

C63.8 Overlapping lesion of male genital organs

Malignant neoplasms of urinary tract (C64–C68)

C64 Malignant neoplasm of kidney, except renal pelvis

C65 Malignant neoplasm of renal pelvis

Pelviureteric junction
Renal calyces

C66 Malignant neoplasm of ureter

C67.– Malignant neoplasm of bladder

C68 Malignant neoplasm of other and unspecified urinary organs

C68.8 Overlapping lesion of urinary organs

Malignant neoplasms of eye, brain and other parts of central nervous system (C69–C72)

C69 Malignant neoplasm of eye and adnexa

Excludes: optic nerve (C72.3)

C69.2 Retina

C69.6 Orbit

Connective tissue of orbit
Extraocular muscle
Peripheral nerves of orbit
Retrobulbar tissue
Retro-ocular tissue

C70 Malignant neoplasm of meninges

Excludes: secondary carcinomatous meningitis (C79.36)

C70.0 Cerebral meninges

C70.1 Spinal meninges

C70.9 Meninges, unspecified

C71 Malignant neoplasm of brain

Excludes: cranial nerves (C72.2–C72.5)
retrobulbar tissue (C69.6)

C71.0 Cerebrum, except lobes and ventricles

C71.00 Corpus callosum
C71.01 Basal ganglia and thalamus
C71.02 Hypothalamus
C71.07 Other parts of cerebrum, except lobes and ventricles
C71.09 Supratentorial, unspecified

C71.1 Frontal lobe

C71.2 Temporal lobe

C71.3 Parietal lobe

C71.4 Occipital lobe

C71.5 Cerebral ventricle
Excludes: fourth ventricle (C71.73)

C71.50 Lateral ventricle
C71.51 Third ventricle

C71.6 Cerebellum

C71.7 Brain stem

C71.70 Midbrain
C71.71 Pons
C71.72 Medulla
C71.73 Fourth ventricle
C71.78 Multiple and overlapping lesion of brain stem
C71.79 Infratentorial, unspecified

C71.8 Overlapping lesion of brain

C71.9 Brain, unspecified

C72 Malignant neoplasm of spinal cord, cranial nerves and other parts of central nervous system

Excludes: meninges (C70.–)
peripheral nerves and autonomic nervous system (C47.–)

C72.0 Spinal cord

C72.00 Cervical spinal cord
C72.01 Cervicothoracic spinal cord
C72.02 Thoracic spinal cord
C72.03 Thoracolumbar spinal cord
C72.04 Lumbar spinal cord
C72.05 Lumbosacral spinal cord
C72.06 Sacral spinal cord
C72.08 Multiple and overlapping lesion of spinal cord

C72.1 Cauda equina

C72.2 Olfactory nerve

C72.20 Olfactory rami
C72.21 Olfactory bulb

C72.3 Optic nerve

C72.30 Retrobulbar optic nerve
C72.31 Optic chiasm

C72.4 Acoustic nerve

C72.5 Other and unspecified cranial nerves
Includes: cranial nerve NOS

C72.50 Oculomotor nerves
C72.500 Oculomotor nerve [3rd cranial nerve]
C72.501 Trochlear nerve [4th cranial nerve]
C72.502 Abducens nerve [6th cranial nerve]
C72.51 Trigeminal nerve [5th cranial nerve]
C72.52 Facial nerve [7th cranial nerve]
C72.53 Glossopharyngeal nerve [9th cranial nerve]
C72.54 Vagus nerve [10th cranial nerve]
C72.55 Accessory nerve [11th cranial nerve]
C72.56 Hypoglossal nerve [12th cranial nerve]
C72.57 Multiple cranial nerves

C72.8 Overlapping lesion of brain and other parts of central nervous system
Malignant neoplasm of brain and other parts of central nervous system whose point of origin cannot be assigned to any one of the categories C70–C72.5

C72.9 Central nervous system, unspecified

Malignant neoplasms of thyroid and other endocrine glands (C73–C75)

C73 Malignant neoplasm of thyroid gland

C74.– Malignant neoplasm of adrenal gland

C75 Malignant neoplasm of other endocrine glands and related structures

C75.0 Parathyroid gland

C75.1 Pituitary gland

C75.2 Craniopharyngeal duct

C75.3 Pineal gland

C75.4 Carotid body

C75.5 Aortic body and other paraganglia

C75.50 Glomus jugulare
C75.51 Glomus tympanicum
C75.57 Other paraganglia

C75.8 Pluriglandular involvement, unspecified

Note: If the sites of multiple involvement are known, they should be coded separately.

C75.9 Endocrine gland, unspecified

Malignant neoplasms of ill-defined sites, secondary and unspecified sites (C76–C80)

C76 Malignant neoplasm of other and ill-defined sites

Excludes: malignant neoplasm of:
- lymphoid, haematopoietic and related tissue (C81–C96)
- unspecified site (C80)

C76.0 Head, face and neck

Cheek NOS
Nose NOS

C77.– Secondary and unspecified malignant neoplasm of lymph nodes

Excludes: malignant neoplasm of lymph nodes, specified as primary (C81–C88, C96.–)

C78.– Secondary malignant neoplasm of respiratory and digestive organs

C79 Secondary malignant neoplasm of other sites

C79.3 Secondary malignant neoplasm of brain and cerebral meninges

C79.30 Cerebral lobes
- C79.300 Frontal lobe
- C79.301 Temporal lobe
- C79.302 Parietal lobe
- C79.303 Occipital lobe

C79.31 Cerebral ventricles
C79.310 Lateral ventricle
C79.311 Third ventricle
C79.32 Basal ganglia and thalamus
C79.33 Hypothalamus
C79.34 Corpus callosum
C79.35 Brain stem
C79.350 Midbrain
C79.351 Pons
C79.352 Medulla
C79.353 Fourth ventricle
C79.358 Multiple or overlapping lesion of brain stem
C79.36 Cerebellum
C79.37 Meninges
C79.370 Cerebral meninges, supratentorial
C79.371 Cerebral meninges, infratentorial
C79.372 Carcinomatous meningitis
C79.38 Multiple or overlapping

C79.4 Secondary malignant neoplasm of other and unspecified parts of nervous system

C79.40 Spinal cord
C79.41 Nerve roots and cauda equina
C79.42 Brachial plexus
C79.43 Lumbosacral plexus
C79.44 Cranial nerves [Garcin]
C79.45 Peripheral nerves of upper limb
C79.46 Peripheral nerves of lower limb
C79.47 Other specified parts of nervous system

C79.5 Secondary malignant neoplasm of bone and bone marro

C80 Malignant neoplasm without specification of site

Malignant cachexia

Malignant neoplasms of lymphoid, haematopoietic and related tissue (C81–C96)

Excludes: secondary and unspecified neoplasm of lymph nodes (C77.–)

C81.– Hodgkin's disease

Includes: morphology codes M965–M966 with behaviour code /3

C82.– Follicular [nodular] non-Hodgkin's lymphoma

Includes: with or without diffuse areas
morphology code M969 with behaviour code /3

C83.– Diffuse non-Hodgkin's lymphoma

Includes: morphology codes M9593, M9595, M967–M968 with behaviour code /3

C84.– Peripheral and cutaneous T-cell lymphomas

Includes: morphology code M970 with behaviour code /3

C85 Other and unspecified types of non-Hodgkin's lymphoma

Includes: morphology codes M9590–M9592, M9594, M971 with behaviour code /3

C85.0 Lymphosarcoma

C88 Malignant immunoproliferative diseases

Includes: morphology code M976 with behaviour code /3

C88.0 Waldenström's macroglobulinaemia

C88.1 Alpha heavy chain disease

C88.2 Gamma heavy chain disease
Franklin's disease

C90 Multiple myeloma and malignant plasma cell neoplasms

Includes: morphology codes M973, M9830 with behaviour code /3

C90.0 Multiple myeloma
Kahler's disease
Myelomatosis
Excludes: solitary myeloma (C90.2)

C90.1 Plasma cell leukaemia

C90.2 Plasmacytoma, extramedullary
Malignant plasma cell tumour NOS
Plasmacytoma NOS
Solitary myeloma

C91.– Lymphoid leukaemia

Includes: morphology codes M982, M9940–M9941 with behaviour code /3

C92.– Myeloid leukaemia

Includes: morphology codes M986–M988, M9930 with behaviour code /3

C93.– Monocytic leukaemia

Includes: morphology code M989 with behaviour code /3

C94.– Other leukaemias of specified cell type

Includes: morphology codes M984, M9850, M9900, M9910, M9931–M9932 with behaviour code /3

C95.– Leukaemia of unspecified cell type

Includes: morphology code M980 with behaviour code /3

C96 Other and unspecified malignant neoplasms of lymphoid, haematopoietic and related tissue

Includes: morphology codes M972, M974 with behaviour code /3

C96.0 Letterer–Siwe disease

Nonlipid:
- reticuloendotheliosis
- reticulosis

C96.1 Malignant histiocytosis

Histiocytic medullary reticulosis

Malignant neoplasms of independent (primary) multiple sites (C97)

C97 Malignant neoplasms of independent (primary) multiple sites

Benign neoplasms (D10–D36)

D10.– Benign neoplasm of mouth and pharynx

D11 Benign neoplasm of major salivary glands

D11.0 **Parotid gland**

D13 Benign neoplasm of other and ill-defined parts of digestive system

D13.7 **Endocrine pancreas**
Islet cell tumour

D14 Benign neoplasm of middle ear and respiratory system

D14.0 **Middle ear, nasal cavity and accessory sinuses**

D14.1 **Larynx**

D15 Benign neoplasm of other and unspecified intrathoracic organs

D15.0 **Thymus**

D15.1 **Heart**

D15.2 **Mediastinum**

D16 Benign neoplasm of bone and articular cartilage

D16.4 **Bones of skull and face**
Excludes: lower jaw bone (D16.5)

D16.5 **Lower jaw bone**

D16.6 **Vertebral column**
Excludes: sacrum and coccyx (D16.8)

D16.7 **Ribs, sternum and clavicle**

D16.8 **Pelvic bones, sacrum and coccyx**

D17 Benign lipomatous neoplasm

D17.7 **Benign lipomatous neoplasm of other sites**

D17.70 Lipoma of cauda equina
D17.71 Lipoma of corpus callosum
D17.78 Lipoma of other parts of nervous system

D18.– Haemangioma and lymphangioma, any site

D20.– Benign neoplasm of soft tissue of retroperitoneum and peritoneum

D21 Other benign neoplasms of connective and other soft tissue

Excludes: peripheral nerves and autonomic nervous system (D36.1)

D21.0 Connective and other soft tissue of head, face and neck

D21.1 Connective and other soft tissue of upper limb, including shoulder

D21.2 Connective and other soft tissue of lower limb, including hip

D21.3 Connective and other soft tissue of thorax

Excludes: heart (D15.1)
mediastinum (D15.2)
thymus (D15.0)

D21.4 Connective and other soft tissue of abdomen

D21.5 Connective and other soft tissue of pelvis

D21.6 Connective and other soft tissue of trunk, unspecified

D21.9 Connective and other soft tissue, unspecified

D31 Benign neoplasm of eye and adnexa

Excludes: optic nerve (D33.31)

D31.2 Retina

D31.6 Orbit, unspecified

Peripheral nerves of orbit

D32 Benign neoplasm of meninges

D32.0 Cerebral meninges

D32.00 Cerebral meninges, supratentorial
D32.01 Cerebral meninges, infratentorial
D32.02 Disseminated benign meningiomatosis

D32.1 Spinal meninges

D32.9 Meninges, unspecified

Meningioma NOS

D33 Benign neoplasm of brain and other parts of central nervous system

Excludes: angioma (D18.–)
meninges (D32.–)
peripheral nerves and autonomic nervous system (D36.1)
retro-ocular tissue (D31.6)

D33.0 Brain, supratentorial

D33.00 Cerebral lobes
D33.000 Frontal lobe
D33.001 Temporal lobe
D33.002 Parietal lobe
D33.003 Occipital lobe
D33.01 Supratentorial ventricle
D33.010 Lateral ventricle
D33.011 Third ventricle
D33.02 Basal ganglia and thalamus
D33.03 Hypothalamus
D33.04 Corpus callosum
D33.08 Multiple or overlapping lesion of brain, supratentorial

D33.1 Brain, infratentorial

D33.10 Brain stem
D33.100 Midbrain
D33.101 Pons
D33.102 Medulla
D33.103 Fourth ventricle
D33.108 Multiple or overlapping lesion of brain stem
D33.11 Cerebellum
D33.18 Multiple or overlapping lesion of brain, infratentorial

D33.2 Brain, unspecified

D33.3 Cranial nerves

D33.30 Olfactory bulb [1st cranial nerve]
D33.31 Optic nerve [2nd cranial nerve] and optic chiasm
D33.32 Oculomotor, trochlear and abducens nerves
D33.320 Oculomotor nerve [3rd cranial nerve]
D33.321 Trochlear nerve [4th cranial nerve]
D33.322 Abducens nerve [6th cranial nerve]
D33.33 Trigeminal nerve [5th cranial nerve]
D33.34 Facial nerve [7th cranial nerve]
D33.35 Acoustic nerve [8th cranial nerve]

D33.36 9th and 10th cranial nerves
- D33.360 Glossopharyngeal nerve [9th cranial nerve]
- D33.361 Vagus nerve [10th cranial nerve]

D33.37 Accessory nerve [11th cranial nerve]
D33.38 Hypoglossal nerve [12th cranial nerve]
D33.39 Multiple cranial nerves

D33.4 Spinal cord

D33.40 Cervical spinal cord
D33.41 Cervicothoracic spinal cord
D33.42 Thoracic spinal cord
D33.43 Thoracolumbar spinal cord
D33.44 Lumbar spinal cord
D33.45 Lumbosacral spinal cord
D33.46 Sacral spinal cord
D33.48 Multiple or overlapping lesion of spinal cord

D33.7 Other specified parts of central nervous system
Cauda equina

D33.9 Central nervous system, unspecified

D34 Benign neoplasm of thyroid gland

D35 Benign neoplasm of other and unspecified endocrine glands

Excludes: thymus (D15.0)

D35.0 Adrenal gland

D35.1 Parathyroid gland

D35.2 Pituitary gland

D35.20 Growth-hormone-secreting
D35.21 Prolactin-secreting
D35.22 Adrenocorticotropic hormone-secreting
D35.23 Thyroid-stimulating hormone-secreting
D35.24 Luteinizing hormone/follicle-stimulating hormone-secreting
D35.25 α-Subunit-secreting
D35.26 Plurihormonal-secreting
D35.27 Non-secreting adenoma
D35.28 Other hormone-secreting benign neoplasms
D35.29 Hormone-secreting benign neoplasm, unspecified

D35.3 Craniopharyngeal duct

D35.4 Pineal gland

D35.5 Carotid body

D35.6 Aortic body and other paraganglia

D35.60 Glomus jugulare
D35.61 Glomus tympanicum
D35.67 Other paraganglia

D35.7 Other specified endocrine glands

D35.8 Pluriglandular involvement

D35.9 Endocrine gland, unspecified

D36 Benign neoplasm of other and unspecified sites

D36.0 Lymph nodes

D36.1 Peripheral nerves and autonomic nervous system

D36.10 Head, face and neck
- D36.100 Cervical nerve roots
- D36.101 Cervical nerves
- D36.102 Cervical sympathetic chain and plexus
- D36.107 Other parts of peripheral and autonomic nervous system of head, face and neck

D36.11 Upper limb, including shoulder
- D36.110 Brachial plexus
- D36.111 Radial nerve and branches
- D36.112 Median nerve and branches
- D36.113 Ulnar nerve and branches
- D36.117 Other parts of peripheral and autonomic nervous system of upper limb

D36.12 Lower limb, including hip
- D36.120 Sciatic nerve
- D36.121 Gluteal nerve
- D36.122 Peroneal nerve and branches
- D36.123 Tibial nerve and branches
- D36.127 Other parts of peripheral and autonomic nervous system of lower limb

D36.13 Thorax
- D36.130 Thoracic nerve root
- D36.131 Thoracic nerves
- D36.132 Thoracic sympathetic chain and plexus

D36.137 Other parts of peripheral and autonomic nervous system of thorax

D36.14 Abdomen

D36.140 Lumbar nerve root

D36.141 Lumbar nerve

D36.142 Lumbar plexus

D36.147 Other parts of peripheral and autonomic nervous system of abdomen

D36.15 Pelvis

D36.150 Sacral nerve root

D36.151 Sacral nerve

D36.152 Pudendal nerve

D36.153 Obturator nerve

D36.157 Other parts of peripheral and autonomic nervous system of pelvis

D36.16 Trunk, unspecified

D36.18 Overlapping lesion of peripheral nerves and autonomic nervous system

D36.7 Other specified sites

Nose NOS

Neoplasms of uncertain or unknown behaviour (D37–D48)

Note: Categories D37–D48 classify by site neoplasms of uncertain or unknown behaviour, i.e. there is doubt whether the neoplasm is malignant or benign. Such neoplasms are assigned behaviour code /1 in the classification of the morphology of neoplasms.

D37 Neoplasm of uncertain or unknown behaviour of oral cavity and digestive organs

D37.0 Lip, oral cavity and pharynx

Major and minor salivary glands

D38 Neoplasm of uncertain or unknown behaviour of middle ear and respiratory and intrathoracic organs

D38.0 Larynx

D38.4 Thymus

D42 Neoplasm of uncertain or unknown behaviour of meninges

D42.0 Cerebral meninges

D42.00 Cerebral meninges, supratentorial
D42.01 Cerebral meninges, infratentorial
D42.02 Disseminated neoplasm of meninges

D42.1 Spinal meninges

D42.9 Meninges, unspecified

D43 Neoplasm of uncertain or unknown behaviour of brain and central nervous system

Excludes: peripheral nerves and autonomic nervous system (D48.2)

D43.0 Brain, supratentorial

D43.00 Cerebral lobes
- D43.000 Frontal lobe
- D43.001 Temporal lobe
- D43.002 Parietal lobe
- D43.003 Occipital lobe

D43.01 Supratentorial ventricle
- D43.010 Lateral ventricle
- D43.011 Third ventricle

D43.02 Basal ganglia and thalamus
D43.03 Hypothalamus
D43.04 Corpus callosum
D43.08 Multiple or overlapping lesion of brain, supratentorial

D43.1 Brain, infratentorial

D43.10 Brain stem
- D43.100 Midbrain
- D43.101 Pons
- D43.102 Medulla
- D43.103 Fourth ventricle
- D43.108 Multiple or overlapping lesion of brain stem

D43.11 Cerebellum
D43.18 Multiple or overlapping lesion of brain, infratentorial

D43.2 Brain, unspecified

D43.3 Cranial nerves

D43.30 Olfactory bulb [1st cranial nerve]
D43.31 Optic nerve [2nd cranial nerve] and optic chiasm
D43.32 Oculomotor, trochlear and abducens nerves
D43.320 Oculomotor nerve [3rd cranial nerve]
D43.321 Trochlear nerve [4th cranial nerve]
D43.322 Abducens nerve [6th cranial nerve]
D43.33 Trigeminal nerve [5th cranial nerve]
D43.34 Facial nerve [7th cranial nerve]
D43.35 Acoustic nerve [8th cranial nerve]
D43.36 9th and 10th cranial nerves
D43.360 Glossopharyngeal nerve [9th cranial nerve]
D43.361 Vagus nerve [10th cranial nerve]
D43.37 Accessory nerve [11th cranial nerve]
D43.38 Hypoglossal nerve [12th cranial nerve]
D43.39 Multiple cranial nerves

D43.4 Spinal cord

D43.40 Cervical spinal cord
D43.41 Cervicothoracic spinal cord
D43.42 Thoracic spinal cord
D43.43 Thoracolumbar spinal cord
D43.44 Lumbar spinal cord
D43.45 Lumbosacral spinal cord
D43.46 Sacral spinal cord
D43.48 Multiple or overlapping lesion of spinal cord

D43.7 Other parts of central nervous system
Cauda equina

D43.9 Central nervous system, unspecified

D44 Neoplasm of uncertain or unknown behaviour of endocrine glands

Excludes: thymus (D38.4)

D44.3 Pituitary gland

D44.4 Craniopharyngeal duct

D44.5 Pineal gland

D44.6 Carotid body

D44.7 Aortic body and other paraganglia

D44.70 Glomus jugulare

D44.71 Glomus tympanicum
D44.77 Other paraganglia

D44.8 Pluriglandular involvement
Multiple endocrine adenomatosis

D44.9 Endocrine gland, unspecified

D45 Polycythaemia vera

Morphology code M9950 with behaviour code /1

D47 Other neoplasms of uncertain or unknown behaviour of lymphoid, haematopoietic and related tissue

D47.2 Monoclonal gammopathy

D47.20 IgM monoclonal gammopathy with anti-myelin-associated glycoprotein activity
D47.200 With kappa light chain
D47.201 With lambda light chain
D47.21 IgM monoclonal gammopathy without anti-myelin-associated glycoprotein activity
D47.210 With kappa light chain
D47.211 With lambda light chain
D47.22 IgG monoclonal gammopathy
D47.220 With kappa light chain
D47.221 With lambda light chain
D47.23 IgA monoclonal gammopathy
D47.27 Other monoclonal gammopathy

D47.3 Essential (haemorrhagic) thrombocythaemia
Idiopathic haemorrhagic thrombocythaemia

D47.9 Neoplasm of uncertain or unknown behaviour of lymphoid, haematopoietic and related tissue, unspecified
Lymphoproliferative disease NOS

D48 Neoplasm of uncertain or unknown behaviour of other and unspecified sites

Excludes: neurofibromatosis (nonmalignant) (Q85.0)

D48.0 Bone and articular cartilage

D48.2 Peripheral nerves and autonomic nervous system

D48.3 Retroperitoneum

D48.4 Peritoneum

D48.5 Skin

D48.6 Breast

D48.7 Other specified sites
Eye
Peripheral nerves of orbit

D48.9 Neoplasm of unknown or uncertain behaviour, unspecified

CHAPTER III

Diseases of the blood and blood-forming organs and certain disorders involving the immune mechanism (D50–D89)

Nutritional anaemias (D50–D53)

D50.– Iron deficiency anaemia

D51 Vitamin B_{12} deficiency anaemia

Excludes: vitamin B_{12} deficiency (E53.8)

D51.0 **Vitamin B_{12} deficiency anaemia due to intrinsic factor deficiency**

D51.1 **Vitamin B_{12} deficiency anaemia due to selective vitamin B_{12} malabsorption with proteinuria**

D51.2 **Transcobalamin II deficiency**

D51.3 **Other dietary vitamin B_{12} deficiency anaemia**

D51.8 **Other vitamin B_{12} deficiency anaemias**

D51.9 **Vitamin B_{12} deficiency anaemia, unspecified**

D52 Folate deficiency anaemia

D52.0 **Dietary folate deficiency anaemia**

D52.1 **Drug-induced folate deficiency anaemia**

D52.8 **Other folate deficiency anaemias**

D52.9 **Folate deficiency anaemia, unspecified**

D53.– Other nutritional anaemias

Includes: megaloblastic anaemia unresponsive to vitamin B_{12} or folate therapy

Haemolytic anaemias (D55–D59)

D55.– Anaemia due to enzyme disorders

D56.– Thalassaemia

D57 Sickle-cell disorders

Excludes: other haemoglobinopathies (D58.–)
sickle-cell beta thalassaemia (D56.–)

D57.0 Sickle-cell anaemia with crisis
Hb-SS disease with crisis

D58.– Other hereditary haemolytic anaemias

Coagulation defects, purpura and other haemorrhagic conditions (D65–D69)

D65 Disseminated intravascular coagulation [defibrination syndrome]

Afibrinogenaemia, acquired
Consumption coagulopathy
Diffuse or disseminated intravascular coagulation [DIC]
Fibrinolytic haemorrhage, acquired
Purpura:
- fibrinolytic
- fulminans

D66 Hereditary factor VIII deficiency

Deficiency factor VIII (with functional defect)
Haemophilia A

D67 Hereditary factor IX deficiency

Christmas disease
Deficiency:
- factor IX (with functional defect)
- plasma thromboplastin component [PTC]

Haemophilia B

D68 Other coagulation defects

D68.0 Von Willebrand's disease

Angiohaemophilia
Factor VIII deficiency with vascular defect
Vascular haemophilia
Excludes: capillary fragility (hereditary) (D69.8)
factor VIII deficiency:
- NOS (D66)
- with functional defect (D66)

D68.1 Hereditary factor XI deficiency

Haemophilia C
Plasma thromboplastin antecedent [PTA] deficiency

D68.2 Hereditary deficiency of other clotting factors

Congenital afibrinogenaemia
Deficiency:
- AC globulin
- proaccelerin

Deficiency of factor:
- I [fibrinogen]
- II [prothrombin]
- V [labile]
- VII [stable]
- X [Stuart–Prower]
- XII [Hageman]
- XIII [fibrin-stabilizing]

Dysfibrinogenaemia (congenital)
Hypoproconvertinaemia
Owren's disease

D68.3 Haemorrhagic disorder due to circulating anticoagulants

Hyperheparinaemia
Increase in:
- antithrombin
- anti-VIIIa
- anti-IXa
- anti-Xa
- anti-XIa

Use additional external cause code (Chapter XX), if desired, to identify any administered anticoagulant.

D68.4 Acquired coagulation factor deficiency

Deficiency of coagulation factor due to:
- liver disease

- vitamin K deficiency

Excludes: vitamin K deficiency of newborn (P53)

D68.8 Other specified coagulation defects

D68.80 Presence of systemic lupus erythematosus [SLE] inhibitor
Lupus anticoagulant

D68.81 Circulating anticoagulants without SLE

D68.82 Protein C deficiency

D68.83 Protein S deficiency

D68.9 Coagulation defect, unspecified

D69 Purpura and other haemorrhagic conditions

Excludes: benign hypergammaglobulinaemic purpura (D89.0)
cryoglobulinaemic purpura (D89.1)
essential (haemorrhagic) thrombocythaemia (D47.3)
purpura fulminans (D65)
thrombotic thrombocytopenic purpura (M31.1)

D69.0 Allergic purpura
Henoch–Schönlein purpura
Vasculitis, allergic

D69.1 Qualitative platelet defects

D69.2 Other nonthrombocytopenic purpura

D69.3 Idiopathic thrombocytopenic purpura
Evans' syndrome

D69.4 Other primary thrombocytopenia

D69.5 Secondary thrombocytopenia
Use additional external cause code (Chapter XX), if desired, to identify cause.

D69.6 Thrombocytopenia, unspecified

D69.8 Other specified haemorrhagic conditions
Capillary fragility (hereditary)

D69.9 Haemorrhagic condition, unspecified

Other diseases of blood and blood-forming organs (D70–D77)

D70 Agranulocytosis

D73 Diseases of spleen

D73.1 Hypersplenism

Excludes: splenomegaly:
- NOS (R16.1)
- congenital (Q89.0)

D74 Methaemoglobinaemia

D74.0 Congenital methaemoglobinaemia

Congenital NADH-methaemoglobin reductase deficiency
Haemoglobin-M [Hb-M] disease
Methaemoglobinaemia, hereditary

D74.8 Other methaemoglobinaemias

Acquired methaemoglobinaemia (with sulfhaemoglobinaemia)
Toxic methaemoglobinaemia

Use additional external cause code (Chapter XX), if desired, to identify cause.

D74.9 Methaemoglobinaemia, unspecified

D75 Other diseases of blood and blood-forming organs

D75.0 Familial erythrocytosis

Polycythaemia:
- benign
- familial

D75.1 Secondary polycythaemia

Excludes: polycythaemia vera (D45)

D75.2 Essential thrombocytosis

Excludes: essential (haemorrhagic) thrombocythaemia (D47.3)

D76 Certain diseases involving lymphoreticular tissue and reticulohistiocytic system

Excludes: Letterer–Siwe disease (C96.0)
malignant histiocytosis (C96.1)
reticuloendotheliosis or reticulosis:
- histiocytic medullary (C96.1)
- leukaemic (C91.–)
- nonlipid (C96.0)

D76.0 Langerhans' cell histiocytosis, not elsewhere classified

Eeosinophilic granuloma
Hand–Schüller–Christian disease
Histiocytosis X (chronic)

D76.1 **Haemophagocytic lymphohistiocytosis**
Familial haemophagocytic reticulosis
Histiocytoses of mononuclear phagocytes other than Langerhans' cells NOS

D76.3 **Other histiocytosis syndromes**
Reticulohistiocytoma (giant-cell)
Sinus histiocytosis with massive lymphadenopathy
Xanthogranuloma

Certain disorders involving the immune mechanism (D80–D89)

Includes: defects in the complement system
immunodeficiency disorders, except human immunodeficiency virus [HIV] disease
sarcoidosis

Excludes: human immunodeficiency virus [HIV] disease (B20–B24)

D86 Sarcoidosis

D86.8 **Sarcoidosis of other and combined sites**

D86.80† Multiple cranial nerve palsies in sarcoidosis (G53.2*)
D86.81 Peripheral nerve disease in sarcoidosis
D86.82 Spinal cord disease in sarcoidosis
D86.83 Meningoencephalitis in sarcoidosis
D86.84 Hydrocephalus in sarcoidosis
D86.88 Other nervous system involvement in sarcoidosis
D86.89 Sarcoidosis of the nervous system, unspecified

D89 Other disorders involving the immune mechanism, not elsewhere classified

D89.0 **Polyclonal hypergammaglobulinaemia**
Benign hypergammaglobulinaemic purpura
Polyclonal gammopathy NOS

D89.1 **Cryoglobulinaemia**

D89.10 Cryoglobulinaemic vasculitis

D89.2 **Hypergammaglobulinaemia, unspecified**
Excludes: monoclonal gammopathies (D47.20–D47.27)

D89.8 Other specified disorders involving the immune mechanism, not elsewhere classified

D89.9 Disorder involving the immune mechanism, unspecified
Immune disease NOS

CHAPTER IV

Endocrine, nutritional and metabolic diseases (E00–E90)

Note: All neoplasms, whether functionally active or not, are classified in Chapter II. Appropriate codes in this chapter (i.e. E05.8, E16–E31, E34.–) may be used, if desired, as additional codes to indicate either functional activity by neoplasms and ectopic endocrine tissue or hyperfunction and hypofunction of endocrine glands associated with neoplasms and other conditions classified elsewhere.

Disorders of thyroid gland (E00–E07)

E00 Congenital iodine-deficiency syndrome

Includes: endemic conditions associated with environmental iodine-deficiency either directly or as a consequence of maternal iodine deficiency. Some of the conditions have no current hypothyroidism but are the consequence of inadequate thyroid hormone secretion in the developing fetus. Environmental goitrogens may be associated.

Use additional code (F70–F79), if desired, to identify associated mental retardation.

Excludes: subclinical iodine-deficiency hypothyroidism (E02)

E00.0 Congenital iodine-deficiency syndrome, neurological type

Endemic cretinism, neurological type

E00.1 Congenital iodine-deficiency syndrome, myxoedematous type

Endemic cretinism:
- hypothyroid
- myxoedematous type

E00.2 Congenital iodine-deficiency syndrome, mixed type

Endemic cretinism, mixed type

E00.9 Congenital iodine-deficiency syndrome, unspecified
Congenital iodine-deficiency hypothyroidism NOS
Endemic cretinism NOS

E01 Iodine-deficiency-related thyroid disorders and allied conditions

Excludes: congenital iodine-deficiency syndrome (E00.–)
subclinical iodine-deficiency hypothyroidism (E02)

E01.0 Iodine-deficiency-related diffuse (endemic) goitre

E01.1 Iodine-deficiency-related multinodular (endemic) goitre

E01.2 Iodine-deficiency-related (endemic) goitre, unspecified
Endemic goitre NOS

E01.8 Other iodine-deficiency-related thyroid disorders and allied conditions
Acquired iodine-deficiency hypothyroidism NOS

E02 Subclinical iodine-deficiency hypothyroidism

E03 Other hypothyroidism

Excludes: iodine-deficiency related hypothyroidism (E00–E02)
myxoedema psychosis (F06.8)
postprocedural hypothyroidism (E89.0)

E03.0 Congenital hypothyroidism with diffuse goitre
Goitre (nontoxic) congenital:
- NOS
- parenchymatous

E03.1 Congenital hypothyroidism without goitre
Aplasia of thyroid (with myxoedema)
Congenital:
- atrophy of thyroid
- hypothyroidism NOS

E03.2 Hypothyroidism due to medicaments and other exogenous substances
Use additional external cause code (Chapter XX), if desired, to identify cause.

E03.3 Postinfectious hypothyroidism

E03.4 Atrophy of thyroid (acquired)
Excludes: congenital atrophy of thyroid (E03.1)

E03.5 Myxoedema coma

E03.8 Other specified hypothyroidism

E03.9 Hypothyroidism, unspecified
Myxoedema NOS

E04.– Other nontoxic goitre

Excludes: congenital goitre:
- NOS (E03.0)
- diffuse (E03.0)
- parenchymatous (E03.0)

iodine-deficiency-related goitre (E00–E02)

E05 Thyrotoxicosis [hyperthyroidism]

Excludes: chronic thyroiditis with transient thyrotoxicosis (E06.2)
neonatal thyrotoxicosis (P72.1)

E05.0 Thyrotoxicosis with diffuse goitre
Dysthyroid ophthalmoplegia† (G73.50*)
Exophthalmic or toxic goitre NOS
Graves' disease
Toxic diffuse goitre
Excludes: euthyroid ophthalmic Graves' disease (H05.22)

E05.1 Thyrotoxicosis with toxic single thyroid nodule

E05.2 Thyrotoxicosis with toxic multinodular goitre

E05.3 Thyrotoxicosis from ectopic thyroid tissue

E05.4 Thyrotoxicosis factitia

E05.5 Thyroid crisis or storm

E05.8 Other thyrotoxicosis
Overproduction of thyroid-stimulating hormone

Use additional external cause code (Chapter XX), if desired, to identify cause.

E05.80 Thyrotoxicosis due to hypersecretion of thyroid-releasing hormone

E05.9 Thyrotoxicosis, unspecified
Hyperthyroidism NOS
Thyrotoxic heart disease† (I43.–*)

E06 Thyroiditis

E06.2 Chronic thyroiditis with transient thyrotoxicosis
Excludes: autoimmune thyroiditis (E06.3)

E06.3 Autoimmune thyroiditis
Hashimoto's thyroiditis
Hashitoxicosis (transient)
Lymphadenoid goitre
Lymphocytic thyroiditis
Struma lymphomatosa

E06.4 Drug-induced thyroiditis
Use additional external cause code (Chapter XX), if desired, to identify drug.

Diabetes mellitus (E10–E14)

Use additional external cause code (Chapter XX), if desired, to identify drug, if drug-induced.

The following fourth-character subdivisions are for use with categories E10–E14:

.0 With coma
.00 ketoacidosis
.01 hyperosmolar nonketotic
.02 hypoglycaemic

.1 With ketoacidosis
Excludes: with coma (.00)

.2 With renal complications

.3† With ophthalmic complications
Diabetic:
- cataract (H28.0*)
- retinopathy (H36.0*)

.4† With neurological complications
Diabetic:
- amyotrophy (G73.0*)
- autonomic neuropathy (G59.0*)
- mononeuropathy (G59.0*)
- polyneuropathy (G63.2*)
- autonomic (G99.0*)

.5 With peripheral circulatory complications

.6† **With other specified complications**
Diabetic arthropathy (M14.2*)
- neuropathic (M14.6*)

.7 **With multiple complications**

.8 **With unspecified complications**

.9 **Without complications**

E10 Insulin-dependent diabetes mellitus

Includes: diabetes (mellitus):
- brittle
- juvenile-onset
- ketosis-prone
- type I

E11 Non-insulin-dependent diabetes mellitus

Includes: diabetes (mellitus)(non-obese)(obese):
- adult-onset
- maturity-onset
- nonketotic
- stable
- type II

non-insulin-dependent diabetes of the young

E12 Malnutrition-related diabetes mellitus

E13 Other specified diabetes mellitus

E14 Unspecified diabetes mellitus

Other disorders of glucose regulation and pancreatic internal secretion (E15–E16)

E15 Nondiabetic hypoglycaemic coma

Drug-induced insulin coma in nondiabetic
Hyperinsulinism with hypoglycaemic coma
Hypoglycaemic coma NOS

Use additional external cause code (Chapter XX), if desired, to identify drug, if drug-induced.

E16 Other disorders of pancreatic internal secretion

E16.0 Drug-induced hypoglycaemia without coma
Use additional external cause code (Chapter XX), if desired, to identify drug.

E16.1 Other hypoglycaemia
Includes: functional nonhyperinsulinaemic hypoglycaemia
hyperinsulinism:
- NOS
- functional

hyperplasia of pancreatic islet beta cells NOS

E16.10 Posthypoglycaemic coma encephalopathy

E16.2 Hypoglycaemia, unspecified

E16.3 Increased secretion of glucagon
Hyperplasia of pancreatic endocrine cells with glucagon excess

E16.8 Other specified disorders of pancreatic internal secretion
Increased secretion from endocrine pancreas of growth hormone-releasing hormone
Zollinger–Ellison syndrome

E16.9 Disorder of pancreatic internal secretion, unspecified
Islet-cell hyperplasia NOS

Disorders of other endocrine glands (E20–E35)

Excludes: galactorrhoea (N64.3)

E20 Hypoparathyroidism

Excludes: postprocedural hypoparathyroidism (E89.2)
tetany NOS (R29.0)

E20.0 Idiopathic hypoparathyroidism

E20.1 Pseudohypoparathyroidism

E20.8 Other hypoparathyroidism

E20.80 Pseudo-pseudohypoparathyroidism
Normocalcaemic pseudohypoparathyroidism

E20.9 Hypoparathyroidism, unspecified
Parathyroid tetany

E21 Hyperparathyroidism and other disorders of parathyroid gland

Excludes: adult osteomalacia (M83.–)

E21.0 Primary hyperparathyroidism

Hyperplasia of parathyroid
Osteitis fibrosa cystica generalisata [von Recklinghausen's disease of bone]

E21.1 Secondary hyperparathyroidism, not elsewhere classified

Excludes: secondary hyperparathyroidism of renal origin (N25.8)

E21.2 Other hyperparathyroidism

E21.3 Hyperparathyroidism, unspecified

E21.4 Other specified disorders of parathyroid gland

E21.5 Disorder of parathyroid gland, unspecified

E22 Hyperfunction of pituitary gland

Excludes: Cushing's syndrome (E24.–)
Nelson's syndrome (E24.1)
overproduction of:
- adrenocorticotropic hormone [ACTH] not associated with Cushing's disease (E27.0)
- pituitary adrenocorticotropic hormone [ACTH] (E24.0)
- thyroid-stimulating hormone (E05.8)

E22.0 Acromegaly and pituitary gigantism

E22.00 Pituitary growth hormone cell hyperplasia
E22.01 Hypersecretion of growth hormone due to excessive production of growth hormone-releasing hormone
E22.02 Hypersecretion of growth hormone associated with ectopic growth hormone-releasing hormone [GHRH] production
E22.08 Other specified causes of hypersecretion of growth hormone

E22.1 Hyperprolactinaemia

Use additional external cause code (Chapter XX), if desired, to identify drug, if drug-induced.

E22.10 With acromegaly
E22.11 With Cushing's syndrome
E22.12 With empty sella syndrome
E22.13 With pituitary stalk section

E22.14 With lymphocytic hypophysitis
E22.18 Hyperprolactinaemia due to other causes

E22.2 Syndrome of inappropriate secretion of antidiuretic hormone

Includes: syndrome of inappropriate vasopressin secretion

E22.20 Hypothalamic hypersecretion of antidiuretic hormone
E22.21 Associated with central nervous system disease outside the hypothalamus
E22.22 Associated with pulmonary infections
E22.23 Ectopic production by tumour
Use additional code, if desired, to identify tumour.
E22.24 Drug-induced
Use additional external cause code (Chapter XX), if desired, to identify drug.
E22.28 Other syndromes of inappropriate secretion of antidiuretic hormone

E22.8 Other hyperfunction of pituitary gland

E22.80 Hypersecretion of growth hormone unassociated with acromegaly or gigantism
Use additional code, if desired, to identify underlying condition.
E22.81 Hypersecretion of luteinizing hormone [LH] and follicle-stimulating hormone [FSH]
Excludes: gonadotropic cell pituitary adenoma (D35.24)

E22.810 Hypersecretion of luteinizing hormone/follicle-stimulating hormone associated with excessive gonadotropin-releasing hormone stimulation of hypothalamic origin
E22.811 Hypersecretion of luteinizing hormone/follicle-stimulating hormone associated with excessive gonadotropin-releasing hormone stimulation of ectopic origin

E22.82 Central precocious puberty

E22.9 Hyperfunction of pituitary gland, unspecified

E23 Hypofunction and other disorders of pituitary gland

Includes: the listed conditions whether the disorder is in the pituitary or the hypothalamus

Excludes: postprocedural hypopituitarism (E89.3)

E23.0 Hypopituitarism

Includes: pituitary insufficiency NOS

Use additional code, if desired, to identify the underlying cause.

E23.00 Panhypopituitarism
Multiple pituitary hormone deficiency [Simmonds]

E23.01 Postpartum pituitary necrosis [Sheehan]

E23.02 Growth hormone deficiency, not due to pituitary tumour
Excludes: psychosocial short stature (E34.3)

E23.020 Isolated deficiency of growth hormone

E23.021 Lorain–Levi dwarfism (short stature)

E23.022 Pituitary dwarfism (short stature)

E23.023 Due to growth hormone-releasing hormone deficiency

E23.03 Isolated prolactin deficiency

E23.04 Isolated thyrotropin deficiency

E23.040 Due to thyrotropin-releasing hormone [TRH] deficiency

E23.041 Due to hyperthyroidism

E23.05 Isolated follicle-stimulating hormone [FSH] and luteinizing hormone [LH] deficiency

E23.050 Due to gonadotropin-releasing hormone deficiency
Use additional code, if desired, to identify tumour.

E23.06 Isolated adrenocorticotropic hormone [ACTH] deficiency

E23.07 Multiple anterior pituitary hormone deficiencies

E23.1 Drug-induced hypopituitarism

Use additional external cause code (Chapter XX), if desired, to identify drug.

E23.10 Drug-induced adrenocorticotropic hormone [ACTH] deficiency

E23.2 Diabetes insipidus

Vasopressin deficiency

Excludes: nephrogenic diabetes insipidus (N25.1)

E23.3 Hypothalamic dysfunction, not elsewhere classified

Excludes: Prader–Willi syndrome (Q87.15)
Russell–Silver syndrome (Q87.17)

E23.30 Diencephalic syndrome

E23.31 Oxytocin deficiency

E23.6 Other disorders of pituitary gland

E23.60 Abscess of pituitary
E23.61 Adiposogenital dystrophy
E23.62 Cyst of Rathke's pouch
E23.63 Pituitary apoplexy

E23.7 Disorder of pituitary gland, unspecified

E24 Cushing's syndrome

E24.0 Pituitary-dependent Cushing's disease

E24.00 Overproduction of corticotropin-releasing hormone
E24.01 Overproduction of adrenocorticotropic hormone [ACTH] with pituitary hyperplasia

E24.1 Nelson's syndrome

E24.2 Drug-induced Cushing's syndrome
Use additional external cause code (Chapter XX), if desired, to identify drug.

E24.3 Ectopic ACTH syndrome

E24.4 Alcohol-induced pseudo-Cushing's syndrome

E24.8 Other Cushing's syndrome

E24.9 Cushing's syndrome, unspecified

E25 Adrenogenital disorders

Includes: adrenogenital syndromes, virilizing or feminizing, whether acquired or due to adrenal hyperplasia consequent on inborn enzyme defects in hormone synthesis

E25.0 Congenital adrenogenital disorders associated with enzyme deficiency

E25.8 Other adrenogenital disorders
Idiopathic adrenogenital disorders

Use additional external cause code (Chapter XX), if desired, to identify drug, if drug-induced.

E25.9 Adrenogenital disorder, unspecified

E26 Hyperaldosteronism

E26.0 Primary hyperaldosteronism
Conn's syndrome
Primary aldosteronism due to adrenal hyperplasia (bilateral)

E26.1 Secondary hyperaldosteronism

E26.8 Other hyperaldosteronism
Bartter's syndrome

E26.9 Hyperaldosteronism, unspecified

E27 Other disorders of adrenal gland

E27.0 Other adrenocortical overactivity
Overproduction of adrenocorticotropic hormone [ACTH], not associated with Cushing's disease
Premature adrenarche
Excludes: Cushing's syndrome (E24.–)

E27.1 Primary adrenocortical insufficiency
Addison's disease
Autoimmune adrenalitis
Excludes: amyloidosis (E85.–)
Waterhouse–Friderichsen syndrome (A39.1)

E27.2 Addisonian crisis
Adrenal or adrenocortical crisis

E27.3 Drug-induced adrenocortical insufficiency
Use additional external cause code (Chapter XX), if desired, to identify drug.

E27.4 Other and unspecified primary adrenocortical insufficiency
Includes: hypoaldosteronism
Excludes: adrenoleukodystrophy [Addison–Schilder] (E71.33)
Waterhouse–Friderichsen syndrome (A39.1)

E27.40 Adrenal haemorrhage
E27.41 Adrenal infarction

E27.5 Adrenomedullary hyperfunction
Catecholamine hypersecretion

E27.8 Other specified disorders of adrenal gland
Abnormality of cortisol-binding globulin

E27.9 Disorder of adrenal gland, unspecified

E28.– Ovarian dysfunction

Excludes: isolated gonadotropin deficiency (E23.04)

E29.– Testicular dysfunction

Excludes: androgen resistance syndrome (E34.5)
isolated gonadotropin deficiency (E23.04)
Klinefelter's syndrome (Q98.0–Q98.2, Q98.4)
testicular feminization (syndrome) (E34.5)

E30 Disorders of puberty, not elsewhere classified

E30.0 Delayed puberty
Constitutional delay of puberty
Delayed sexual development

E30.1 Precocious puberty
Excludes: Albright(–McCune)(–Sternberg) syndrome (Q78.1)

E30.8 Other disorders of puberty
Premature thelarche

E30.9 Disorder of puberty, unspecified

E31 Polyglandular dysfunction

Excludes: ataxia telangiectasia [Louis–Bar] (G11.30)
dystrophia myotonica [Steinert] (G71.12)
pseudohypoparathyroidism (E20.1)

E31.0 Autoimmune polyglandular failure
Schmidt's syndrome

E32 Diseases of thymus

Excludes: myasthenia gravis (G70.0)

E32.0 Persistent hyperplasia of thymus
Hypertrophy of thymus

E32.1 Abscess of thymus

E32.8 Other diseases of thymus

E32.9 Diseases of thymus, unspecified

E34 Other endocrine disorders

Excludes: pseudohypoparathyroidism (E20.1)

E34.0 Carcinoid syndrome
Note: May be used as an additional code, if desired, to identify functional activity associated with a carcinoid tumour.

E34.1 Other hypersecretion of intestinal hormones

E34.2 Ectopic hormone secretion, not elsewhere classified

E34.3 Short stature, not elsewhere classified
Short stature:
- NOS
- constitutional
- Laron-type
- psychosocial

Excludes: progeria (E34.8)
Russell–Silver syndrome (Q87.17)
short stature:
- achondroplastic (Q77.4)
- in specific dysmorphic syndromes — code to syndrome
- pituitary (E23.012)

E34.5 Androgen resistance syndrome
Male pseudohermaphroditism with androgen resistance
Testicular feminization (syndrome)

E34.8 Other specified endocrine disorders
Pineal gland dysfunction
Progeria

E34.9 Endocrine disorder, unspecified
Disturbance:
- endocrine NOS
- hormone NOS

E35* Disorders of endocrine glands in diseases classified elsewhere

E35.0* Disorders of thyroid gland in diseases classified elsewhere
Tuberculosis of thyroid gland (A18.8†)

E35.1* Disorders of adrenal gland in diseases classified elsewhere
Waterhouse–Friderichsen syndrome (meningococcal) (A39.1†)

Malnutrition (E40–E46)

E40 Kwashiorkor

Severe malnutrition with nutritional oedema with dyspigmentation of skin and hair.

E41 Nutritional marasmus

Severe malnutrition with marasmus

E42 **Marasmic kwashiorkor**
Severe protein–energy malnutrition:
- intermediate form
- with signs of both kwashiorkor and marasmus

E43 **Unspecified severe protein–energy malnutrition**
Starvation oedema

E44.– **Protein–energy malnutrition of moderate and mild degree**

E45 **Retarded development following protein–energy malnutrition**
Nutritional:
- short stature
- stunting

Physical retardation due to malnutrition

E46 **Unspecified protein–energy malnutrition**
Malnutrition NOS

Other nutritional deficiencies (E50–E64)

Excludes: nutritional anaemias (D50–D53)

E50 **Vitamin A deficiency**
Excludes: sequelae of vitamin A deficiency (E64.1)

E50.5 **Vitamin A deficiency with night blindness**

E51 **Thiamine deficiency**
Excludes: sequelae of thiamine deficiency (E64.8)

E51.1 **Beriberi**

E51.2 **Wernicke's encephalopathy**
Wernicke's superior haemorrhagic polioencephalitis syndrome

E51.8 **Other manifestations of thiamine deficiency**

E51.9 **Thiamine deficiency, unspecified**

E52 **Niacin deficiency [pellagra]**
Deficiency:
- niacin(-tryptophan)

• nicotinamide
Pellagra (alcoholic)
Excludes: sequelae of niacin deficiency (E64.8)

E53 Deficiency of other B group vitamins

Excludes: sequelae of vitamin B deficiency (E64.8)
vitamin B_{12} deficiency anaemia (D51.–)

E53.0 Riboflavin deficiency

Ariboflavinosis

E53.1 Pyridoxine deficiency

Vitamin B_6 deficiency

E53.8 Deficiency of other specified B group vitamins

E53.80† Vitamin B_{12} [cyanocobalamin] deficiency
Encephalopathy due to vitamin B_{12} deficiency (G94.82*)
Myelopathy due to vitamin B_{12} deficiency (G99.2*)
Polyneuropathy due to vitamin B_{12} deficiency (G63.4*)

E53.81 Folate (folic acid) deficiency

E53.82 Biotin deficiency

E53.83 Pantothenic acid deficiency

E54 Ascorbic acid deficiency

Deficiency of vitamin C
Scurvy

E55 Vitamin D deficiency

Excludes: osteomalacia (M83.–)
osteoporosis (M80–M81)
sequelae of rickets (E64.3)

E55.0 Rickets, active

Infantile osteomalacia
Juvenile osteomalacia

E56.– Other vitamin deficiencies

Excludes: sequelae of other vitamin deficiencies (E64.8)

E58 Dietary calcium deficiency

Excludes: disorders of calcium metabolism (E83.5)
sequelae of calcium deficiency (E64.8)

E61 Deficiency of other nutrient elements

Use additional external cause code (Chapter XX), if desired, to identify drug, if drug-induced.

Excludes: disorders of mineral metabolism (E83.–)
iodine-deficiency-related thyroid disorders (E00–E02)
sequelae of malnutrition and other nutritional deficiencies (E64.–)

E61.0 Copper deficiency

E61.1 Iron deficiency
Excludes: iron deficiency anaemia (D50.–)

E64 Sequelae of malnutrition and other nutritional deficiencies

[See Section II, note 1.5, coding of late effects]

E64.0 Sequelae of protein–energy malnutrition
Excludes: retarded development following protein–energy malnutrition (E45)

E64.1 Sequelae of vitamin A deficiency

E64.2 Sequelae of vitamin C deficiency

E64.3 Sequelae of rickets

E64.8 Sequelae of other nutritional deficiencies

E64.9 Sequelae of unspecified nutritional deficiency

Obesity and other hyperalimentation (E65–E68)

E66 Obesity

Excludes: adiposogenital dystrophy (E23.61)
Prader–Willi syndrome (Q87.15)

E66.2 Extreme obesity with alveolar hypoventilation
Pickwickian syndrome

E67 Other hyperalimentation

Excludes: hyperalimentation NOS (R63.2)

E67.0 Hypervitaminosis A

E67.1 Hypercarotenaemia

E67.2 Megavitamin-B_6 syndrome

Metabolic disorders (E70–E90)

E70 Disorders of aromatic amino-acid metabolism

E70.0 Classical phenylketonuria

E70.00 Severe phenylalanine 4-monooxygenase [phenylalanine hydroxylase] deficiency (classical phenylketonuria)
E70.01 Partial phenylalanine 4-monooxygenase [phenylalanine hydroxylase] deficiency (benign phenylketonuria variant)
E70.02 Dihydropteridine reductase deficiency
E70.03 Dihydrobiopterin synthetase deficiency
E70.04 Guanosine triphosphate cyclohydrolase I deficiency
E70.08 Other specified disorders of phenylalanine metabolism

E70.1 Other hyperphenylalaninaemias

E70.10 4-Hydroxyphenylpyruvate dioxygenase deficiency [hawkinsuria]

E70.2 Disorders of tyrosine metabolism

Excludes: transitory tyrosinaemia of newborn (P74.5)

E70.20 Fumarylacetoacetase deficiency (tyrosinaemia type I)
E70.21 Oculocutaneous tyrosinaemia (tyrosinaemia type II)
E70.22 Alkaptonuria (homogentisic acid defects)
E70.23 Alkaptonuric ochranosis (ochronosis)

E70.3 Albinism

E70.30 Oculocutaneous albinism
E70.31 Ocular albinism
E70.32 Tyrosinase deficiency [Chediak(–Steinbrinck)–Higashi]
E70.33 Cross' syndrome
E70.34 Hermansky–Pudlak syndrome

E70.8 Other disorders of aromatic amino-acid metabolism

E70.80 Disorders of histidine metabolism
- E70.800 Histidine ammonia-lyase [histidase] [histidinase] deficiency
- E70.801 Carnosinase deficiency
- E70.802 Imidazole deficiency
- E70.803 β-Alanine transaminase deficiency [β-alaninaemia]

E70.804 Glutamate formiminotransferase deficiency
E70.808 Other specified disorders of histidine metabolism

E70.81 Disorders of tryptophan metabolism

E70.810 Hartnup's disease
E70.811 Tryptophanaemia
E70.812 Kynureninase deficiency [hydroxykynureninuria]
E70.818 Other specified disorders of tryptophan metabolism

E70.82 Wardenburg–Klein syndrome

E70.83 Indicanuria

E70.9 Disorder of aromatic amino-acid metabolism, unspecified

E71 Disorders of branched-chain amino-acid metabolism and fatty-acid metabolism

E71.0 Maple-syrup-urine disease

E71.00 Severe branched-chain keto-acid dehydrogenase deficiency
Classic maple-syrup-urine disease

E71.01 Partial branched-chain keto-acid dehydrogenase deficiency
Intermediate and intermittent maple-syrup-urine disease

E71.02 Branched-chain keto-acid dihydrolipoyltransacetylase deficiency

E71.08 Other specified disorders of branched-chain dehydrogenase metabolism

E71.1 Other disorders of branched-chain amino-acid metabolism

E71.10 Hyperleucine-isoleucinaemia

E71.11 Isovaleric acidaemia
Isovaleryl-CoA dehydrogenase deficiency

E71.12 Methylmalonic acidaemia
Coenzyme A mutase deficiency
Methylmalonyl-CoA mutase deficiency
Partial L-methylmalonyl-CoA mutase deficiency
Disorders of cobalamin metabolism

E71.13 Propionic acidaemia
Propionyl-CoA carboxylase deficiency

E71.14 Valine dehydrogenase ($NADP^+$) deficiency [valinaemia] [hypervalinaemia]

E71.15 Isoleucine and leucine transaminase deficiency [leucinosis]

E71.16 Leucine-induced hypoglycinaemia
E71.18 Other specified disorders of branched-chain amino-acid metabolism

E71.2 Disorder of branched-chain amino-acid metabolism, unspecified

E71.3 Disorders of fatty-acid metabolism
Excludes: coenzyme A mutase deficiency (E71.12)
methylmalonic acidaemia (E71.12)
Refsum's disease (G60.1)
Schilder's disease (G37.0)
Zellweger's syndrome (Q87.82)

E71.30 Coenzyme A lyase deficiency
Excludes: hydroxymethylglutaryl-CoA lyase deficiency (E88.820)
E71.31 Disorders of carnitine metabolism
E71.310 Carnitine *O*-acetyltransferase deficiency
E71.311 Carnitine *O*-palmitoyltransferase deficiency
E71.312 Muscle carnitine deficiency
E71.313 Systemic carnitine deficiency
E71.314 Carnitine deficiency NOS
E71.32 Adrenoleukodystrophy
Includes: adrenomyeloleukodystrophy
adrenomyeloneuropathy
E71.320 Adult type [Addison–Schilder]
E71.321 Neonatal type
E71.38 Other specified disorders of fatty-acid metabolism

E72 Other disorders of amino-acid metabolism

Excludes: abnormal findings without manifest disease (R70–R89)
disorders of:
- aromatic amino-acid metabolism (E70.–)
- branched-chain amino-acid metabolism (E71.0–E71.2)
- fatty-acid metabolism (E71.3)
- purine and pyrimidine metabolism (E79.–)

gout (M10.–)

E72.0 Disorders of amino-acid transport
Excludes: disorders of tryptophan metabolism (E70.81)

E72.00 Lowe's syndrome
E72.01 Lysinuric protein intolerance

E72.02 Cystinosis
E72.03 Oasthouse disease
E72.04 Fanconi(–de Toni)(–Debré) syndrome
E72.05 Hartnup's disease
E72.06 Cystinuria
E72.08 Other specified disorders of amino-acid transport

E72.1 Disorders of sulfur-bearing amino-acid metabolism
Excludes: transcobalamin II deficiency (D51.2)

E72.10 Homocystinuria
E72.100 Cystathionine β-synthase deficiency [type I (classical) homocystinuria]
E72.101 Homocystinuria, type II
E72.102 Homocystinuria, type III
E72.108 Other specified homocystinuria
E72.11 Sulfite oxidase deficiency
E72.12 Cystathioninuria
E72.13 Methioninaemia
E72.18 Other specified disorders of sulfur-bearing amino-acid metabolism

E72.2 Disorders of urea cycle metabolism
Excludes: disorders of ornithine metabolism (E72.4)

E72.20 Argininosuccinate lyase deficiency [argininosuccinic aciduria]
E72.21 Argininosuccinate synthetase deficiency [citrullinaemia]
E72.22 Carbamoylphosphate synthetase I deficiency
E72.23 Arginase deficiency
E72.24 *N*-Acetyltransferase [*N*-acetylglutamate synthetase] deficiency
E72.25 Argininaemia
E72.26 Hyperammonaemia
E72.28 Other specified disorders of urea cycle metabolism

E72.3 Disorders of lysine and hydroxylysine metabolism

E72.30 Glutaric aciduria, type I
Glutaryl-CoA dehydrogenase deficiency
E72.31 Hydroxylysinaemia
E72.32 Hyperlysinaemia
E72.38 Other specified disorders of lysine and hydroxylysine metabolism

E72.4 Disorders of ornithine metabolism

E72.40 Ornithine carbamoyltransferase [ornithine transcarbamylase] deficiency
E72.41 Ornithine–ketoacid aminotransferase deficiency
E72.42 Hyperornithinaemia, type I
E72.43 Hyperornithinaemia, type II
E72.48 Other specified disorders of ornithine metabolism

E72.5 Disorders of glycine metabolism

E72.50 Hyperhydroxyprolinaemia
E72.51 Hyperprolinaemia, type I
E72.52 Hyperprolinaemia, type II
E72.53 Non-ketotic hyperglycinaemia, type I [glycine dehydrogenase (decarboxylating) deficiency]
E72.54 Sarcosinaemia
E72.55 Non-ketotic hyperglycinaemia, type II [aminomethyltransferase deficiency]
E72.58 Other specified disorders of glycine metabolism

E72.8 Other specified disorders of amino-acid metabolism

E72.80 Disorders of β-amino-acid metabolism
E72.81 Disorders of glutamic acid and γ-glutamyl cycle metabolism

E72.810 Glutamate–cysteine ligase deficiency
E72.811 5-Oxoprolinase deficiency [pyroglutamate hydrolase deficiency]
E72.812 Glutathione synthetase deficiency [pyroglutamic acidaemia]
E72.813 γ-Glutamyltransferase deficiency
E72.814 Glutamate decarboxylase deficiency
E72.815 Succinate-semialdehyde dehydrogenase deficiency [γ-hydroxybutyric acidaemia]
E72.818 Other specified disorders of glutamic acid and γ-glutamyl cycle metabolism

E72.9 Disorder of amino-acid metabolism, unspecified

E73 Lactose intolerance

E73.0 Congenital lactase deficiency

E73.1 Secondary lactase deficiency

E73.8 Other lactose intolerance

E73.9 Lactose intolerance, unspecified

E74 Other disorders of carbohydrate metabolism

Excludes: diabetes mellitus (E10–E14)
hypoglycaemia NOS (E16.2)
increased secretion of glucagon (E16.3)
mucopolysaccharidosis (E76.0–E76.3)

E74.0 Glycogen storage disease

E74.00 Glucose-6-phosphatase deficiency [glycogen storage disease, type I] [von Gierke]

E74.01 Lysosomal α-glucosidase deficiency [glycogen storage disease, type II]

- E74.010 Infantile onset [Pompe]
- E74.011 Juvenile onset
- E74.012 Adult onset

E74.02 Amylo-1,6-glucosidase (debrancher) deficiency [glycogen storage disease, type III] [Cori] [Forbes]

E74.03 1,4-α-Glucan branching enzyme deficiency [glycogen storage disease, type IV] [Andersen]

E74.04 Glycogen storage disease, type V [McArdle]

- E74.040 Muscle phosphorylase deficiency
- E74.041 Muscle phosphorylase kinase deficiency

E74.05 Liver phosphorylase deficiency [glycogen storage disease, type IV] [Hers]
Liver phosphorylase b deficiency

E74.06 6-Phosphofructokinase deficiency [glycogen storage disease, type VII] [Tauri]

E74.08 Other specified disorders of glycogen metabolism

E74.1 Disorders of fructose metabolism

E74.10 Fructokinase deficiency [essential fructosuria]

E74.11 Fructose-bisphosphate aldolase deficiency [hereditary fructose intolerance]

E74.12 Fructose-bisphosphatase deficiency

E74.18 Other specified disorders of fructose metabolism

E74.2 Disorders of galactose metabolism

E74.20 UTP-hexose-1-phosphate uridylyl transferase [galactose-1-phosphate uridydyl transferase] deficiency [classical galactosaemia]

E74.21 Galactokinase deficiency

E74.22 Uridine diphosphogalactose-4-epimerase deficiency

E74.28 Other specified disorders of galactose metabolism

E74.3 Other disorders of intestinal carbohydrate absorption

Glucose–galactose malabsorption

Sucrose-α-glucosidase deficiency
Excludes: lactose intolerance (E73.–)

E74.4 Disorders of pyruvate metabolism and gluconeogenesis

E74.40 Disorders of pyruvate metabolism
E74.400 Pyruvate dehydrogenase deficiency
E74.401 [Pyruvate dehydrogenase (lipoamide)]-phosphatase deficiency
E74.402 Dihydrolipoamide dehydrogenase deficiency
E74.408 Other specified disorders of pyruvate metabolism
E74.41 Disorders of gluconeogenesis
Excludes: fructose-bisphosphatase deficiency (E74.12)
- with anaemia (D55.–)

E74.410 Pyruvate carboxylase deficiency
E74.411 Phosphoenolpyruvate carboxykinase deficiency
E74.418 Other specified disorders of gluconeogenesis

E74.8 Other specified disorders of carbohydrate metabolism

E74.80 Essential pentosuria
E74.81 Hyperoxaluria, type II
Glycerate dehydrogenase deficiency
Excludes: hyperoxaluria, type I (E80.311)
E74.82 Renal glycosuria
E74.83 Mannose-6-phosphate isomerase deficiency
E74.84 Phosphoglycerate mutase deficiency
E74.85 Phosphoglycerate kinase deficiency
E74.86 Muscle lactate dehydrogenase deficiency
E74.88 Other specified disorders of glycolysis

E74.9 Disorder of carbohydrate metabolism, unspecified

E75 Disorders of sphingolipid metabolism and other lipid storage disorders

Excludes: mucolipidosis, types I–III (E77.0–E77.1)
Refsum's disease (G60.1)

E75.0 GM_2 gangliosidosis

E75.00 Infantile β-hexosaminidase A deficiency [infantile GM_2 gangliosidosis] [Tay–Sachs]
E75.01 Juvenile β-hexosaminidase A deficiency [juvenile GM_2 gangliosidosis]
E75.02 Adult β-hexosaminidase A deficiency [adult GM_2 gangliosidosis]

E75.03 Sandhoff's disease [β-hexosaminidase A and B deficiencies]
E75.08 Other GM_2 gangliosidosis

E75.1 Other gangliosidosis

E75.10 Acid β-gangliosidase deficiency [GM_1 gangliosidosis]
E75.100 Infantile GM_1 gangliosidosis
E75.101 Juvenile GM_1 gangliosidosis
E75.102 Adult GM_1 gangliosidosis
E75.108 Other GM_1 gangliosidosis
E75.11 Gangliosidosis NOS
E75.12 GM_3 gangliosidosis
E75.13 Mucolipidosis, type IV

E75.2 Other sphingolipidosis

E75.20 Glucocerebrosidase deficiency [Gaucher]
E75.200 Type I Gaucher's disease (adult)
E75.201 Type II Gaucher's disease (infantile)
E75.202 Type III Gaucher's disease (juvenile)
E75.21 Galactocerebroside β-galactosidase deficiency [Krabbe]
E75.210 Type I Krabbe's disease (infantile)
E75.211 Type II Krabbe's disease (late-onset)
E75.22 α-Galactosidase deficiency [Fabry(–Anderson)]
E75.23 Aryl-sulphatase A deficiency [metachromatic leukodystrophy]
E75.230 Late infantile metachromatic leukodystrophy
E75.231 Juvenile metachromatic leukodystrophy
E75.232 Late-onset metachromatic leukodystrophy
E75.24 Multiple sulfatase deficiency
E75.25 Farber's syndrome
E75.26 Sphingomyelin phosphodiesterase deficiency [Niemann–Pick]
E75.260 Type A Niemann–Pick disease (infantile)
E75.261 Type B Niemann–Pick disease
E75.262 Type C Niemann–Pick disease (late infantile)
E75.263 Type D Niemann–Pick disease (Nova Scotia variant)

E75.3 Sphingolipidosis, unspecified

E75.4 Neuronal ceroid lipofuscinosis

Includes: Batten's disease

E75.40 Infantile [Haltia–Santavouri type]
E75.41 Late infantile [Bielschowsky–Jansky type]

E75.42 Juvenile [Spielmeyer–Vogt type]
E75.43 Adult [Kufs' type]
E75.48 Other specified neuronal ceroid lipofuscinosis

E75.5 Other lipid storage disorders
Excludes: Refsum's disease (G60.1)

E75.50 Cerebrotendinous cholesterosis [cerebrotendinous xanthomatosis] [van Bogaert–Scherer–Epstein]
E75.51 Cholesterol ester hydrolase deficiency [Wolman]
E75.52 Multiple system lipid storage with ichthyosis [Chanarin]
E75.53 Multiple system lipid storage without ichthyosis [Jordan]

E75.6 Lipid storage disorder, unspecified

E76 Disorders of glycosaminoglycan metabolism

E76.0 Mucopolysaccharidosis, type I
Includes: L-iduronidase deficiency

E76.00 Type I–H [Hurler]
E76.01 Type I–H/S [Hurler–Scheie]
E76.02 Type I–S [Scheie]

E76.1 Mucopolysaccharidosis, type II
Hunter's syndrome

E76.2 Other mucopolysaccharidoses

E76.20 Mucopolysaccharidosis, type III [Sanfilippo]
E76.200 Heparan-*N*-sulfatase deficiency [mucopolysaccharidosis, type IIIA]
E76.201 α-*N*-Acetylglucosaminidase deficiency [mucopolysaccharidosis, type IIIB]
E76.202 Acetyl CoA-α-glucosaminide *N*-acetyltransferase deficiency [mucopolysaccharidosis, type IIIC]
E76.203 *N*-Acetyl-α-D-glucosaminide-6-sulfatase deficiency [mucopolysaccharidosis, type IIID]
E76.21 Mucopolysaccharidosis, type IV [Morquio]
E76.210 Galactosamine-6-sulfate sulfatase deficiency [mucopolysaccharidosis, type IVA]
E76.211 β-Galactosidase deficiency [mucopolysaccharidosis, type IVB]
E76.22 *N*-Acetyl-galactosamine-4-sulfatase deficiency
E76.23 Mucopolysaccharidosis, type VI
E76.24 β-Glucuronidase deficiency [mucopolysaccharidosis, type VII] [Sly]
E76.28 Other specified mucopolysaccharidosis

E76.3 Mucopolysaccharidosis, unspecified

E76.8 Other disorders of glycosaminoglycan metabolism

E76.9 Disorder of glycosaminoglycan metabolism, unspecified

E77 Disorders of glycoprotein metabolism

E77.0 Defects in post-translational modification of lysosomal enzymes

E77.00 *N*-Acetylglucosaminephosphotransferase deficiency [mucolipidosis II] [I-cell disease]
E77.01 Mucolipidosis III [pseudo-Hurler polydystrophy]

E77.1 Defects in glycoprotein degradation

E77.10 α-Mannosidase deficiency [mannosidosis]
  E77.100 α-D-Mannosidase deficiency, type I
  E77.101 α-D-Mannosidase deficiency, type II
E77.11 α-L-Fucosidase deficiency [fucosidosis]
  E77.110 α-L-Fucosidase deficiency, type I
  E77.111 α-L-Fucosidase deficiency, type II
E77.12 Exo-α-sialidase deficiency [sialidosis] [mucolipidosis I]
  E77.120 α-Neuraminidase deficiency, type I
  E77.121 α-Neuraminidase deficiency, type II
E77.13 β-Aspartyl-*N*-acetylglucosaminidase deficiency [aspartylglucosaminuria]
E77.18 Other defects in glycoprotein degradation

E77.8 Other disorders of glycoprotein metabolism

E77.9 Disorder of glycoprotein metabolism, unspecified

E78 Disorders of lipoprotein metabolism and other lipidaemias

Excludes: sphingolipidosis (E75.0–E75.3)

E78.0 Pure hypercholesterolaemia

E78.00 Familial hypercholesterolaemia
E78.01 Fredrickson's hyperlipoproteinaemia, type IIa
E78.02 Hyperbetalipoproteinaemia
E78.03 Hyperlipidaemia, group A
E78.04 Low-density-lipoprotein-type [LDL] hyperlipoproteinaemia
E78.08 Other pure hypercholesterolaemia

E78.1 Pure hyperglyceridaemia

E78.10 Endogenous hyperglyceridaemia
E78.11 Fredrickson's hyperlipoproteinaemia, type IV
E78.12 Hyperlipidaemia, group B
E78.13 Hyperprebetalipoproteinaemia
E78.14 Very-low-density-lipoprotein-type [VLDL] hyperlipoproteinaemia
E78.18 Other pure hyperglyceridaemia

E78.2 Mixed hyperlipidaemia

Excludes: cerebrotendinous cholesterosis [van Bogaert–Scherer–Epstein] (E75.50)

E78.20 Broad- or floating-betalipoproteinaemia
E78.21 Fredrickson's hyperlipoproteinaemia, type IIb or III
E78.22 Hyperbetalipoproteinaemia with prebetalipoproteinaemia
E78.23 Hypercholesterolaemia with endogenous hyperglyceridaemia
E78.24 Hyperlipidaemia, group C
E78.25 Tubero-eruptive xanthoma
E78.26 Xanthoma tuberosum
E78.28 Other mixed hyperlipidaemia

E78.3 Hyperchylomicronaemia

E78.30 Fredrickson's hyperlipoproteinaemia, type I or V
E78.31 Hyperlipidaemia, group D
E78.32 Mixed hyperglyceridaemia
E78.38 Other hyperchylomicronaemia

E78.4 Other hyperlipidaemia

Familial combined hyperlipidaemia

E78.5 Hyperlipidaemia, unspecified

E78.6 Lipoprotein deficiency

E78.60 Analphaliproteinaemia [Tangier disease]
E78.61 Hypoalphalipoproteinaemia
E78.62 Abetalipoproteinaemia [Bassen–Kornzweig]
E78.63 Familial hypobetalipoproteinaemia
E78.64 High-density lipoprotein deficiency
E78.65 Lecithin–cholesterol acyltransferase deficiency
E78.68 Other lipoprotein deficiency

E78.8 Other disorders of lipoprotein metabolism

E78.9 Disorder of lipoprotein metabolism, unspecified

E79 Disorders of purine and pyrimidine metabolism

Excludes: gout (M10.–)
xeroderma pigmentosum (Q82.1)

E79.1 Lesch–Nyhan syndrome
Hypoxanthine phosphoribosyltransferase deficiency

E79.8 Other disorders of purine and pyrimidine metabolism

E79.80 Hereditary xanthinuria
E79.81 Orotate phosphoribosyl transferase deficiency [orotic acidaemia, type I]
E79.82 Orotidine-5′-phosphate decarboxylase deficiency [orotic acidaemia, type II]
E79.83 Myoadenylate deaminase deficiency

E79.9 Disorder of purine and pyrimidine metabolism, unspecified

E80 Disorders of porphyrin and bilirubin metabolism

Includes: defects of catalase and peroxidase

E80.0 Hereditary erythropoietic porphyria

E80.00 Uroporphyrinogen-III synthase deficiency [congenital erythropoietic porphyria]
E80.01 Ferrochelatase deficiency [erythropoietic protoporphyria]
E80.08 Other hereditary erythropoietic porphyria

E80.1 Porphyria cutanea tarda
Uroporphyrinogen decarboxylase deficiency

E80.2 Other porphyria
Use additional external cause code (Chapter XX), if desired, to identify cause.

E80.20 Hydroxymethylbilane synthase [porphobilinogen deaminase] deficiency [acute intermittent porphyria]
E80.21 Coproporphyrinogen oxidase deficiency [hereditary coproporphyria]
E80.22 Protoporphyrinogen oxidase or ferrochetalase deficiency [variegate porphyria]

E80.3 Defects of catalase and peroxidase
Excludes: adrenoleukodystrophy (E71.33):
- neonatal (E71.331)

hyperoxaluria, type II (E74.81)
Refsum's disease (G60.1)
Zellweger's syndrome (Q87.82)

E80.30 Peroxisomal disorders, perioxisomes reduced or absent with multiple enzyme defects

E80.300 Infantile Refsum's disease

E80.301 Hyperpipecolic acidaemia

E80.31 Peroxisomal disorders, single enzyme defects of peroxisomes

E80.310 Acatalasaemia
Acatalasia [Takahara]

E80.311 Hyperoxaluria type I
Alanine–glyoxylate transaminase deficiency

E80.312 3-Oxoacyl-CoA thiolase deficiency [pseudo-Zellweger]

E80.313 Acyl-CoA oxidase deficiency

E80.314 Bifunctional enzyme deficiency

E80.315 Dihydroxyacetone phosphate acyl transferase deficiency

E80.32 Peroxisomal disorder, peroxisomes present with abnormal structures and multiple enzyme deficiencies
Excludes: chondrodysplasia punctata (Q77.3)

E80.38 Other defects of catalase and peroxidase

E80.4 Gilbert's syndrome

E80.5 Crigler–Najjar syndrome

E80.6 Other disorders of bilirubin metabolism

E80.60 Dubin–Johnson syndrome

E80.61 Rotor's syndrome

E80.7 Disorder of bilirubin metabolism, unspecified

E83 Disorders of mineral metabolism

Excludes: dietary mineral deficiency (E58–E61)
parathyroid disorders (E20–E21)
vitamin D deficiency (E55.–)

E83.0 Disorders of copper metabolism

E83.00 Menkes' (kinky hair)(steely hair) disease

E83.01 Wilson's disease [hepatolenticular degeneration]

E83.08 Other disorders of copper metabolism

E83.1 Disorders of iron metabolism
Excludes: iron deficiency anaemia (D50.–)

E83.10 Haemochromatosis
E83.18 Other disorders of iron metabolism

E83.2 Disorders of zinc metabolism

E83.20 Acrodermatitis enteropathica
E83.28 Other disorders of zinc metabolism

E83.3 Disorders of phosphorus metabolism
Excludes: adult osteomalacia (M83.–)
osteoporosis (M80–M81)

E83.30 Acid phosphatase deficiency
E83.31 Familial hypophosphataemia
E83.32 Hypophosphatasia
E83.33 Vitamin-D-resistant rickets
E83.38 Other disorders of phosphorus metabolism

E83.4 Disorders of magnesium metabolism

E83.40 Hypermagnesaemia
E83.41 Hypomagnesaemia
Excludes: neonatal hypomagnesaemia (P71.2)
E83.48 Other disorders of magnesium metabolism

E83.5 Disorders of calcium metabolism
Excludes: hyperparathyroidism (E21.0–E21.3)

E83.50 Familial hypocalciuric hypercalcaemia
E83.51 Idiopathic hypercalciuria

E83.8 Other disorders of mineral metabolism

E83.9 Disorder of mineral metabolism, unspecified

E84 Cystic fibrosis

E84.0 Cystic fibrosis with pulmonary manifestations

E84.1 Cystic fibrosis with intestinal manifestations

E84.8 Cystic fibrosis with other manifestations

E84.9 Cystic fibrosis, unspecified

E85 Amyloidosis

Includes: cerebral amyloid angiopathy† (I68.0*)
non-hereditary cerebral amyloidosis (congophilic or amyloid angiopathy)† (I68.0*)

E85.0 Non-neuropathic heredofamilial amyloidosis

E85.00 Familial Mediterranean fever
E85.01 Familial oculoleptomeningeal amyloidosis
E85.08 Other non-neuropathic heredofamilial amyloidosis

E85.1 Neuropathic heredofamilial amyloidosis

E85.10 Familial amyloid polyneuropathy, type I [Andrade type]
E85.11 Familial amyloid polyneuropathy, type II (Indiana) [Rukavina type]
E85.12 Familial amyloid polyneuropathy, type III (Iowa) [Van Allen type]
E85.13 Familial amyloid polyneuropathy, type IV [cranial neuropathy with corneal lattice dystrophy] [Meretoja type]
E85.18 Other neuropathic heredofamilial amyloidosis

E85.2 Heredofamilial amyloidosis, unspecified

E85.3 Secondary systemic amyloidosis

E85.30 Immunocytic amyloidosis (AL protein)
E85.31 Reactive amyloidosis (AA protein)
E85.32 Tumour-associated amyloidosis (associated with hypernephroma)
E85.33 Haemodialysis-associated amyloidosis
E85.38 Other secondary systemic amyloidosis

E85.4 Organ-limited amyloidosis

Excludes: cerebral amyloidosis in:
- Alzheimer's disease (G30.–)
- Creutzfeldt–Jakob disease (A81.0)
- Down's syndrome (Q90.–)
- Gerstmann–Straussler–Scheinker disease (A81.81)
- kuru (A81.80)

cranial neuropathy with corneal lattice dystrophy (E85.13)

E85.8 Other amyloidosis

Amyloidosis of skin

E85.9 Amyloidosis, unspecified

E86 Volume depletion

Dehydration
Depletion of volume of plasma or extracellular fluid
Hypovolaemia

Excludes: dehydration of newborn (P74.1)
hypovolaemic shock:
- NOS (R57.1)
- postoperative (T81.1)
- traumatic (T79.4)

E87 Other disorders of fluid, electrolyte and acid–base balance

E87.0 Hyperosmolality and hypernatraemia
Sodium [Na] excess
Sodium [Na] overload

E87.1 Hyposmolality and hyponatraemia
Excludes: syndrome of inappropriate secretion of antidiuretic hormone (E22.2)

E87.10 Sodium [Na] deficiency

E87.2 Acidosis
Excludes: diabetic acidosis (E10–E14 with common fourth character .1)

E87.20 Metabolic acidosis
E87.21 Respiratory acidosis
Excludes: renal tubular acidosis (N25.8)
E87.22 Lactic acidosis

E87.3 Alkalosis

E87.30 Metabolic alkalosis
E87.31 Respiratory alkalosis

E87.4 Mixed disorder of acid–base balance

E87.5 Hyperkalaemia
Potassium [K] excess
Potassium [K] overload

E87.6 Hypokalaemia
Potassium [K] deficiency

E87.7 Fluid overload

E87.8 Other disorders of electrolyte and fluid balance, not elsewhere classified
Electrolyte imbalance NOS
Hyperchloraemia
Hypochloraemia

E88 Other metabolic disorders

Use additional external cause code (Chapter XX), if desired, to identify drug, if drug-induced.

E88.0 Disorders of plasma-protein metabolism, not elsewhere classified

α-1-Antitrypsin deficiency
Bisalbuminaemia

Excludes: disorders of lipoprotein metabolism (E78.–)
monoclonal gammopathy (D47.2)
polyclonal hypergammaglobulinaemia (D89.0)
Waldenström's macroglobulinaemia (C88.0)

E88.8 Other specified metabolic disorders

E88.80 Launois–Bensaude adenolipomatosis

E88.81 Trimethylaminuria

E88.82 Organic acidaemias, not elsewhere classified

Excludes: glutaric aciduria type I (E72.30)
hyperpipecolic acidaemia (E80.301)
isovaleric acidaemia (E71.11)
lactic acidosis (E87.23)
methylmalonic acidaemia (E71.12)
orotic acidaemia (E79.81, E79.82)
propionic acidaemia (E71.13)

E88.820 Disorders of intermediary branched chain keto-acid metabolism

Hydroxymethylglutaryl-CoA lyase deficiency
3-Methyl-crotonyl-CoA carboxylase deficiency
Acetyl-CoA *C*-acyltransferase deficiency
Multiple acyl-CoA dehydrogenase deficiency [glutaric acidaemia, type II]

E88.821 Multiple carboxylase deficiency

E88.822 Biotinidase deficiency

E88.83 Defects of mitochondrial respiratory chain

Excludes: mitochondrial myopathy (G71.3)

E88.830 NADH-coenzyme Q reductase deficiency

E88.831 Succinate-coenzyme Q reductase deficiency

E88.832 Reduced coenzyme Q-cytochrome c reductase deficiency

E88.833 Deletion of mitochondrial DNA

E88.838 Other specified defect of mitochondrial respiratory chain

E88.9 Metabolic disorder, unspecified

E89 Postprocedural endocrine and metabolic disorders, not elsewhere classified

E89.0 Postprocedural hypothyroidism

E89.00 Postirradiation hypothyroidism
E89.01 Postsurgical hypothyroidism

E89.1 Postprocedural hypoinsulinaemia

E89.10 Postpancreatectomy hypoinsulinaemia
E89.11 Postsurgical hypoinsulinaemia

E89.2 Postprocedural hypoparathyroidism
Parathyroprival tetany

E89.3 Postprocedural hypopituitarism

E89.30 Postirradiation hypopituitarism
E89.31 Postsurgical hypopituitarism

E89.8 Other postprocedural endocrine and metabolic disorders

E90* Nutritional and metabolic disorders in diseases classified elsewhere

CHAPTER V

Mental and behavioural disorders (F00–F99)

Organic, including symptomatic, mental disorders (F00–F09)

This block comprises a range of mental disorders grouped together on the basis of their having in common a demonstrable etiology in cerebral disease, brain injury, or other insult leading to cerebral dysfunction. The dysfunction may be primary, as in diseases, injuries, and insults that affect the brain directly and selectively; or secondary, as in systemic diseases and disorders that attack the brain only as one of the multiple organs or systems of the body that are involved.

Dementia (F00–F03) is a syndrome due to disease of the brain, usually of a chronic or progressive nature, in which there is disturbance of multiple higher cortical functions, including memory, thinking, orientation, comprehension, calculation, learning capacity, language, and judgement. Consciousness is not clouded. The impairments of cognitive function are commonly accompanied, and occasionally preceded, by deterioration in emotional control, social behaviour, or motivation. This syndrome occurs in Alzheimer's disease, in cerebrovascular disease, and in other conditions primarily or secondarily affecting the brain.

Use additional code, if desired, to identify the underlying disease.

F00* Dementia in Alzheimer's disease (G30.–†)

Alzheimer's disease is a primary degenerative cerebral disease of unknown etiology with characteristic neuropathological and neurochemical features. The disorder is usually insidious in onset and develops slowly but steadily over a period of several years.

F00.0* **Dementia in Alzheimer's disease with early onset (G30.0†)**

Dementia in Alzheimer's disease with onset before the age of 65, with a relatively rapid deteriorating course and with marked multiple disorders of the higher cortical functions.

Alzheimer's disease, type 2
Presenile dementia, Alzheimer's type
Primary degenerative dementia of the Alzheimer's type, presenile onset

F00.1* Dementia in Alzheimer's disease with late onset (G30.1†)
Dementia in Alzheimer's disease with onset after the age of 65, usually in the late 70s or thereafter, with a slow progression, and with memory impairment as the principal feature.

Alzheimer's disease, type 1
Primary degenerative dementia of the Alzheimer's type, senile onset
Senile dementia, Alzheimer's type

F00.2* Dementia in Alzheimer's disease, atypical or mixed type (G30.8†)
Atypical dementia, Alzheimer's type

F00.9* Dementia in Alzheimer's disease, unspecified (G30.9†)

F01 Vascular dementia

Vascular dementia is the result of infarction of the brain due to vascular disease, including hypertensive cerebrovascular disease. The infarcts are usually small but cumulative in their effect. Onset is usually in later life.

Includes: arteriosclerotic dementia

Use additional code(s) (I60–I69), if desired, to identify the cause(s) or underlying conditions.

F01.0 Vascular dementia of acute onset
Usually develops rapidly after a succession of strokes from cerebrovascular thrombosis, embolism, or haemorrhage. In rare cases, a single large infarction may be the cause.

F01.1 Multi-infarct dementia
Gradual in onset, following a number of transient ischaemic episodes that produce an accumulation of infarcts in the cerebral parenchyma.

Predominantly cortical dementia

F01.2 Subcortical vascular dementia
Includes cases with a history of hypertension and foci of ischaemic destruction in the deep white matter of the cerebral hemispheres. The cerebral cortex is usually preserved and this contrasts with the clinical picture which may closely resemble that of dementia in Alzheimer's disease.

F01.3 Mixed cortical and subcortical vascular dementia

F01.8 Other vascular dementia

F01.9 Vascular dementia, unspecified

F02* Dementia in other diseases classified elsewhere

Cases of dementia due, or presumed to be due, to causes other than Alzheimer's disease or cerebrovascular disease. Onset may be at any time in life, though rarely in old age.

F02.0* Dementia in Pick's disease (G31.00†)

A progressive dementia, commencing in middle age, characterized by early, slowly progressing changes of character and social deterioration, followed by impairment of intellect, memory, and language functions, with apathy, euphoria, and, occasionally, extrapyramidal phenomena.

F02.1* Dementia in Creutzfeldt–Jakob disease (A81.0†)

A progressive dementia with extensive neurological signs, due to specific neuropathological changes that are presumed to be caused by a transmissible agent. Onset is usually in middle or later life, but may be at any adult age. The course is subacute, leading to death within one to two years.

F02.2* Dementia in Huntington's disease (G10.–†)

A dementia occurring as part of a widespread degeneration of the brain. The disorder is transmitted by a single autosomal dominant gene. Symptoms typically emerge in the third and fourth decade. Progression is slow, leading to death usually within 10 to 15 years.

Dementia in Huntington's chorea

F02.3* Dementia in Parkinson's disease (G20.–†)

A dementia developing in the course of established Parkinson's disease. No particular distinguishing clinical features have yet been demonstrated.

Dementia in:
- paralysis agitans
- parkinsonism

F02.4* Dementia in human immunodeficiency virus [HIV] disease (B22.0†)

Dementia developing in the course of HIV disease, in the absence of a concurrent illness or condition other than HIV infection that could explain the clinical features.

F02.8* Dementia in other specified diseases classified elsewhere

Dementia in:
- adult ceroid lipofuscinosis [Kufs] (E75.43†)
- carbon monoxide poisoning (T58†)
- circumscribed brain atrophy (G31.0†)
- epilepsy (G40.–†)
- head injury, including "dementia pugilistica" (S06–S07†)
- hepatolenticular degeneration (E83.01†)
- hypercalcaemia (E83.5†)
- hypothyroidism, acquired (E01.–†, E03.–†)
- intoxications (T36–T65†)

- Lewy body disease (G31.85†)
- multiple sclerosis (G35.–†)
- neurosyphilis (A52.1†)
- niacin deficiency [pellagra] (E52†)
- polyarteritis nodosa (M30.0†)
- systemic lupus erythematosus (M32.–†)
- trypanosomiasis (B56.–†, B57.–†)
- vitamin B_{12} deficiency (E53.80†)

F03 Dementia, unspecified

Presenile:
- dementia NOS
- psychosis NOS

Primary degenerative dementia NOS
Senile:
- dementia:
  - NOS
  - depressed or paranoid type
- psychosis NOS

Excludes: senile dementia with delirium or acute confusional state (F05.1)
senility NOS (R54)

F04 Organic amnesic syndrome, not induced by alcohol and other psychoactive substances

A syndrome of prominent impairment of recent and remote memory while immediate recall is preserved, with reduced ability to learn new material and disorientation in time. Confabulation may be a marked feature, but perception and other cognitive functions, including the intellect, are usually intact. The prognosis depends on the course of the underlying lesion.

Korsakov's psychosis or syndrome, nonalcoholic
Excludes: amnesia:
- NOS (R41.3)
- anterograde (R41.1)
- dissociative (F44.0)
- retrograde (R41.2)

Korsakov's syndrome:
- alcohol-induced or unspecified (F10.6)
- induced by other psychoactive substances (F11–F19 with common fourth character .6)

F05 Delirium, not induced by alcohol and other psychoactive substances

An etiologically nonspecific organic cerebral syndrome characterized by concurrent disturbances of consciousness and attention, perception, thinking, memory, psychomotor behaviour, emotion, and the sleep–wake schedule. The duration is variable and the degree of severity ranges from mild to very severe.

Includes: acute or subacute:
- brain syndrome
- confusional state (nonalcoholic)
- infective psychosis
- organic reaction
- psycho-organic syndrome

Excludes: delirium tremens, alcohol-induced (F10.4)

F05.0 Delirium, not superimposed on dementia, so described

F05.1 Delirium, superimposed on dementia, so described

Conditions meeting the above criteria but developing in the course of a dementia (F00–F03).

F05.8 Other delirium

Delirium of mixed origin

F05.9 Delirium, unspecified

F06 Other mental disorders due to brain damage and dysfunction and to physical disease

Includes miscellaneous conditions causally related to brain disorder due to primary cerebral disease, to systemic disease affecting the brain secondarily, to exogenous toxic substances or hormones, to endocrine disorders, or to other somatic illnesses.

Use additional code, if desired, to identify the underlying cause or disorder.

Excludes: associated with:
- delirium (F05.–)
- dementia as classified in F00–F03

resulting from use of alcohol and other psychoactive substances (F10–F19)

F06.0 Organic hallucinosis

A disorder of persistent or recurrent hallucinations, usually visual or auditory, that occur in clear consciousness and may or may not be recognized by the subject as such. Delusional elaboration of the hallucinations may occur, but delusions do not dominate the clinical picture; insight may be preserved.

Organic hallucinatory state (nonalcoholic)

Excludes: alcoholic hallucinosis (F10.5)

F06.1 Organic catatonic disorder

A disorder of diminished (stupor) or increased (excitement) psychomotor activity associated with catatonic symptoms. The extremes of psychomotor disturbance may alternate.

Excludes: stupor:
- NOS (R40.1)
- dissociative (F44.2)

F06.2 Organic delusional [schizophrenia-like] disorder

A disorder in which persistent or recurrent delusions dominate the clinical picture. The delusions may be accompanied by hallucinations. Some features suggestive of schizophrenia, such as bizarre hallucinations or thought disorder, may be present.

Paranoid and paranoid-hallucinatory organic states
Schizophrenia-like psychosis in epilepsy
Excludes: psychotic drug-induced disorders (F11–F19 with common fourth character .5)

F06.3 Organic mood [affective] disorders

Disorders characterized by a change in mood or affect, usually accompanied by a change in the overall level of activity, depressive, hypomanic, manic or bipolar (see F30–F32), but arising as a consequence of an organic disorder.

F06.30 Organic manic disorder
F06.31 Organic bipolar disorder
F06.32 Organic depressive disorder
F06.33 Organic mixed affective disorder

F06.4 Organic anxiety disorder

A disorder characterized by the features of a generalized anxiety disorder, a panic disorder, or a combination of both, but arising as a consequence of an organic disorder.

F06.5 Organic dissociative disorder

A disorder characterized by a partial or complete loss of the normal integration between memories of the past, awareness of identity and immediate sensations, and control of bodily movements (see F44.–), but arising as a consequence of an organic disorder.

Excludes: dissociative [conversion] disorders, nonorganic or unspecified (F44.–)

F06.6 Organic emotionally labile [asthenic] disorder

A disorder characterized by emotional incontinence or lability, fatiguability, and a variety of unpleasant physical sensations (e.g. dizziness) and pains, but arising as a consequence of an organic disorder.

Excludes: somatoform disorders, nonorganic or unspecified (F45.–)

F06.7 Mild cognitive disorder

A disorder characterized by impairment of memory, learning difficulties, and reduced ability to concentrate on a task for more than brief periods. There is often a marked feeling of mental fatigue when mental tasks are attempted, and new learning is found to be subjectively difficult even when objectively successful. None of these symptoms is so severe that a diagnosis of either dementia (F00–F03) or delirium (F05.–) can be made. This diagnosis should be made only in association with a specified physical disorder, and should not be made in the presence of any of the mental or behavioural disorders classified to F10–F99. The disorder may precede, accompany, or follow a wide variety of infections and physical disorders, both cerebral and systemic, but direct evidence of cerebral involvement is not necessarily present. It can be differentiated from postencephalitic syndrome (F07.1) and postconcussional syndrome (F07.2) by its different etiology, more restricted range of generally milder symptoms, and usually shorter duration.

F06.8 Other specified mental disorders due to brain damage and dysfunction and to physical disease

F06.9 Unspecified mental disorder due to brain damage and dysfunction and to physical disease

F07 Personality and behavioural disorders due to brain disease, damage and dysfunction

Alteration of personality and behaviour can be a residual or concomitant disorder of brain disease, damage, or dysfunction.

F07.0 Organic personality disorder

A disorder characterized by a significant alteration of the habitual patterns of behaviour displayed by the subject premorbidly, involving the expression of emotions, needs, and impulses. Impairment of cognitive and thought functions and altered sexuality may also be part of the clinical picture.

Organic:
- pseudopsychopathic personality
- pseudoretarded personality

Syndrome:
- frontal lobe
- limbic epilepsy personality
- lobotomy
- postleucotomy

Excludes: postencephalitic syndrome (F07.1)

F07.1 Postencephalitic syndrome

Residual nonspecific and variable behavioural change following recovery from either viral or bacterial encephalitis. The principal difference between this disorder and the organic personality disorders is that it is reversible.

Excludes: organic personality disorder (F07.0)

F07.2 Postconcussional syndrome

A syndrome that occurs following head trauma (usually sufficiently severe to result in loss of consciousness) and includes a number of disparate symptoms such as headache, dizziness, fatigue, irritability, difficulty in concentration and performing mental tasks, impairment of memory, insomnia, and reduced tolerance to stress, emotional excitement, or alcohol.

Postcontusional syndrome (encephalopathy)
Post-traumatic brain syndrome, nonpsychotic

F07.8 Other organic personality and behavioural disorders due to brain disease, damage and dysfunction

Right hemispheric organic affective disorder

F07.9 Unspecified organic personality and behavioural disorders due to brain disease, damage and dysfunction

Organic psychosyndrome

F09 Unspecified organic or symptomatic mental disorder

Organic psychosis NOS

Mental and behavioural disorders due to psychoactive substance use (F10–F19)

This block contains a wide variety of disorders that differ in severity and clinical form but that are all attributable to the use of one or more psychoactive substances, which may or may not have been medically prescribed. The third character of the code identifies the substance involved, and the fourth character specifies the clinical state. The codes should be used, as required, for each substance specified, but it should be noted that not all four-character codes are applicable to all substances.

Identification of the psychoactive substance should be based on as many sources of information as possible. These include self-report data, analysis of blood and other body fluids, characteristic physical and psychological symptoms, clinical signs and behaviour, and other evidence such as a drug being in the patient's possession or reports from informed third parties. Many drug users take more than one type of substance. The principal diagnosis should be classified, whenever possible, according to the substance or class of substances that has caused or contributed most to the presenting clinical syndrome. Other diagnoses should be coded when other psychoactive substances have been taken in intoxicating amounts (common fourth character .0) or to the extent of causing harm (common fourth character .1), dependence (common fourth character .2), or other disorders (common fourth character .3–.9).

Only in cases in which patterns of psychoactive substance-taking are chaotic and indiscriminate, or in which the contributions of different psychoactive substances are inextricably mixed, should the diagnosis of disorders resulting from multiple drug use (F19.–) be used.

Excludes: abuse of non-dependence producing substances (F55)

The following fourth-character subdivisions are for use with categories F10–F19:

F1*x*.0 Acute intoxication

A condition that follows the administration of a psychoactive substance resulting in disturbances in level of consciousness, cognition, perception, affect or behaviour, or other psychophysiological functions and responses. The disturbances are directly related to the acute pharmacological effects of the substance and resolve with time, with complete recovery, except where tissue damage or other complications have arisen. Complications may include trauma, inhalation of vomitus, delirium, coma, convulsions, and other medical complications. The nature of these complications depends on the pharmacological class of substance and mode of administration.

Includes: acute drunkenness in alcoholism
"bad trips" (drugs)
drunkenness NOS
pathological intoxication
trance and possession disorders in psychoactive substance intoxication

F1*x*.00 Uncomplicated
F1*x*.01 With trauma or other bodily injury
F1*x*.02 With other medical complication
F1*x*.03 With delirium
F1*x*.04 With perceptual distortions
F1*x*.05 With coma
F1*x*.06 With convulsions
F1*x*.07 Pathological intoxication

F1*x*.1 Harmful use

A pattern of psychoactive substance use that is causing damage to health. The damage may be physical (as in cases of hepatitis from the self-administration of injected psychoactive substances) or mental (e.g. episodes of depressive disorder secondary to heavy consumption of alcohol).

Includes: psychoactive substance abuse

F1*x*.10 Mild
F1*x*.11 Moderate
F1*x*.12 Severe

F1*x*.2 Dependence syndrome

A cluster of behavioural, cognitive, and physiological phenomena that develop after repeated psychoactive substance use and that typically include a strong desire to take the drug, difficulties in controlling its use, persisting in its use despite harmful consequences, a higher priority given to drug use than to other activities and obligations, increased tolerance, and sometimes a physical withdrawal state.

The dependence syndrome may be present for a specific substance (e.g. tobacco, alcohol, or diazepam), for a class of substances (e.g. opioid drugs), or for a wider range of pharmacologically different psychoactive substances.

Includes: chronic alcoholism
dipsomania
drug addiction

F1*x*.20 Currently abstinent
F1*x*.21 Currently abstinent, but in a protected environment
F1*x*.22 Currently on a clinically supervised maintenance or replacement regime [controlled dependence]
F1*x*.23 Currently abstinent, but receiving treatment with aversive or blocking drugs
F1*x*.24 Currently using the substance [active dependence]
F1*x*.25 Continuous use
F1*x*.26 Episodic use [dipsomania]

F1*x*.3 Withdrawal state

A group of symptoms of variable clustering and severity occurring on absolute or relative withdrawal of a psychoactive substance after persistent use of that substance. The onset and course of the withdrawal state are time-limited and are related to the type of psychoactive substance and dose being used immediately before cessation or reduction of use. The withdrawal state may be complicated by convulsions.

F1*x*.30 Uncomplicated
F1*x*.31 With convulsions

F1*x*.4 Withdrawal state with delirium

A condition where the withdrawal state as defined in the common fourth character .3 is complicated by delirium as defined in F05.–. Convulsions may also occur. When organic factors are also considered to play a role in the etiology, the condition should be classified to F05.8.

Includes: delirium tremens (alcohol-induced)

F1*x*.40 Without convulsions
F1*x*.41 With convulsions

F1*x*.5 Psychotic disorder

A cluster of psychotic phenomena that occur during or following psychoactive substance use but that are not explained on the basis of acute intoxication alone and do not form part of a withdrawal state. The disorder is characterized by hallucinations (typically auditory, but often in more than one sensory modality), perceptual distortions, delusions (often of a paranoid or persecutory nature), psychomotor disturbances (excitement or stupor), and an abnormal affect, which may range from intense fear to ecstasy. The sensorium is usually clear but some degree of clouding of consciousness, though not severe confusion, may be present.

Includes: alcoholic:
- hallucinosis
- jealousy
- paranoia
- psychosis NOS

Excludes: alcohol- or other psychoactive substance-induced residual and late-onset psychotic disorder (F10–F19 with common fourth character .7)

F1*x*.50 Schizophrenia-like
F1*x*.51 Predominantly delusional
F1*x*.52 Predominantly hallucinatory
F1*x*.53 Predominantly polymorphic
F1*x*.54 Predominantly depressive symptoms
F1*x*.55 Predominantly manic symptoms
F1*x*.56 Mixed

F1*x*.6 Amnesic syndrome

A syndrome associated with chronic prominent impairment of recent and remote memory. Immediate recall is usually preserved and recent memory is characteristically more disturbed than remote memory. Disturbances of time sense and ordering of events are usually evident, as are difficulties in learning new material. Confabulation may be marked but it is not invariably present. Other cognitive functions are usually relatively well preserved and amnesic defects are out of proportion to other disturbances.

Amnestic disorder, alcohol- or drug-induced
Korsakov's psychosis or syndrome, alcohol- or other psychoactive substance-induced or unspecified

Excludes: nonalcoholic Korsakov's psychosis or syndrome (F04)

F1*x*.7 Residual and late-onset psychotic disorder

A disorder in which alcohol- or psychoactive substance-induced changes of cognition, affect, personality, or behaviour persist beyond the period during which a direct psychoactive substance-related effect might reasonably be assumed to be operating. Onset of the disorder should be directly related to the use of the psychoactive substance. Cases in which initial onset of the state occurs later than episode(s) of such substance use should be coded here only where clear and strong evidence is available to attribute the state to the residual effect of the psychoactive substance. Flashbacks may be distinguished from psychotic state partly by their episodic nature, frequently of very short duration, and by their duplication of previous alcohol- or psychoactive substance-related experiences.

Excludes: alcohol- or psychoactive substance-induced:
- Korsakov's syndrome (F10–F19 with common fourth character .6)
- psychotic state (F10–F19 with common fourth character .5)

F1*x*.70 Flashbacks
F1*x*.71 Personality or behaviour disorder
F1*x*.72 Residual affective disorder
F1*x*.73 Dementia
F1*x*.74 Other persisting cognitive impairment
F1*x*.75 Late-onset psychotic disorder

F1*x*.8 Other mental and behavioural disorders

F1*x*.9 Unspecified mental and behavioural disorder

F10.– Mental and behavioural disorders due to use of alcohol

[See pages 133–136 for subdivisions]

F11.– Mental and behavioural disorders due to use of opioids

[See pages 133–136 for subdivisions]

F12.– Mental and behavioural disorders due to use of cannabinoids

[See pages 133–136 for subdivisions]

F13.– Mental and behavioural disorders due to use of sedatives or hypnotics

[See pages 133–136 for subdivisions]

F14.– Mental and behavioural disorders due to use of cocaine

[See pages 133–136 for subdivisions]

F15.– Mental and behavioural disorders due to use of other stimulants, including caffeine

[See pages 133–136 for subdivisions]

F16.– Mental and behavioural disorders due to use of hallucinogens

[See pages 133–136 for subdivisions]

F17.– Mental and behavioural disorders due to use of tobacco

[See pages 133–136 for subdivisions]

F18.– Mental and behavioural disorders due to use of volatile solvents

[See pages 133–136 for subdivisions]

F19.– Mental and behavioural disorders due to multiple drug use and use of other psychoactive substances

[See pages 133–136 for subdivisions]

This category should be used when two or more substances are known to be involved, but it is impossible to assess which substance is contributing most to the disorders. It should also be used when the exact identity of some or even all the substances being used is uncertain or unknown, since many multiple drug users themselves often do not know the details of what they are taking.

Includes: misuse of drugs NOS

Mood [affective] disorders (F30–F39)

This block contains disorders in which the fundamental disturbance is a change in affect or mood to depression (with or without associated anxiety) or to elation. The mood change is usually accompanied by a change in the overall level of activity; most of the other symptoms are either secondary to, or easily understood in the context of, the change in mood and activity. Most of these disorders tend to be recurrent and the onset of individual episodes can often be related to stressful events or situations.

F30 Manic episode

All the subdivisions of this category should be used only for a single episode. Hypomanic or manic episodes in individuals who have had one or more previous affective episodes (depressive, hypomanic, manic, or mixed) should be coded as bipolar affective disorder (F31.–).

Includes: bipolar disorder, single manic episode

F30.0 Hypomania

A disorder characterized by a persistent mild elevation of mood, increased energy and activity, and usually marked feelings of well-being and both physical and mental efficiency. Increased sociability, talkativeness, overfamiliarity, increased sexual energy, and a decreased need for sleep are often present but not to the extent that they lead to severe disruption of work or result in social rejection. Irritability, conceit and boorish behaviour may take the place of the more usual euphoric sociability. The disturbances of mood and behaviour are not accompanied by hallucinations or delusions.

F30.1 Mania without psychotic symptoms

Mood is elevated out of keeping with the patient's circumstances and may vary from carefree joviality to almost uncontrollable excitement. Elation is accompanied by increased energy, resulting in overactivity, pressure of speech, and a decreased need for sleep. Attention cannot be sustained, and there is often marked distractibility. Self-esteem is often inflated with grandiose ideas and overconfidence. Loss of normal social inhibitions may result in behaviour that is reckless, foolhardy, or inappropriate to the circumstances, and out of character.

F30.2 Mania with psychotic symptoms

In addition to the clinical picture described in F30.1, delusions (usually grandiose) or hallucinations (usually of voices speaking directly to the patient) are present, or the excitement, excessive motor activity, and flight of ideas are so extreme that the patient is incomprehensible or inaccessible to ordinary communication.

Mania with:
- mood-congruent psychotic symptoms
- mood-incongruent psychotic symptoms

Manic stupor

F30.8 Other manic episodes

F30.9 Manic episode, unspecified

Mania NOS

F31 Bipolar affective disorder

A disorder characterized by two or more episodes in which the patient's mood and activity levels are significantly disturbed, this disturbance consisting on some occasions of an elevation of mood and increased energy and activity (hypomania or mania) and on others of a lowering of mood and decreased energy and activity (depression). Repeated episodes of hypomania or mania only are classified as bipolar (F31.8).

Includes: manic–depressive:
- illness
- psychosis
- reaction

Excludes: bipolar disorder, simple manic episode (F30.–)
cyclothymia (F34.0)

F31.0 Bipolar affective disorder, current episode hypomanic

The patient is currently hypomanic, and has had at least one other affective episode (hypomanic, manic, depressive, or mixed) in the past.

F31.1 Bipolar affective disorder, current episode manic without psychotic symptoms

The patient is currently manic, without psychotic symptoms (as in F30.1), and has had at least one other affective episode (hypomanic, manic, depressive, or mixed) in the past.

F31.2 Bipolar affective disorder, current episode manic with psychotic symptoms

The patient is currently manic, with psychotic symptoms (as in F30.2), and has had at least one other affective episode (hypomanic, manic, depressive, or mixed) in the past.

F31.3 Bipolar affective disorder, current episode mild or moderate depression

The patient is currently depressed, as in a depressive episode of either mild or moderate severity (F32.0 or F32.1), and has had at least one authenticated hypomanic, manic, or mixed affective episode in the past.

F31.4 Bipolar affective disorder, current episode severe depression without psychotic symptoms

The patient is currently depressed, as in severe depressive episode without psychotic symptoms (F32.2), and has had at least one authenticated hypomanic, manic, or mixed affective episode in the past.

F31.5 Bipolar affective disorder, current episode severe depression with psychotic symptoms

The patient is currently depressed, as in severe depressive episode with psychotic symptoms (F32.3), and has had at least one authenticated hypomanic, manic, or mixed affective episode in the past.

F31.6 Bipolar affective disorder, current episode mixed

The patient has had at least one authenticated hypomanic, manic, depressive, or mixed affective episode in the past, and currently exhibits either a mixture or a rapid alteration of manic and depressive symptoms.

Excludes: single mixed affective episode (F38.0)

F31.7 Bipolar affective disorder, currently in remission

The patient has had at least one authenticated hypomanic, manic, or mixed affective episode in the past, and at least one other affective episode (depressive, hypomanic, manic, or mixed) in addition, but is not currently suffering from any significant mood disturbance, and has not done so for several months. Periods of remission while receiving prophylactic treatment should be coded here.

F31.8 Other bipolar affective disorders

Bipolar II disorder
Recurrent manic episodes

F31.9 Bipolar affective disorder, unspecified

F32 Depressive episode

In typical mild, moderate, or severe depressive episodes, the patient suffers from lowering of mood, reduction of energy, and decrease in activity. Capacity for enjoyment, interest, and concentration is reduced, and marked tiredness after even minimum effort is common. Sleep is usually disturbed and appetite diminished. Self-esteem and self-confidence are almost always reduced and, even in the mild form, some ideas of guilt or worthlessness are often present. The lowered mood varies little from day to day, is unresponsive to circumstances, and may be accompanied by so-called "somatic" symptoms, such as loss of interest and pleasurable feelings, waking in the morning several hours before the usual time, depression worst in the morning, marked psychomotor retardation, agitation, loss of appetite, weight loss, and loss of libido. Depending upon the number and severity of the symptoms, a depressive episode may be specified as mild, moderate or severe.

Includes: single episodes of:
- depressive reaction
- psychogenic depression
- reactive depression

Excludes: recurrent depressive disorder (F33.–)

F32.0 Mild depressive episode

Two or three of the above symptoms are usually present. The patient is usually distressed by these but will probably be able to continue with most activities.

F32.1 Moderate depressive episode

Four or more of the above symptoms are usually present and the patient is likely to have great difficulty in continuing with ordinary activities.

F32.2 Severe depressive episode without psychotic symptoms

An episode of depression in which several of the symptoms are marked and distressing, typically loss of self-esteem and ideas of worthlessness or guilt. Suicidal thoughts and acts are common and a number of "somatic" symptoms are usually present.

Agitated depression } single episode without psychotic symptoms
Major depression } single episode without psychotic symptoms
Vital depression } single episode without psychotic symptoms

F32.3 Severe depressive episode with psychotic symptoms

An episode of depression as described in F32.2, but with the presence of hallucinations, delusions, psychomotor retardation, or stupor so severe that ordinary social activities are impossible; there may be danger to life from suicide, dehydration, or starvation. The hallucinations and delusions may or may not be mood-congruent.

Single episodes of:
- major depression with psychotic symptoms
- psychogenic depressive psychosis
- psychotic depression
- reactive depressive psychosis

F32.8 Other depressive episodes

Atypical depression
Single episodes of "masked" depression NOS

F32.9 Depressive episode, unspecified

Depression NOS
Depressive disorder NOS

F33 Recurrent depressive disorder

A disorder characterized by repeated episodes of depression, as described for depressive episode (F32.–), without any history of independent episodes of mood elevation and increased energy (mania). There may, however, be brief episodes of mild mood elevation and overactivity (hypomania) immediately after a depressive episode, sometimes precipitated by antidepressant treatment. The more severe forms of recurrent depressive disorder (F33.2 and F33.3) have much in common with earlier concepts such as manic–depressive depression, melancholia, vital depression, and endogenous depression. The first episode may occur at any age from childhood to old age, the onset may be either acute or insidious, and the duration varies from a few weeks to many months. The risk that a patient with recurrent depressive disorder will have an episode of mania never disappears completely, however many depressive episodes have been experienced. If such an episode does occur, the diagnosis should be changed to bipolar affective disorder (F31.–).

Includes: recurrent episodes of:
- depressive reaction
- psychogenic depression
- reactive depression

seasonal depressive disorder

Excludes: recurrent brief depressive episodes (F38.1)

F33.0 Recurrent depressive disorder, current episode mild

A disorder characterized by repeated episodes of depression, the current episode being mild, as in F32.0, and without any history of mania.

F33.1 Recurrent depressive disorder, current episode moderate

A disorder characterized by repeated episodes of depression, the current episode being of moderate severity, as in F32.1, and without any history of mania.

F33.2 Recurrent depressive disorder, current episode severe without psychotic symptoms

A disorder characterized by repeated episodes of depression, the current episode being severe without psychotic symptoms, as in F32.2, and without any history of mania.

Endogenous depression without psychotic symptoms
Major depression, recurrent without psychotic symptoms
Manic–depressive psychosis, depressed type without psychotic symptoms
Vital depression, recurrent without psychotic symptoms

F33.3 Recurrent depressive disorder, current episode severe with psychotic symptoms

A disorder characterized by repeated episodes of depression, the current episode being severe with psychotic symptoms, as in F32.3, and with no previous episodes of mania.

Endogenous depression with psychotic symptoms
Manic–depressive psychosis, depressed type with psychotic symptoms
Recurrent severe episodes of:
- major depression with psychotic symptoms
- psychogenic depressive psychosis
- psychotic depression
- reactive depressive psychosis

F33.4 Recurrent depressive disorder, currently in remission

The patient has had two or more depressive episodes as described in F33.0–F33.3, in the past, but has been free from depressive symptoms for several months.

F33.8 Other recurrent depressive disorders

F33.9 Recurrent depressive disorder, unspecified

Monopolar depression NOS

F34 Persistent affective disorders

Persistent and usually fluctuating disorders of mood in which the majority of the individual episodes are not sufficiently severe to warrant being described as hypomanic or mild depressive episodes. Because they last for many years, and sometimes for the greater part of the patient's adult life, they involve considerable distress and disability. In some instances, recurrent or single manic or depressive episodes may become superimposed on a persistent affective disorder.

F34.0 Cyclothymia

A persistent instability of mood involving numerous periods of depression and mild elation (hypomania), none of which is sufficiently severe or prolonged to justify a diagnosis of bipolar affective disorder (F31.–) or recurrent depressive disorder (F33.–). This disorder is frequently found in the relatives of patients with bipolar affective disorder. Some patients with cyclothymia eventually develop bipolar affective disorder.

Affective personality disorder
Cycloid personality
Cyclothymic personality

F34.1 Dysthymia

A chronic depression of mood, lasting at least several years, which is not sufficiently severe, or in which individual episodes are not sufficiently prolonged, to justify a diagnosis of severe, moderate, or mild recurrent depressive disorder (F33.–).

Depressive:
- neurosis
- personality disorder

Neurotic depression
Persistent anxiety depression

F34.8 Other persistent mood [affective] disorders

F34.9 Persistent mood [affective] disorder, unspecified

F38 Other mood [affective] disorders

Any other mood disorders that do not justify classification to F30–F34 because they are not of sufficient severity or duration.

F38.0 Other single mood [affective] disorders

Mixed affective episode

F38.1 Other recurrent mood [affective] disorders

Recurrent brief depressive episodes

F38.8 Other mood [affective] disorders

F39 Unspecified mood [affective] disorder

Affective psychosis NOS

Neurotic, stress-related and somatoform disorders (F40–F48)

F42.– Obsessive–compulsive disorder

The essential feature is recurrent obsessional thoughts or compulsive acts. Obsessional thoughts are ideas, images, or impulses that enter the patient's mind again and again in a stereotyped form. They are almost invariably distressing and the patient often tries, unsuccessfully, to resist them. They are, however, recognized as his or her own thoughts, even though they are involuntary and often repugnant. Compulsive acts or rituals are stereotyped behaviours that are repeated again and again. They are not inherently enjoyable, nor do they result in the completion of inherently useful tasks. Their function is to prevent some objectively unlikely event, often involving harm to or caused by the patient, which he or she fears might otherwise occur. Usually, this behaviour is recognized by the patient as pointless or ineffectual and repeated attempts are made to resist. Anxiety is almost invariably present. If compulsive acts are resisted the anxiety gets worse.

F44 Dissociative [conversion] disorders

The common themes that are shared by dissociative or conversion disorders are a partial or complete loss of the normal integration between memories of the past, awareness of identity and immediate sensations, and control of bodily movements. All types of dissociative disorders tend to remit after a few weeks or months, particularly if their onset is associated with a traumatic life event. More chronic disorders, particularly paralyses and anaesthesias, may develop if the onset is associated with insoluble problems or interpersonal difficulties. These disorders have previously been classified as various types of "conversion hysteria". They are presumed to be psychogenic in origin, being associated closely in time with traumatic events, insoluble and intolerable problems, or disturbed relationships. The symptoms often represent the patient's concept of how a physical illness would be manifest. Medical examination and investigation do not reveal the presence of any known physical or neurological disorder. In addition, there is evidence that the loss of function is an expression of emotional conflicts or needs. The symptoms may develop in close relationship to psychological stress, and often appear suddenly. Only disorders of physical functions normally under voluntary control and loss of sensations are included here. Disorders involving pain and other complex physical sensations mediated by the autonomic nervous system are classified under somatization disorder (F45.0). The possibility of the later appearance of serious physical or psychiatric disorders should always be kept in mind.

Includes: conversion:
- hysteria
- reaction

hysteria
hysterical psychosis

Excludes: malingering [conscious simulation] (Z76.5)

F44.0 Dissociative amnesia

The main feature is loss of memory, usually of important recent events, that is not due to organic mental disorder, and is too great to be explained by ordinary forgetfulness or fatigue. The amnesia is usually centred on traumatic events, such as accidents or unexpected bereavements, and is usually partial and selective. Complete and generalized amnesia is rare, and is usually part of a fugue (F44.1). If this is the case, the disorder should be classified as such. The diagnosis should not be made in the presence of organic brain disorders, intoxication, or excessive fatigue.

Excludes: alcohol- or other psychoactive substance-induced amnesic disorder (F10–F19 with common fourth character .6)
nonalcoholic organic amnesic disorder (F04)
postictal amnesia in epilepsy (G40.–)

F44.1 Dissociative fugue

Dissociative fugue has all the features of dissociative amnesia, plus purposeful travel beyond the usual everyday range. Although there is amnesia for the period of the fugue, the patient's behaviour during this time may appear completely normal to independent observers.

Excludes: postictal fugue in epilepsy (G40.–)

F44.2 Dissociative stupor

Dissociative stupor is diagnosed on the basis of a profound diminution or absence of voluntary movement and normal responsiveness to external stimuli such as light, noise, and touch, but examination and investigation reveal no evidence of a physical cause. In addition, there is positive evidence of psychogenic causation in the form of recent stressful events or problems.

Excludes: organic catatonic disorder (F06.1)
stupor:
- NOS (R40.1)
- depressive (F31–F33)
- manic (F30.2)

F44.3 Trance and possession disorders

Disorders in which there is a temporary loss of the sense of personal identity and full awareness of the surroundings. Include here only trance states that are involuntary or unwanted, occurring outside religious or culturally accepted situations.

Excludes: states associated with:
- organic personality disorder (F07.0)
- postconcussional syndrome (F07.2)
- psychoactive substance intoxication (F10–F19 with common fourth character .0)

F44.4 Dissociative motor disorders

In the commonest varieties there is loss of ability to move the whole or a part of a limb or limbs. There may be close resemblance to almost any variety of ataxia, apraxia, akinesia, aphonia, dysarthria, dyskinesia, seizures, or paralysis.

Hysterical tremor
Psychogenic:
- aphonia
- dysphonia
- parkinsonism† (G22.–3*)

F44.5 Dissociative convulsions

Dissociative convulsions may mimic epileptic seizures very closely in terms of movements, but tongue-biting, bruising due to falling, and incontinence of urine are rare, and consciousness is maintained or replaced by a state of stupor or trance.

Hysterical tetany
Pseudoseizures

F44.6 Dissociative anaesthesia and sensory loss

Anaesthetic areas of skin often have boundaries that make it clear that they are associated with the patient's ideas about bodily functions, rather than medical knowledge. There may be differential loss between the sensory modalities which cannot be due to a neurological lesion. Sensory loss may be accompanied by complaints of paraesthesia. Loss of vision and hearing is rarely total in dissociative disorders.

Psychogenic:
- anaesthesia
- blindness
- deafness

F44.7 Mixed dissociative [conversion] disorders

Combination of disorders specified in F44.0–F44.6

F44.8 Other dissociative [conversion] disorders

Includes: psychogenic:
- confusion
- twilight state

F44.80 Ganser's syndrome
F44.81 Multiple personality disorder
F44.82 Transient dissociative [conversion] disorders occurring in childhood and adolescence
F44.88 Other specified dissociative [conversion] disorders

F44.9 Dissociative [conversion] disorder, unspecified

F45 Somatoform disorders

The main feature is repeated presentation of physical symptoms together with persistent requests for medical investigations, in spite of repeated negative findings and reassurances by doctors that the symptoms have no physical basis. If any physical disorders are present, they do not explain the nature and extent of the symptoms or the distress and preoccupation of the patient.

Excludes: dissociative disorders (F44.–)
hair-plucking (F98.4)
lalling (F80.0)
lisping (F80.8)
nail-biting (F98.8)
thumb-sucking (F98.8)
tic disorders (in childhood and adolescence) (F95.–)
Tourette's syndrome (F95.2)

F45.0 Somatization disorder

The main features are multiple, recurrent, and frequently changing physical symptoms of at least two years' duration. Most patients have a long and complicated history of contact with both primary and specialist medical care services, during which many negative investigations or fruitless exploratory operations may have been carried out. Symptoms may be referred to any part or system of the body. The course of the disorder is chronic and fluctuating, and is often associated with disruption of social, interpersonal, and family behaviour. Short-lived (less than two years) and less striking symptom patterns should be classified under undifferentiated somatoform disorder (F45.1).

Multiple psychosomatic disorder
Excludes: malingering [conscious simulation] (Z76.5)

F45.1 Undifferentiated somatoform disorder

When somatoform complaints are multiple, varying, and persistent, but the complete and typical clinical picture of somatization disorder is not fulfilled, the diagnosis of undifferentiated somatoform disorders should be considered.

Undifferentiated psychosomatic disorder

F45.2 Hypochondriacal disorder

The essential feature is a persistent preoccupation with the possibility of having one or more serious and progressive physical disorders. Patients manifest persistent somatic complaints or a persistent preoccupation with their physical appearance. Normal or commonplace sensations and appearances are often interpreted by the patient as abnormal and distressing, and attention is usually focused upon only one or two organs or systems of the body. Marked depression and anxiety are often present, and may justify additional diagnoses.

Body dysmorphic disorder
Dysmorphophobia (nondelusional)
Hypochondriacal neurosis
Hypochondriasis
Nosophobia

F45.3 Somatoform autonomic dysfunction

Symptoms are presented by the patient as if they were due to a physical disorder of a system or organ that is largely or completely under autonomic innervation and control, i.e. the cardiovascular, gastrointestinal, respiratory, and urogenital systems. The symptoms are usually of two types, neither of which indicates a physical disorder of the organ or system concerned. First, there are complaints based upon objective signs of autonomic arousal, such as palpitations, sweating, flushing, tremor, and expression of fear and distress about the possibility of a physical disorder. Second, there are subjective complaints of a nonspecific or changing nature such as fleeting aches and pains, sensations of burning, heaviness, tightness, and feelings of being bloated or distended, which are referred by the patient to a specific organ or system.

Neurocirculatory asthenia
Psychogenic:
- hiccough
- hyperventilation

F45.4 Persistent somatoform pain disorder

The predominant complaint is of persistent, severe, and distressing pain, which cannot be explained fully by a physiological process or a physical disorder, and which occurs in association with emotional conflict or psychosocial problems that are sufficient to allow the conclusion that they are the main causative influences. The result is usually a marked increase in support and attention, either personal or medical. Pain presumed to be of psychogenic origin occurring during the course of depressive disorders or schizophrenia should not be included here.

Psychalgia
Psychogenic:
- backache
- headache

Somatoform pain disorder

Excludes: backache NOS (M54.9)
pain:
- NOS (R52.9)
- acute (R52.0)
- chronic (R52.2)
- intractable (R52.1)

tension headache (G44.2)

F45.8 Other somatoform disorders

Any other disorders of sensation, function, and behaviour, not due to physical disorders, which are not mediated through the autonomic nervous system, which are limited to specific systems or parts of the body, and which are closely associated in time with stressful events or problems.

Psychogenic:
- dysmenorrhoea
- dysphagia, including "globus hystericus"
- pruritus
- torticollis

Teeth-grinding

Excludes: tic disorders (F95.–)

F45.9 Somatoform disorder, unspecified

Psychosomatic disorder NOS

F48 Other neurotic disorders

F48.0 Neurasthenia

Considerable cultural variations occur in the presentation of this disorder, and two main types occur, with substantial overlap. In one type, the main feature is a complaint of increased fatigue after mental effort, often associated with some decrease in occupational performance or coping efficiency in daily tasks. The mental fatiguability is typically described as an unpleasant intrusion of distracting associations or recollections, difficulty in concentrating, and generally inefficient thinking. In the other type, the emphasis is on feelings of bodily or physical weakness and exhaustion after only minimal effort, accompanied by a feeling of muscular aches and pains and inability to relax. In both types a variety of other unpleasant physical feelings is common, such as dizziness, tension headaches, and feelings of general instability. Worry about decreasing mental and bodily well-being, irritability, anhedonia, and varying minor degrees of both depression and anxiety are all common. Sleep is often disturbed in its initial and middle phases but hypersomnia may also be prominent.

Fatigue syndrome

Use additional code, if desired, to identify previous physical illness.

Excludes: asthenia NOS (R53)
burn-out (Z73.0)
malaise and fatigue (R53)
postviral fatigue syndrome (G93.3)
psychasthenia (F48.83)

F48.1 Depersonalization–derealization syndrome

A rare disorder in which the patient complains spontaneously that his or her mental activity, body, and surroundings are changed in their quality, so as to be unreal, remote, or automatized. Among the varied phenomena of the syndrome, patients complain most frequently of loss of emotions and feelings of estrangement or detachment from their thinking, their body, or the real world. In spite of the dramatic nature of the experience, the patient is aware of the unreality of the change. The sensorium is normal and the capacity for emotional expression intact. Depersonalization–derealization symptoms may occur as part of a diagnosable schizophrenic, depressive, phobic, or obsessive–compulsive disorder. In such cases the diagnosis should be that of the main disorder.

F48.8 Other specified neurotic disorders

F48.80 Briquet's disorder
F48.81 Dhat syndrome
F48.82 Occupational neurosis, including writer's cramp
Excludes: occupational dystonia of organic type (G24.–)
F48.83 Psychasthenia
Psychasthenic neurosis
F48.84 Psychogenic syncope
F48.88 Other neurotic disorders
Excludes: compensation neurosis (F68.0)

F48.9 Neurotic disorder, unspecified
Neurosis NOS

Behavioural syndromes associated with physiological disturbances and physical factors (F50–F59)

F51 Nonorganic sleep disorders

In many cases, a disturbance of sleep is one of the symptoms of another disorder, either mental or physical. Whether a sleep disorder in a given patient is an independent condition or simply one of the features of another disorder classified elsewhere, either in this chapter or in other chapters, should be determined on the basis of its clinical presentation and course as well as on the therapeutic considerations and priorities at the time of the consultation. Generally, if the sleep disorder is one of the major complaints and is perceived as a condition in itself, the present code should be used along with other pertinent diagnoses describing the psychopathology and pathophysiology involved in a given case. This category includes only those sleep disorders in which emotional causes are considered to be a primary factor, and which are not due to identifiable physical disorders classified elsewhere.

Excludes: sleep disorders (organic) (G47.–)

F51.0 Nonorganic insomnia

A condition of unsatisfactory quantity and quality of sleep, which persists for a considerable period of time, including difficulty falling asleep, difficulty staying asleep, or early final wakening. Insomnia is a common symptom of many mental and physical disorders, and should be classified here in addition to the basic disorder only if it dominates the clinical picture.

Excludes: insomnia (organic) (G47.0)

F51.1 Nonorganic hypersomnia

Hypersomnia is defined as a condition of either excessive daytime sleepiness and sleep attacks (not accounted for by an inadequate amount of sleep) or prolonged transitions to the fully aroused state upon awakening. In the absence of an organic factor for the occurrence of hypersomnia, this condition is usually associated with mental disorders.

Excludes: hypersomnia (organic) (G47.1)
narcolepsy (G47.4)

F51.2 Nonorganic disorder of the sleep–wake schedule

A lack of synchrony between the sleep–wake schedule and the desired sleep–wake schedule for the individual's environment, resulting in a complaint of either insomnia or hypersomnia.

Psychogenic inversion of:
- circadian } rhythm
- nyctohemeral } rhythm
- sleep } rhythm

Excludes: disorders of the sleep–wake schedule (organic) (G47.2)

F51.3 Sleepwalking [somnambulism]

A state of altered consciousness in which phenomena of sleep and wakefulness are combined. During a sleepwalking episode the individual arises from bed, usually during the first third of nocturnal sleep, and walks about, exhibiting low levels of awareness, reactivity, and motor skill. Upon awakening, there is usually no recall of the event.

F51.4 Sleep terrors [night terrors]

Nocturnal episodes of extreme terror and panic associated with intense vocalization, motility, and high levels of autonomic discharge. The individual sits up or gets up, usually during the first third of nocturnal sleep, with a panicky scream. Quite often he or she rushes to the door as if trying to escape, although very seldom leaves the room. Recall of the event, if any, is very limited (usually to one or two fragmentary mental images).

F51.5 Nightmares

Dream experiences loaded with anxiety or fear. There is very detailed recall of the dream content. The dream experience is very vivid and usually includes themes involving threats to survival, security, or self-esteem. Quite often there is a recurrence of the same or similar frightening nightmare themes. During a typical episode there is a degree of autonomic discharge but no appreciable vocalization or body motility. Upon awakening the individual rapidly becomes alert and oriented.

Dream anxiety disorder

F51.8 Other nonorganic sleep disorders

F51.9 Nonorganic sleep disorder, unspecified
Emotional sleep disorder NOS

Disorders of adult personality and behaviour (F60–F69)

F68 Other disorders of adult personality and behaviour

F68.0 Elaboration of physical symptoms for psychological reasons
Physical symptoms compatible with and originally due to a confirmed physical disorder, disease, or disability become exaggerated or prolonged due to the psychological state of the patient. The patient is commonly distressed by this pain or disability, and is often preoccupied with worries, which may be justified, of the possibility of prolonged or progressive disability or pain.

Compensation neurosis

F68.1 Intentional production or feigning of symptoms or disabilities, either physical or psychological [factitious disorder]
The patient feigns symptoms repeatedly for no obvious reason and may even inflict self-harm in order to produce symptoms or signs. The motivation is obscure and presumably internal, with the aim of adopting the sick role. The disorder is often combined with marked disorders of personality and relationships.

Hospital hopper syndrome
Münchhausen's syndrome
Peregrinating patient
Excludes: person feigning illness (with obvious motivation) (Z76.5)

F68.8 Other specified disorders of adult personality and behaviour
Character disorder NOS
Relationship disorder NOS

F69 Unspecified disorder of adult personality and behaviour

Mental retardation (F70–F79)

A condition of arrested or incomplete development of the mind, which is especially characterized by impairment of skills manifested during the developmental period, skills which contribute to the overall level of intelligence, i.e. cognitive, language, motor, and social abilities. Retardation can occur with or without any other mental or physical condition.

Degrees of mental retardation are conventionally estimated by standardized intelligence tests. These can be supplemented by scales assessing social adaptation in a given environment. These measures provide an approximate indication of the degree of mental retardation. The diagnosis will also depend on the overall assessment of intellectual functioning by a skilled diagnostician.

Intellectual abilities and social adaptation may change over time, and, however poor, may improve as a result of training and rehabilitation. Diagnosis should be based on the current levels of functioning.

The following fourth-character subdivisions are for use with categories F70–F79 to identify the extent of the impairment of behaviour:

F7*x*.0 With the statement of no, or minimal, impairment of behaviour

F7*x*.1 Significant impairment of behaviour requiring attention or treatment

F7*x*.8 Other impairments of behaviour

F7*x*.9 Without mention of impairment of behaviour

Use additional code, if desired, to identify associated conditions such as autism, other developmental disorders, epilepsy, conduct disorders, or severe physical handicap.

F70 Mild mental retardation

Approximate IQ range of 50 to 69 (in adults, mental age from 9 to under 12 years). Likely to result in some learning difficulties in school. Many adults will be able to work, make and maintain good social relationships, and contribute to society.

Includes: feeble-mindedness
mild mental subnormality

F71 Moderate mental retardation

Approximate IQ range of 35 to 49 (in adults, mental age from 6 to under 9 years). Likely to result in marked developmental delays in childhood, but most can learn to develop some degree of independence in self-care and acquire adequate communication and academic skills. Adults will need varying degrees of support to live and work in the community.

Includes: moderate mental subnormality

F72 Severe mental retardation

Approximate IQ range of 20 to 34 (in adults, mental age from 3 to under 6 years). Likely to result in continuous need of support.

Includes: severe mental subnormality

F73 Profound mental retardation

IQ under 20 (in adults, mental age below 3 years). Results in severe limitation in self-care, continence, communication, and mobility.

Includes: profound mental subnormality

F78 Other mental retardation

F79 Unspecified mental retardation

Includes: mental:
- deficiency NOS
- subnormality NOS

Disorders of psychological development (F80–F89)

The disorders included in this block have in common: (a) onset invariably during infancy or childhood; (b) impairment or delay in development of functions that are strongly related to biological maturation of the central nervous system; and (c) a steady course without remissions and relapses. In most cases, the functions affected include language, visuo-spatial skills, and motor coordination. Usually, the delay or impairment has been present from as early as it could be detected reliably and will diminish progressively as the child grows older, although milder deficits often remain in adult life.

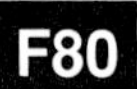

Specific developmental disorders of speech and language

Disorders in which normal patterns of language acquisition are disturbed from the early stages of development. The conditions are not directly attributable to neurological or speech mechanism abnormalities, sensory impairments, mental retardation, or environmental factors. Specific developmental disorders of speech and language are often followed by associated problems, such as difficulties in reading and spelling, abnormalities in interpersonal relationships, and emotional and behavioural disorders.

F80.0 Specific speech articulation disorder

A specific developmental disorder in which the child's use of speech sounds is below the appropriate level for its mental age, but in which there is a normal level of language skills.

Developmental:
- phonological disorder
- speech articulation disorder

Dyslalia
Functional speech articulation disorder
Lalling

Excludes: speech articulation disorder (due to):
- aphasia (R47.0)
- apraxia (R48.2)
- hearing loss (H90–H91)
- mental retardation (F70–F79)
- with language developmental disorder:
  - expressive (F80.1)
  - receptive (F80.2)

F80.1 Expressive language disorder

A specific developmental disorder in which the child's ability to use expressive spoken language is markedly below the appropriate level for its mental age, but in which language comprehension is within normal limits. There may or may not be abnormalities in articulation.

Developmental dysphasia or aphasia, expressive type

Excludes: acquired aphasia with epilepsy [Landau–Kleffner] (F80.3)
developmental dysphasia or aphasia, receptive type (F80.2)
dysphasia and aphasia NOS (R47.0)
mental retardation (F70–F79)
pervasive developmental disorders (F84.–)

F80.2 Receptive language disorder

A specific developmental disorder in which the child's understanding of language is below the appropriate level for its mental age. In virtually all cases expressive language will also be markedly affected and abnormalities in word-sound production are common.

Congenital auditory imperception
Developmental:
- dysphasia or aphasia, receptive type
- Wernicke's aphasia

Word deafness

Excludes: acquired aphasia with epilepsy [Landau–Kleffner] (F80.3)
autism (F84.0–F84.1)
language delay due to deafness (H90–H91)
mental retardation (F70–F79)
Wernicke's receptive aphasia (R47.01)

F80.3 Acquired aphasia with epilepsy [Landau–Kleffner]

A disorder in which the child, having previously made normal progress in language development, loses both receptive and expressive language skills but retains general intelligence; the onset of the disorder is accompanied by paroxysmal abnormalities on the EEG, and in the majority of cases also by epileptic seizures. Usually the onset is between the ages of three and seven years, with skills being lost over days or weeks. The temporal association between the onset of seizures and loss of language is rather variable, with one preceding the other (either way round) by a few months to two years. An inflammatory encephalitic process has been suggested as a possible cause of this disorder. About two-thirds of the patients are left with a more or less severe receptive language deficit.

Excludes: aphasia (due to):
- NOS (R47.0)
- autism (F84.0–F84.1)
- disintegrative disorders of childhood (F84.2–F84.3)

F80.8 Other developmental disorders of speech and language

Lisping

F80.9 Developmental disorder of speech and language, unspecified

Language disorder NOS

F81 Specific developmental disorders of scholastic skills

Disorders in which the normal patterns of skill acquisition are disturbed from the early stages of development. This is not simply a consequence of a lack of opportunity to learn, it is not solely a result of mental retardation, and it is not due to any form of acquired brain trauma or disease.

F81.0 Specific reading disorder

The main feature is a specific and significant impairment in the development of reading skills that is not solely accounted for by low mental age, visual acuity problems, or inadequate schooling. Reading comprehension skill, reading word recognition, oral reading skill, and performance of tasks requiring reading may all be affected. Spelling difficulties are frequently associated with specific reading disorder and often remain into adolescence even after some progress in reading has been made. Specific developmental disorders of reading are commonly preceded by a history of disorders in speech or language development. Associated emotional and behavioural disturbances are common during the school age period.

"Backward reading"
Developmental dyslexia
Specific reading retardation
Excludes: alexia NOS (R48.0)
dyslexia NOS (R48.0)

F81.1 Specific spelling disorder

The main feature is a specific and significant impairment in the development of spelling skills in the absence of a history of specific reading disorder, which is not solely accounted for by low mental age, visual acuity problems, or inadequate schooling. The ability to spell orally and to write out words correctly are both affected.

Specific spelling retardation (without reading disorder)
Excludes: agraphia NOS (R48.81)
spelling difficulties associated with a reading disorder (F81.0)

F81.2 Specific disorder of arithmetical skills

Involves a specific impairment in arithmetical skills that is not solely explicable on the basis of general mental retardation or of inadequate schooling. The deficit concerns mastery of basic computational skills of addition, subtraction, multiplication, and division rather than of the more abstract mathematical skills involved in algebra, trigonometry, geometry, or calculus.

Developmental:
- acalculia
- arithmetical disorder
- Gerstmann's syndrome

Excludes: acalculia NOS (R48.8)
arithmetical difficulties associated with a reading or spelling disorder (F81.3)

F81.3 Mixed disorder of scholastic skills

An ill-defined residual category of disorders in which both arithmetical and reading or spelling skills are significantly impaired, but in which the disorder is not solely explicable in terms of general mental retardation or of inadequate schooling. It should be used for disorders meeting the criteria for both F81.2 and either F81.0 or F81.1.

Excludes: specific:
- disorder of arithmetical skills (F81.2)
- reading disorder (F81.0)
- spelling disorder (F81.1)

F81.8 Other developmental disorders of scholastic skills
Developmental expressive writing disorder

F81.9 Developmental disorder of scholastic skills, unspecified
Knowledge acquisition disability NOS
Learning:
- disability NOS
- disorder NOS

F82 Specific developmental disorder of motor function

A disorder in which the main feature is a serious impairment in the development of motor coordination that is not solely explicable in terms of general intellectual retardation or of any specific congenital or acquired neurological disorder. Nevertheless, in most cases a careful clinical examination shows marked neurodevelopmental immaturities such as choreiform movements of unsupported limbs or mirror movements and other associated motor features, as well as signs of impaired fine and gross motor coordination.

Clumsy child syndrome
Developmental:
- coordination disorder
- dyspraxia

Excludes: abnormalities of gait and mobility (R26.–)
lack of coordination (R27.–)
- secondary to mental retardation (F70–F79)

F83 Mixed specific developmental disorders

A residual category for disorders in which there is some admixture of specific developmental disorders of speech and language, of scholastic skills, and of motor function, but in which none predominates sufficiently to constitute the prime diagnosis. This mixed category should be used only when there is a major overlap between each of these specific developmental disorders. They are usually, but not always, associated with some degree of general impairment of cognitive functions. Thus, the category should be used when there are dysfunctions meeting the criteria for two or more of F80.–, F81.– and F82.

F84 Pervasive developmental disorders

A group of disorders characterized by qualitative abnormalities in reciprocal social interactions and in patterns of communication, and by a restricted, stereotyped, repetitive repertoire of interests and activities. These qualitative abnormalities are a pervasive feature of the individual's functioning in all situations.

Use additional code, if desired, to identify any associated medical condition and mental retardation.

F84.0 Childhood autism

A type of pervasive developmental disorder that is defined by: (a) the presence of abnormal or impaired development that is manifest before the age of three years, and (b) the characteristic type of abnormal functioning in all the three areas of psychopathology: reciprocal social interaction, communication, and restricted, stereotyped, repetitive behaviour. In addition to these specific diagnostic features, a range of other nonspecific problems are common, such as fear and phobias, sleeping and eating disturbances, temper tantrums, and (self-directed) aggression.

Autistic disorder
Infantile:
- autism
- psychosis

Kanner's syndrome
Excludes: autistic psychopathy (F84.5)

F84.1 Atypical autism

A type of pervasive developmental disorder that differs from childhood autism either in age of onset or in failing to fulfil all three sets of diagnostic criteria. This subcategory should be used when there is abnormal and impaired development that is present only after age three years, and a lack of sufficient demonstrable abnormalities in one or two of the three areas of psychopathology required for the diagnosis of autism (namely, reciprocal social interactions, communication, and restricted, stereotyped, repetitive behaviour) in spite of characteristic abnormalities in the other area(s). Atypical autism arises most often in profoundly retarded individuals and in individuals with a severe specific developmental disorder of receptive language.

Atypical childhood psychosis
Mental retardation with autistic features

Use additional code (F70–F79), if desired, to identify mental retardation.

F84.2 Rett's syndrome

A condition, so far found only in girls, in which apparently normal early development is followed by partial or complete loss of speech and of skills in locomotion and use of hands, together with deceleration in head growth, usually with an onset between seven and 24 months of age. Loss of purposive hand movements, hand-wringing stereotypies, and hyperventilation are characteristic. Social and play development are arrested but social interest tends to be maintained. Trunk ataxia and apraxia start to develop by age four years and choreoathetoid movements frequently follow. Severe mental retardation almost invariably results.

F84.3 Other childhood disintegrative disorder

A type of pervasive developmental disorder that is defined by a period of entirely normal development before the onset of the disorder, followed by a definite loss of previously acquired skills in several areas of development over the course of a few months. Typically, this is accompanied by a general loss of interest in the environment, by stereotyped, repetitive motor mannerisms, and by autistic-like abnormalities in social interaction and communication. In some cases the disorder can be shown to be due to some associated encephalopathy but the diagnosis should be made on the behavioural features.

Dementia infantilis
Disintegrative psychosis
Heller's syndrome
Symbiotic psychosis

Use additional code, if desired, to identify any associated neurological condition.

Excludes: Rett's syndrome (F84.2)

F84.4 Overactive disorder associated with mental retardation and stereotyped movements

An ill-defined disorder of uncertain nosological validity. The category is designed to include a group of children with severe mental retardation (IQ below 34) who show major problems in hyperactivity and in attention, as well as stereotyped behaviours. They tend not to benefit from stimulant drugs (unlike those with an IQ in the normal range) and may exhibit a severe dysphoric reaction (sometimes with psychomotor retardation) when given stimulants. In adolescence, the overactivity tends to be replaced by underactivity (a pattern that is not usual in hyperkinetic children with normal intelligence). This syndrome is also often associated with a variety of developmental delays, either specific or global. The extent to which the behavioural pattern is a function of low IQ or of organic brain damage is not known.

F84.5 Asperger's syndrome

A disorder of uncertain nosological validity, characterized by the same type of qualitative abnormalities of reciprocal social interaction that typify autism, together with a restricted, stereotyped, repetitive repertoire of interests and activities. It differs from autism primarily in the fact that there is no general delay or retardation in language or in cognitive development. This disorder is often associated with marked clumsiness. There is a strong tendency for the abnormalities to persist into adolescence and adult life. Psychotic episodes occasionally occur in early adult life.

Autistic psychopathy
Schizoid disorder of childhood

F84.8 Other pervasive developmental disorders

F84.9 Pervasive developmental disorder, unspecified

F88 Other disorders of psychological development

Developmental agnosia

F89 Unspecified disorder of psychological development

Developmental disorder NOS

Behavioural and emotional disorders with onset usually occurring in childhood and adolescence (F90–F98)

F90 Hyperkinetic disorders

A group of disorders characterized by an early onset (usually in the first five years of life), lack of persistence in activities that require cognitive involvement, and a tendency to move from one activity to another without completing any one, together with disorganized, ill-regulated, and excessive activity. Several other abnormalities may be associated. Hyperkinetic children are often reckless and impulsive, prone to accidents, and find themselves in disciplinary trouble because of unthinking breaches of rules rather than deliberate defiance. Their relationships with adults are often socially disinhibited, with a lack of normal caution and reserve. They are unpopular with other children and may become isolated. Impairment of cognitive functions is common, and specific delays in motor and language development are disproportionately frequent. Secondary complications include dissocial behaviour and low self-esteem.

F90.0 Disturbance of activity and attention

Attention deficit:
- disorder with hyperactivity
- hyperactivity disorder
- syndrome with hyperactivity

Excludes: hyperkinetic disorder associated with conduct disorder (F90.1)

F90.1 Hyperkinetic conduct disorder

Hyperkinetic disorder associated with conduct disorder

F90.8 Other hyperkinetic disorders

F90.9 Hyperkinetic disorder, unspecified

Hyperkinetic reaction of childhood or adolescence NOS
Hyperkinetic syndrome NOS

F95 Tic disorders

Syndromes in which the predominant manifestation is some form of tic. A tic is an involuntary, rapid, recurrent, nonrhythmic motor movement (usually involving circumscribed muscle groups) or vocal production that is of sudden onset and that serves no apparent purpose. Tics tend to be experienced as irresistible but usually they can be suppressed for varying periods of time, are exacerbated by stress, and disappear during sleep.

Common simple motor tics include eye-blinking, neck-jerking, shoulder-shrugging, and facial grimacing. Common simple vocal tics include throat-clearing, barking, sniffing, and hissing. Common complex tics include hitting oneself, jumping, and hopping. Common complex vocal tics include the repetition of particular words, and sometimes the use of socially unacceptable (often obscene) words (coprolalia), and the repetition of one's own sounds or words (palilalia).

F95.0 Transient tic disorder

Meets the general criteria for a tic disorder but the tics do not persist longer than 12 months. The tics usually take the form of eye-blinking, facial grimacing, or head-jerking.

F95.1 Chronic motor or vocal tic disorder

Meets the general criteria for a tic disorder, in which there are motor or vocal tics (but not both), that may be either single or multiple (but usually multiple) and last for more than a year.

F95.2 Combined vocal and multiple motor tic disorder [de la Tourette]

A form of tic disorder in which there are, or have been, multiple motor tics and one or more vocal tics, although these need not have occurred concurrently. The disorder usually worsens during adolescence and tends to persist into adult life. The vocal tics are often multiple with explosive repetitive vocalizations, throat-clearing, and grunting, and there may be the use of obscene words or phrases. Sometimes there is associated gestural echopraxia which also may be of an obscene nature (copropraxia).

Tourette's disorder

F95.8 Other tic disorders

F95.9 Tic disorder, unspecified

Tic NOS

F98 Other behavioural and emotional disorders with onset usually occurring in childhood and adolescence

A heterogeneous group of disorders that share the characteristic of an onset in childhood but otherwise differ in many respects. Some of the conditions represent well-defined syndromes but others are no more than symptom complexes that need inclusion because of their frequency and association with psychosocial problems, and because they cannot be incorporated into other syndromes.

Excludes: breath-holding spells (R06.81)
Kleine–Levin syndrome (G47.84)

F98.0 Nonorganic enuresis

A disorder characterized by involuntary voiding of urine, by day and by night, which is abnormal in relation to the individual's mental age, and which is not a consequence of a lack of bladder control due to any neurological disorder, to epileptic attacks, or to any structural abnormality of the urinary tract. The enuresis may have been present from birth or it may have arisen following a period of acquired bladder control. The enuresis may or may not be associated with a more widespread emotional or behavioural disorder.

Functional enuresis
Psychogenic enuresis
Urinary incontinence of nonorganic origin
Excludes: enuresis NOS (R32)

F98.1 Nonorganic encopresis

Repeated, voluntary or involuntary passage of faeces, usually of normal or near-normal consistency, in places not appropriate for that purpose in the individual's own sociocultural setting. The condition may represent an abnormal continuation of normal infantile incontinence, it may involve a loss of continence following the acquisition of bowel control, or it may involve the deliberate deposition of faeces in inappropriate places in spite of normal physiological bowel control. The condition may occur as a monosymptomatic disorder, or it may be associated with a more widespread emotional or behavioural disorder.

Functional encopresis
Incontinence of faeces of nonorganic origin
Psychogenic encopresis

Use additional code, if desired, to identify the cause of any coexisting constipation.

Excludes: encopresis NOS (R15)

F98.4 Stereotyped movement disorders

Voluntary, repetitive, stereotyped, nonfunctional (and often rhythmic) movements that do not form part of any recognized psychiatric or neurological condition. When such movements occur as symptoms of some other disorder, only the overall disorder should be coded (i.e. F98.4 should not be coded). The movements that are of a non-self-injurious variety include: body-rocking, head-rocking, hair-plucking, hair-twisting, finger-flicking mannerisms, and hand-flapping. Stereotyped self-injurious behaviour includes repetitive head-banging, face-slapping, eye-poking, and biting of hands, lips, or other body parts. All the stereotyped movement disorders occur most frequently in association with mental retardation (when this is the case, both should be recorded). If eye-poking occurs in a child with visual impairment, both should be coded: eye-poking under this category and the visual condition under the appropriate somatic disorder code.

Stereotype/habit disorder
Excludes: abnormal involuntary movements (R25.–)
movement disorders of organic origin (G20–G25)
tic disorders (F95.–)

F98.5 Stuttering [stammering]

Speech that is characterized by frequent repetition or prolongation of sounds or syllables or words, or by frequent hesitations or pauses that disrupt the rhythmic flow of speech. It should be classified as a disorder only if its severity is such as to markedly disturb the fluency of speech.

Excludes: cluttering (F98.6)
stuttering of organic origin (R47.80)
tic disorders (F95.–)

F98.6 Cluttering

A rapid rate of speech with breakdown in fluency, but no repetitions or hesitations, of a severity to give rise to diminished speech intelligibility. Speech is erratic and dysrhythmic, with rapid jerky spurts that usually involve faulty phrasing patterns.

Excludes: cluttering of organic origin (R47.81)
stuttering (F98.5)
tic disorders (F95.–)

F98.8 Other specified behavioural and emotional disorders with onset usually occurring in childhood and adolescence

Attention deficit disorder without hyperactivity

Unspecified mental disorder (F99)

F99 Mental disorder, not otherwise specified

Mental illness NOS

Excludes: organic mental disorder NOS (F06.9)

CHAPTER VI

Diseases of the nervous system (G00–G99)

Excludes: certain conditions originating in the perinatal period (P00–P96)
certain infectious and parasitic diseases (A00–B99)
complications of pregnancy, childbirth and the puerperium (O00–O99)
congenital malformations, deformations and chromosomal abnormalities (Q00–Q99)
endocrine, nutritional and metabolic diseases (E00–E90)
injury, poisoning and certain other consequences of external causes (S00–T98)
neoplasms (C00–D48)
symptoms, signs and abnormal clinical and laboratory findings, not elsewhere classified (R00–R99)

Inflammatory diseases of the central nervous system (G00–G09)

G00 Bacterial meningitis, not elsewhere classified

Includes: bacterial:
- arachnoiditis
- leptomeningitis
- meningitis
- pachymeningitis

Excludes: bacterial:
- meningoencephalitis (G04.2)
- meningomyelitis (G04.2)

G00.0 Haemophilus meningitis
Meningitis due to *Haemophilus influenzae*

G00.1 Pneumococcal meningitis

G00.2 Streptococcal meningitis

G00.3 Staphylococcal meningitis

G00.30 Meningitis due to *Staphylococcus aureus*
G00.31 Meningitis due to *Staphylococcus epidermidis*
G00.38 Other staphylococcal meningitis

G00.8 Other bacterial meningitis

G00.80 Anaerobic bacterial meningitis

G00.800 Meningitis due to *Bacteroides fragilis*

G00.801 Meningitis due to *Fusobacterium* species

G00.802 Meningitis due to *Propionibacterium* species

G00.803 Meningitis due to *Peptococcus* species [*Peptostreptococcus*]

G00.804 Meningitis due to *Clostridium* species

G00.805 Meningitis due to *Actinomyces* species

G00.81 Facultative anaerobic bacterial meningitis

G00.811 Meningitis due to *Citrobacter* species

G00.812 Meningitis due to *Enterobacter* species

G00.82 Meningitis due to *Acinetobacter* species

G00.83 Meningitis due to *Escherichia coli*

G00.84 Meningitis due to *Klebsiella* species

G00.840 Meningitis due to *Klebsiella pneumoniae*
Friedländer bacillus

G00.848 Meningitis due to other *Klebsiella* species

G00.85 Meningitis due to *Nocardia* species

G00.86 Meningitis due to *Pasteurella multocida*

G00.87 Meningitis due to *Proteus* species

G00.88 Meningitis due to *Pseudomonas* species

G00.89 Meningitis due to *Serratia* species

G00.9 Bacterial meningitis, unspecified

Includes: meningitis:
- purulent NOS
- pyogenic NOS
- suppurative NOS

G00.90 Gram-negative meningitis NOS

G00.91 Gram-positive meningitis NOS

G01* Meningitis in bacterial diseases classified elsewhere

Meningitis (in):
- anthrax(A22.8†)
- gonococcal (A54.8†)
- leptospiral (A27.–†)
- listerial (A32.1†)
- Lyme disease (A69.2†)
- meningococcal (A39.0†)
- neurosyphilis (A52.1†)
- salmonella infection (A02.2†)

- syphilis:
  - congenital (A50.4†)
  - secondary (A51.4†)
- tuberculous (A17.0†)
- typhoid fever (A01.0†)

G02* Meningitis in other infectious and parasitic diseases classified elsewhere

G02.0* Meningitis in viral diseases classified elsewhere

Meningitis (due to):
- adenoviral (A87.1†)
- arenaviral haemorrhagic fever (A96.–†)
- cytomegaloviral disease (B25.–†)
- enteroviral (A87.0†)
- herpesviral [herpes simplex] (B00.3†)
- HIV disease resulting in infectious and parasitic diseases (B20.–†)
- infectious mononucleosis (B27.–†)
- Kyasanur Forest disease (A98.2†)
- lymphocytic choriomeningitis (A87.2†)
- measles (B05.1†)
- mumps (B26.1†)
- rubella (B06.0†)
- varicella [chickenpox] (B01.0†)
- zoster (B02.1†)

G02.1* Meningitis in mycoses classified elsewhere

Meningitis (in):
- candidal (B37.5†)
- coccidioidomycosis (B38.4†)
- cryptococcal (B45.1†)

G02.8* Meningitis in other specified infectious and parasitic diseases classified elsewhere

Meningitis due to:
- African trypanosomiasis (B56.–†)
- Chagas' disease (chronic) (B57.4†)

G03 Meningitis due to other and unspecified causes

Includes: arachnoiditis, leptomeningitis, meningitis, pachymeningitis } due to other and unspecified causes

Excludes: meningoencephalitis (G04.–)
meningomyelitis (G04.–)

G03.0 Nonpyogenic meningitis
Nonbacterial meningitis

G03.1 Chronic meningitis

G03.2 Benign recurrent meningitis [Mollaret]

G03.8 Meningitis due to other specified causes
Use additional code, if desired, to identify the associated condition or cause, e.g. Behçet's disease (M35.2); Harada's disease [Vogt–Koyanagi–Harada] (H30.8).

Excludes: carcinomatous meningitis (C79.362)
meningoencephalomyelitis in sarcoidosis (D86.83)

G03.9 Meningitis, unspecified
Arachnoiditis (spinal) NOS

G04 Encephalitis, myelitis and encephalomyelitis

Includes: acute ascending myelitis
meningoencephalitis
meningomyelitis

Excludes: benign myalgic encephalomyelitis (G93.3)
encephalopathy:
- NOS (G93.4)
- alcoholic (G31.21)
- toxic (G92.–)

multiple sclerosis (G35.–)
myelitis:
- acute transverse (G37.3)
- subacute necrotizing (G37.4)

G04.0 Acute disseminated encephalitis
Use additional external cause code (Chapter XX), if desired, to identify vaccine.

Excludes: acute disseminated demyelination (G36.–)

G04.00 Postimmunization encephalitis
G04.01 Postimmunization encephalomyelitis

G04.1 Tropical spastic paraplegia

G04.10 Associated with HTLV-1 infection [HTLV-1-associated myelopathy] [HAM]
G04.11 Associated with HTLV-2 infection
G04.12 Not associated with HTLV infection

G04.2 Bacterial meningoencephalitis and meningomyelitis, not elsewhere classified

G04.8 Other encephalitis, myelitis and encephalomyelitis
Use additional code, if desired, to identify the infectious agent.
Excludes: postimmunization:
- encephalitis (G04.00)
- encephalomyelitis (G04.01)

G04.80 Postinfectious encephalitis
G04.81 Postinfectious encephalomyelitis

G04.9 Encephalitis, myelitis and encephalomyelitis, unspecified
Ventriculitis (cerebral) NOS

G05* Encephalitis, myelitis and encephalomyelitis in diseases classified elsewhere

Includes: meningoencephalitis and meningomyelitis in diseases classified elsewhere

G05.0* Encephalitis, myelitis and encephalomyelitis in bacterial diseases classified elsewhere
Includes: encephalitis, myelitis or encephalomyelitis (in):
- listerial (A32.1†)
- meningococcal (A39.8†)
- syphilis:
  - congenital (A50.4†)
  - late (A52.1†)
- tuberculous (A17.8†)

late syphilitic general paresis (A52.1†)

G05.00* Encephalitis in bacterial diseases classified elsewhere
G05.01* Myelitis in bacterial diseases classified elsewhere
Tabes dorsalis
G05.02* Encephalomyelitis in bacterial diseases classified elsewhere

G05.1* **Encephalitis, myelitis and encephalomyelitis in viral diseases classified elsewhere**

Includes: encephalitis, myelitis or encephalomyelitis (in):
- adenoviral (A85.1†)
- cytomegaloviral (B25.8†)
- enteroviral (A85.0†)
- herpesviral [herpes simplex] (B00.4†)
- HIV (B23.8†)
- influenza (J10.8+, J11.8†)
- measles (B05.0†)
- mosquito-borne (A83.–†)
- mumps (B26.2†)
- postchickenpox (B01.1†)
- rubella (B06.0†)
- zoster (B02.0†)

G05.10* Encephalitis in viral diseases classified elsewhere
G05.11* Myelitis in viral diseases classified elsewhere
G05.12* Encephalomyelitis in viral diseases classified elsewhere

G05.2* **Encephalitis, myelitis and encephalomyelitis in other infectious and parasitic diseases classified elsewhere**

Includes: encephalitis, myelitis or encephalomyelitis (in):
- African trypanosomiasis (B56.–†)
- amoebic (B60.2†)
- Chagas' disease (chronic) (B57.4†)
- Lyme disease (A69.2†)
- naegleriasis (B60.2†)
- toxoplasmosis (B58.2†)

eosinophilic meningoencephalitis (B83.2†)

G05.20* Encephalitis in other infectious and parasitic diseases classified elsewhere
G05.21* Myelitis in other infectious and parasitic diseases classified elsewhere
G05.22* Encephalomyelitis in other infectious and parasitic diseases classified elsewhere

G05.8* **Encephalitis, myelitis and encephalomyelitis in other diseases classified elsewhere**

G05.80* Encephalitis in other diseases classified elsewhere
Encephalitis in systemic lupus erythematosus (M32.1†)
G05.81* Myelitis in other diseases classified elsewhere

G05.82* Encephalomyelitis in other diseases classified elsewhere

G06 Intracranial and intraspinal abscess and granuloma

Use additional code (B95–B97), if desired, to identify infectious agent.

Excludes: abscess of pituitary (E23.60)

G06.0 Intracranial abscess and granuloma

Use seventh character, if desired, to identify origin:

G06.0xx0 Embolic
G06.0xx1 Direct implantation
G06.0xx2 Spread from scalp
G06.0xx3 Spread from middle ear
G06.0xx4 Spread from paranasal air sinuses
G06.0xx8 Spread from other adjacent structure

G06.00 Cerebellar
G06.01 Cerebral hemisphere, cortical
G06.010 Frontal
G06.011 Parietal
G06.012 Temporal
G06.013 Occipital
G06.02 Cerebral hemisphere, deep
G06.020 Basal ganglia
G06.021 Thalamus
G06.022 Hypothalamus
G06.023 Centrum semiovale
G06.03 Corpus callosum
G06.04 Brainstem
G06.040 Midbrain
G06.041 Pons
G06.042 Medulla
G06.05 Intracranial epidural (extradural) abscess and granuloma
G06.06 Intracranial subdural abscess and granuloma
G06.07 Multiple or widespread intracranial abscess and granuloma

G06.1 Intraspinal abscess and granuloma

G06.10 Spinal cord
G06.11 Epidural (extradural)
Epiduritis
G06.12 Subdural

G06.2 Extradural and subdural abscess, unspecified

G07* Intracranial and intraspinal abscess and granuloma in diseases classified elsewhere

Abscess of brain:
- amoebic (A06.6†)
- cryptococcal (B45.1†)
- gonococcal (A54.8†)
- salmonella (A02.2†)
- tuberculous (A17.8†)

Cryptococcoma of brain (B45.1†)
Schistosomiasis granuloma of brain (B65.–†)
Tuberculoma of:
- brain (A17.8†)
- meninges (A17.1†)

G08 Intracranial and intraspinal phlebitis and thrombophlebitis

Includes: septic:
- embolism
- endophlebitis
- phlebitis
- thrombophlebitis
- thrombosis

} of intracranial or intraspinal venous sinuses and veins

Excludes: intracranial phlebitis and thrombophlebitis:
- complicating:
  - abortion or ectopic or molar pregnancy (O08.7)
  - pregnancy, childbirth and the puerperium (O22.5, O87.3)
- of nonpyogenic origin (I67.6)

nonpyogenic intraspinal phlebitis and thrombophlebitis (G95.1)

G08.–0 Sagittal sinus
G08.–1 Straight sinus
G08.–2 Sigmoid sinus
G08.–3 Cavernous sinus
G08.–4 Cortical vein
G08.–5 Great cerebral vein
G08.–6 Spinal veins
G08.–7 Multiple or diffuse

G09 Sequelae of inflammatory diseases of central nervous system

Note: This category is to be used to indicate conditions whose primary classification is to G00–G08 (i.e. excluding those marked with an asterisk (*)) as the cause of sequelae, themselves classifiable elsewhere. The "sequelae" include conditions specified as such or as late effects, or those present one year or more after onset of the causal condition. For use of this category reference should be made to the relevant coding rules and guidelines (see Section II, note 1.5, coding of late effects).

Systemic atrophies primarily affecting the central nervous system (G10–G13)

G10 Huntington's disease

Includes: Huntington's chorea

G10.–0 Huntington's disease, typical (age of onset between 20 and 50 years)
G10.–1 Juvenile onset (before age 20 years)
G10.–2 Late onset (after age 50 years)
G10.–3 Akinetic–rigid form with onset before age 20 years
G10.–4 Akinetic–rigid form with onset after age 20 years
G10.–5 Huntington's disease without dementia
G10.–6 Huntington's disease without chorea
G10.–8 Other specified types of Huntington's disease

G11 Hereditary ataxia

Excludes: hereditary and idiopathic neuropathy (G60.–)
infantile cerebral palsy (G80.–)
metabolic disorders (E70–E90)

Use additional sixth character, if desired, to indicate inheritance:

G11.*xx*0 Autosomal dominant
G11.*xx*1 Autosomal recessive
G11.*xx*2 X-linked recessive
G11.*xx*3 X-linked dominant
G11.*xx*4 Maternal inheritance
G11.*xx*5 Familial without clear inheritance pattern
G11.*xx*6 Non-inherited (sporadic)
G11.*xx*8 Other specified inheritance

G11.0 Congenital nonprogressive ataxia

G11.00 Cerebellar dysplasia and aplasia
G11.01 Congenital cerebellar ataxia
G11.02 Congenital ataxic diplegia
G11.03 Congenital cerebellar vermis agenesis [Joubert]
G11.04 Granular cell hypoplasia
G11.05 Congenital ataxia, mental retardation and partial aniridia [Gillespie]
G11.06 Congenital dysequilibrium syndrome
G11.08 Other specified congenital nonprogressive ataxias

G11.1 Early-onset cerebellar ataxia

Note: Onset usually before the age of 20 years.

G11.10 Early-onset cerebellar ataxia with retained tendon reflexes
G11.11 Ataxia with decreased tendon reflexes [Friedreich]
G11.12 Ataxia with hypogonadism [Holmes]
G11.13 Ataxia with myoclonus
Dyssynergia cerebellaris myoclonica [(Ramsay–)Hunt]
Excludes: baltic myoclonus [Unverricht–Lundborg] (G40.37)
G11.14 Ataxia with pigmentary retinopathy/optic atrophy
G11.15 Ataxia with cataracts [Marinesco–Sjögren]
G11.16 Ataxia with deafness and mental retardation
G11.17 Ataxia with extrapyramidal features/essential tremor
G11.18 Other specified early onset spinocerebellar degeneration

G11.2 Late-onset cerebellar ataxia

Note: Onset usually after the age of 20 years.

G11.20 Progressive cerebellar ataxia [olivopontocerebellar atrophy]
G11.21 Periodic ataxia
G11.22 Olivopontocerebellar atrophy with slow eye movement
Indian [Wadia]
Cuban [Orozco–Diaz]
G11.23 Olivopontocerebellar atrophy with blindness [Sanger–Brown ataxia]
G11.24 Imbalance with fasciculations and basal ganglia signs [(Machado–)Joseph]
G11.25 Progressive spinocerebellar ataxia with decreased tendon reflexes
G11.26 Progressive spinocerebellar ataxia with retained tendon reflexes

G11.27 Progressive cerebellar ataxia with palatal myoclonus
G11.28 Other specified late-onset cerebellar ataxia

G11.3 Cerebellar ataxia with defective DNA repair
Excludes: Cockayne's syndrome (Q87.11)
xeroderma pigmentosum (Q82.1)

G11.30 Ataxia–telangiectasia [Louis–Bar]

G11.4 Hereditary spastic paraplegia

G11.40 Without involvement of other parts of the nervous system
G11.41 With specified involvement of other parts of the nervous system

G11.8 Other hereditary ataxias

G11.9 Hereditary ataxia, unspecified
Hereditary cerebellar:
- ataxia NOS
- degeneration
- disease
- syndrome

G12 Spinal muscular atrophy and related syndromes

G12.0 Infantile spinal muscular atrophy, type I [Werdnig–Hoffmann]

G12.1 Other inherited spinal muscular atrophy

G12.10 Proximal and diffuse spinal muscular atrophy
G12.100 Late infantile spinal muscular atrophy
Childhood form, type II
G12.101 Juvenile form, type III [Kugelberg–Welander]
G12.102 Adult onset spinal muscular atrophy
G12.11 Focal and localized spinal muscular atrophy
G12.110 Progressive bulbar palsy of childhood [Fazio–Londe]
G12.111 Distal form of spinal muscular atrophy
G12.112 Scapuloperoneal form of spinal muscular atrophy
G12.113 Facioscapulohumeral form of spinal muscular atrophy
G12.114 Facioscapulohumeral form of spinal muscular atrophy with sensory loss [Davidenkow]
G12.115 Scapulohumeral form of spinal muscular atrophy
G12.116 Oculopharyngeal form of spinal muscular atrophy

G12.117 Ryukyu type of spinal muscular atrophy
G12.118 Bulbospinal muscular atrophy [Kennedy]

G12.2 Motor neuron disease

Excludes: paraneoplastic motor neuron disease (G13.12)
progressive post-polio muscular atrophy (B91.–0)

G12.20 Amyotrophic lateral sclerosis (ALS) [Charcot]
G12.21 Primary lateral sclerosis
G12.22 Progressive bulbar palsy
G12.23 Progressive pseudobulbar palsy
G12.24 Progressive muscular atrophy
G12.25 Pseudopolyneuritic form of ALS [Patrikios]
G12.26 Western Pacific type motor neuron disease

Excludes: parkinsonism–dementia–amyotrophic lateral sclerosis complex (G23.84)

G12.260 Guamanian type motor neuron disease
G12.261 Motor neuron disease of Kii Peninsula
G12.262 Motor neuron disease of West New Guinea

G12.27 Madras type motor neuron disease
G12.28 Benign monomelic amyotrophy
Segmental motor neuron disease
G12.29 Other motor neuron disease
Use additional code, if desired, to identify any associated condition, e.g. motor neuron disease (in) (with):

- autoimmune disease including increased anti-GM1 ganglioside antibody (R76.84)
- Creutzfeldt–Jakob disease (A81.0)
- dysproteinemia and gammopathy (D89.–)
- hereditary spastic paraplegia (G11.4)
- herpes zoster (B02.2)
- Huntington's disease (G10.–)
- hyperparathyroidism (E21.–)
- hyperthyroidism (E05.–)
- irradiation of the spinal cord (G95.82)
- lead intoxication (T56.0)
- (Machado–)Joseph disease (G11.24)
- multi-system atrophy [Shy–Drager] (G90.31)
- parkinsonism (G20.–, G21.–)

G12.8 Other spinal muscular atrophies and related syndromes

G12.9 Spinal muscular atrophy, unspecified

G13* Systemic atrophies primarily affecting central nervous system in diseases classified elsewhere

Note: In ICD-10 this category also includes disorders affecting the peripheral nervous system.

G13.0* Paraneoplastic neuromyopathy and neuropathy [C00–D48†]
Includes: carcinomatous neuromyopathy (C00–C97†)

G13.00* Paraneoplastic sensory-motor neuropathy
G13.01* Paraneoplastic sensory neuropathy [Denny-Brown]
Sensorial paraneoplastic neuropathy
G13.08* Other paraneoplastic neuromyopathy and neuropathy

G13.1* Other systemic atrophy primarily affecting central nervous system in neoplastic disease (C00–D48†)

G13.10* Paraneoplastic limbic encephalopathy
G13.11* Paraneoplastic cerebellar degeneration
G13.12* Paraneoplastic motor neuron disease

G13.2* Systemic atrophy primarily affecting central nervous system in myxoedema (E00.1†, E03.–†)

G13.20* Cerebellar degeneration in hypothyroidism (E00.1†, E03.–†)

G13.8* Systemic atrophy primarily affecting central nervous system in other diseases classified elsewhere

Extrapyramidal and movement disorders (G20–G26)

G20 Parkinson's disease

Includes: idiopathic parkinsonism
paralysis agitans
Excludes: Guamanian-type parkinsonism–dementia complex (G23.84)
diffuse Lewy body disease (dementia) (G31.85)

G20.–0 Classical type
G20.–1 Akinetic type
G20.–2 Tremor type
G20.–3 Postural instability–gait difficulty (PIGD) type
G20.–4 Hemiparkinsonism

Use additional sixth character, if desired, to indicate:

G20.–*x*0 Sporadic
G20.–*x*1 Familial

G21 Secondary parkinsonism

Excludes: parkinsonism in diseases classified elsewhere (G22.–)

G21.0 Malignant neuroleptic syndrome

Use additional external cause code (Chapter XX), if desired, to identify drug.

G21.1 Other drug-induced secondary parkinsonism

Includes: drug-induced akathisia

Use additional external cause code (Chapter XX), if desired, to identify drug, e.g. dopamine receptor-blockers (neuroleptics (Y49.3–Y49.5), antiemetic drugs (Y43.0)), dopamine depleters (reserpine tetrabenazine (T46.5)), lithium (T43.5), flunarizine (T46.7), cinnarizine (T45.0), diltiazem (T46.1).

Excludes: akathisia, not related to drugs (G25.88)

G21.10 Acute drug reaction
G21.11 Tardive drug reaction

G21.2 Secondary parkinsonism due to other external agents

Use additional external cause code (Chapter XX), if desired, to identify external agent, e.g. manganese (T57.2), carbon monoxide (T58), cyanide (T57.3), methanol (T51.1), carbon disulfide (T65.4), 1-methyl-4-phenyl-1,2,3,6-tetrahydropyridine [MPTP] (T40.94).

G21.3 Postencephalitic parkinsonism

G21.30 Parkinsonism associated with encephalitis lethargica
G21.38 Other postinfectious parkinsonism
Excludes: slow virus or prion infection of central nervous system (A81.–)

G21.8 Other secondary parkinsonism

Use additional code, if desired, to identify cause, e.g. head injury (S06.–), sequelae of intracranial injury (T90.5).

Excludes: psychogenic parkinsonism (F44.4)

G21.9 Secondary parkinsonism, unspecified

G22* Parkinsonism in diseases classified elsewhere

G22.–0* Parkinsonism in sporadic degenerative diseases classified elsewhere

Parkinsonism in:
- Alzheimer's disease (G30.–†)
- corticobasal ganglionic degeneration (G23.81†)
- dentato-rubral-pallido-luysian atrophy [DRPLA] (G23.83†)
- diffuse Lewy body disease (dementia) (G31.85†)
- Guamanian-type parkinsonism–dementia complex (G23.84†)
- Hallervorden–Spatz disease (G23.0†)
- multi-system degeneration with dysautonomia [multiple system atrophy] [MSA] (G90.3†)
- olivopontocerebellar degeneration (G11.22–G11.23†)
- pallidopyramidal dentatoluysian degeneration (G23.82†)
- progressive supranuclear ophthalmoplegia (idiopathic) [Steele–Richardson–Olszewski] (G23.10†)
- Shy–Drager syndrome (G90.31†)
- striatonigral degeneration (G23.2†)

Excludes: parkinsonism associated with calcification of the basal ganglia (G23.85)

G22.–1* Parkinsonism in familial degenerative and metabolic disorders classified elsewhere

Parkinsonism in:
- dopa-responsive dystonia (G24.13†)
- Huntington's disease (G10.–†)
- subacute necrotizing encephalopathy [Leigh] (G31.81†)
- Wilson's disease [hepatolenticular degeneration] (E83.01†)

Excludes: hereditary juvenile parkinsonism–dystonia complex (G24.17)

G22.–2* Parkinsonism in infectious diseases classified elsewhere

Parkinsonism in:
- acquired immunodeficiency syndrome [AIDS] (B24†)
- Creutzfeldt–Jakob disease (A81.0†)
- Gerstmann–Straüssler–Scheinker disease or syndrome (A81.81†)

- subacute sclerosing panencephalitis (A81.1†)
- syphilis (A52.1†)

G22.–3* Parkinsonism in other diseases classified elsewhere

Parkinsonism (in):

- brain tumour (C71.–†, C79.3†, D33.–†)
- cerebrovascular disease (I60.–†, I67.–†)
- non-communicating (obstructive) hydrocephalus (G91.1†)
- normal pressure hydrocephalus (G91.2†)
- paraneoplastic (C00–D48†)
- psychogenic (F44.4†)
- syringomesencephalia (G95.0*x*3†)

G23 Other degenerative diseases of basal ganglia

G23.0 Hallervorden–Spatz disease

G23.00 Pigmentary pallidal degeneration
G23.08 Other specified pallidal degeneration
G23.09 Pallidal degeneration, unspecified

G23.1 Progressive supranuclear ophthalmoplegia

Includes: progressive supranuclear ophthalmoparesis
progressive supranuclear palsy [PSNP]

G23.10 Idiopathic [Steele–Richardson–Olszewski]
G23.11 Vascular [multi-infarct]

G23.2 Striatonigral degeneration

G23.8 Other specified degenerative diseases of basal ganglia

Excludes: multi-system degeneration with dysautonomia [Shy–Drager] (G90.31)
olivopontocerebellar degeneration (G11.22–G11.23)
Wilson's disease [hepatolenticular degeneration] (E83.01)

G23.80 Hemiparkinson–hemiatrophy syndrome
G23.81 Corticobasal ganglionic degeneration
Corticodentatonigral degeneration with neuronal achromasia
G23.82 Pallidopyramidal dentatoluysian atrophy
G23.83 Dentatorubral pallidoluysian atrophy [DRPLA]
G23.84 Guamanian-type parkinsonism–dementia complex
Parkinsonism–dementia–amyotrophic lateral sclerosis complex of Guam

Excludes: Western Pacific type motor neuron disease (G12.26)
Guamanian-type Alzheimer's disease (G30.80)

G23.85 Parkinsonism associated with calcification of the basal ganglia

G23.850 Idiopathic sporadic [Fahr]
G23.851 With hypoparathyroidism
G23.852 With pseudohypoparathyroidism
G23.853 Familial basal ganglia calcification

G23.9 Degenerative disease of basal ganglia, unspecified

G24 Dystonia

Includes: dyskinesia
Excludes: athetoid cerebral palsy (G80.3)

G24.0 Drug-induced dystonia

Use additional external cause code (Chapter XX), if desired, to identify the drug or toxic agent, e.g. manganese (T57.2), carbon dioxide (T59.7), carbon disulfide (T65.4), cyanide (T57.3).

G24.00 Acute drug-induced dystonia
G24.01 Acute drug-induced dyskinesia
G24.02 Tardive dystonia
G24.03 Tardive dyskinesia
G24.04 Other specified drug-induced dystonia
Drug-induced oculogyric crises

G24.1 Idiopathic familial dystonia

G24.10 Classic autosomal dominant dystonia (with DYT1 gene on 9q34)
G24.11 Non-classic dystonia
G24.12 Atypical dystonia
G24.13 Dopa-responsive dystonia [DRD]
Idiopathic diurnal dystonia or Segawa variant
G24.14 Myoclonic dystonia
G24.15 Rapid-onset dystonia
G24.16 X-linked recessive dystonia–parkinsonism complex [Lubag]
G24.17 Hereditary juvenile dystonia–parkinsonism complex
G24.18 Familial dystonia with other specified inheritance

Use additional sixth (and seventh) character, if desired, to indicate the localization of the dystonia:

G24.1*x*0 Generalized dystonia, familial
G24.1*x*1 Hemidystonia, familial
G24.1*x*2 Axial dystonia, familial
G24.1*x*3 Cranial dystonia, familial
G24.1x30 Ocular dystonia, familial
G24.1x31 Orofacial dystonia, familial
G24.1*x*4 Laryngeal dystonia, familial
G24.1*x*5 Cervical dystonia, familial
G24.1*x*6 Limb dystonia, familial
G24.1x60 Arm/hand dystonia, familial
G24.1x61 Leg/foot dystonia, familial
G24.1*x*7 Multiple or combined types of idiopathic familial dystonia
G24.1*x*8 Other types of idiopathic familial dystonia

G24.2 Idiopathic nonfamilial dystonia
Excludes: idiopathic cervical dystonia (G24.3)

G24.20 Generalized dystonia, nonfamilial
G24.21 Hemidystonia, nonfamilial
G24.22 Axial dystonia, nonfamilial
G24.23 Other cranial dystonia, nonfamilial
Excludes: blepharospasm (G24.5)
idiopathic orofacial dystonia (G24.4)
G24.230 Ocular dystonia, nonfamilial
Idiopathic oculogyric crisis
Excludes: drug-induced (G24.04)
G24.24 Laryngeal dystonia, nonfamilial
Isolated spasmodic dysphonia
G24.25 Limb dystonia, nonfamilial
G24.250 Arm/hand dystonia, nonfamilial
Writer's/musician's/other occupational cramps or palsies
Excludes: writer's and occupational cramps of psychogenic origin (F44.4)
G24.251 Leg/foot dystonia, nonfamilial
G24.27 Multiple or combined types of idiopathic nonfamilial dystonia
G24.28 Other types of idiopathic nonfamilial dystonia

G24.3 Spasmodic torticollis
Includes: idiopathic cervical dystonia

Excludes: familial cervical dystonia (G24.1*x*5)
torticollis NOS (M43.6)

G24.30 Spasmodic torticollis
G24.31 Spasmodic retrocollis
G24.32 Spasmodic anterocollis
G24.33 Spasmodic laterocollis
G24.38 Other specified cervical dystonia

G24.4 Idiopathic orofacial dystonia
Excludes: familial orofacial dystonia (G24.1*x*31)

G24.40 Orofacial dyskinesia
G24.41 Edentulous orofacial dyskinesia
G24.42 Isolated oromandibular dystonia

G24.5 Blepharospasm
Idiopathic cranial dystonia
Meige's blepharospasm

G24.8 Other dystonia
Excludes: atlantoaxial subluxation (M43.3–M43.4)
congenital muscular contractions (Q79.8)
seizure-induced twisting postures (G40.–)

G24.80 Paroxysmal dystonias
G24.800 Sporadic kinesigenic dystonia
G24.801 Familial kinesigenic dystonia
G24.802 Sporadic non-kinesigenic dystonia
G24.803 Familial non-kinesigenic dystonia
G24.804 Tonic spasms of multiple sclerosis
G24.805 Paroxysmal nocturnal dystonia
G24.81 Sandifer's syndrome
Anteroflexion associated with gastroesophageal reflux in young children.
G24.82 Secondary dystonia, unspecified
G24.83 Pseudodystonia, unspecified

G24.9 Dystonia, unspecified
Dyskinesia NOS

G25 Other extrapyramidal and movement disorders

G25.0 Essential tremor
Excludes: isolated rest tremor (G25.26)
tremor NOS (R25.1)

G25.00 Isolated head tremor
G25.01 Isolated facial tremor
G25.02 Isolated vocal tremor
G25.03 Isolated hand tremor
G25.04 Shuddering attacks of childhood
G25.07 Multiple site tremor

Use additional sixth character, if desired, to indicate:

G25.0*x*0 Sporadic
G25.0*x*1 Familial

G25.1 Drug-induced tremor

Use additional external cause code (Chapter XX), if desired, to identify drug.

G25.2 Other specified forms of tremor

G25.20 Kinetic [intention] tremor
G25.21 Physiological tremor
G25.22 Dystonic tremor
G25.23 Orthostatic tremor
G25.24 Task-specific (e.g. handwriting) tremor
G25.25 Midbrain-type tremor
G25.26 Isolated rest tremor

G25.3 Myoclonus

Use additional external cause code (Chapter XX), if desired, to identify drug, if drug-induced.

Excludes: ataxia with myoclonus (G11.13)
epilepsia partialis continua [Kozhevnikof] (G40.50)
facial myokymia (G51.4)
hemifacial spasm (G51.3)
myoclonic epilepsy (G40.–)

G25.30 Cortical type diffuse myoclonus
G25.31 Focal or multifocal cortical type myoclonus
G25.32 Essential myoclonus [Friedreich's paramyoclonus multiplex]
G25.33 Oculopalatal myoclonus
G25.34 Segmental spinal myoclonus
G25.35 Propriospinal myoclonus
G25.36 Peripheral myoclonus
G25.37 Sleep (hypnic) myoclonus

G25.38 Post-anoxic action myoclonus [Lance–Adams]
G25.39 Other specified myoclonic disorders

G25.4 Drug-induced chorea

Use additional external cause code (Chapter XX), if desired, to identify drug, e.g. dopamine receptor-blockers (neuroleptics (Y49.3–Y49.5)), antiemetic drugs (Y43.0), dopaminergic (antiparkinsonism and antiepileptic) drugs (Y46.–), psychostimulants (Y49.7), toxins (T51–T65).

G25.5 Other chorea

Includes: chorea NOS
Excludes: chorea NOS with heart involvement (I02.0)
Huntington's chorea (G10)
rheumatic chorea (I02.–)
Sydenham's chorea (I02.–)

G25.50 Chorea gravidarum
G25.51 Chorea associated with hormone therapy
G25.52 Hemichorea
G25.53 Neuroacanthocytosis [choreoacanthocytosis]
G25.54 Benign hereditary chorea
G25.55 Senile chorea
G25.56 Kinesigenic choreathetosis

G25.6 Drug-induced tics and other tics of organic origin

Excludes: de la Tourette's syndrome (F95.2)
tics NOS (F95.9)

G25.60 Drug-induced tics
Use additional external cause code (Chapter XX), if desired, to identify drug.
G25.61 Tics of organic origin not related to drugs
Secondary tic NOS

G25.8 Other specified extrapyramidal and movement disorders

G25.80 Paroxysmal nocturnal limb movement disorder
G25.81 Painful legs (or arms), moving toes (or fingers) syndrome
G25.82 Sporadic restless legs syndrome [Ekbom]
G25.83 Familial restless legs syndrome with or without periodic movements
G25.84 Stiff-person syndrome
Stiff-man syndrome

G25.85 Ballism/hemiballism
Use additional code (I63.–), if desired, when of vascular origin.

G25.86 Opsoclonus–myoclonus syndrome
Dancing eyes, dancing feet syndrome

G25.87 Stereotypies
Excludes: de la Tourette syndrome (F95.2)
edentulous orofacial dyskinesia (G24.41)
epileptic automatisms (G40.–)
orofacial dyskinesia (G24.40)
psychogenic stereotypies (F98.4)
restless legs syndrome (G25.82)
stereotyped movement disorder (F98.4)
tardive dyskinesia (G24.03)

G25.88 Akathisia, not related to drugs
Excludes: akathisia, drug-induced (G21.1)

G25.9 Extrapyramidal and movement disorder, unspecified

G26* Extrapyramidal and movement disorders in diseases classified elsewhere

G26.–0* Dystonia in diseases classified elsewhere
Dyskinesia in diseases classified elsewhere
Dystonia in:
- ataxia–telangectasia [Louis–Bar] (G11.30†)
- corticobasal ganglionic degeneration (G23.81†)
- Hallervorden–Spatz disease (G23.0†)
- hereditary spastic paraplegia (G11.4†)
- Huntington's disease (G10†)
- Joseph's disease (G11.24†)
- juvenile neuronal ceroid lipofuscinosis (E75.42†)
- Lesch–Nyhan syndrome (E79.1†)
- multiple sclerosis (G35†)
- multi-system degeneration with dysautonomia (G90.31†)
- neuroacanthocytosis (G25.53†)
- Niemann–Pick disease, type C (E75.262†)
- pallidal degeneration (G23.82–G23.83†)
- Parkinson's disease (G20†)
- progressive supranuclear ophthalmoparesis [Steele–Richardson–Olszewski] (G23.10†)

- reflex sympathetic dystrophy (G90.83†)
- Rett's syndrome (F84.2†)
- Shy–Drager syndrome (G90.31†)
- subacute necrotizing encephalopathy [Leigh] (G31.81†)
- Wilson's disease [hepatolenticular degeneration] (E83.01†)

Hemidystonia in diseases classified elsewhere

G26.–1* Chorea in diseases classified elsewhere

Chorea in:
- hyperthyroidism (E05.–†)
- neuroacanthocytosis (G25.53†)
- systemic lupus erythematosus (M32.–†)

Hemichorea in diseases classified elsewhere

Excludes: chorea NOS with heart involvement (I02.0)
chorea gravidarum (G25.50)
Huntington's chorea (G10)
rheumatic chorea (I02.–)
Sydenham's chorea (I02.–)

G26.–2* Tremor in diseases classified elsewhere

Tremor in:
- brain tumour (C71.–†, C79.3†, D33.–†)
- cerebrovascular disease (I60–I67†)
- head injury (S06.–†)

G26.–3* Myoclonus in diseases classified elsewhere

Myoclonus in:
- Alzheimer's disease (G30.–†)
- brain tumour (C71.–†, C79.3†, D33.–†)
- Creutzfeldt–Jakob disease (A81.0†)
- cerebrovascular disease (I60–I67†)
- dyssynergia cerebellaris myoclonica [(Ramsay–)Hunt] (G11.13†)
- head injury (S06.–†)
- metabolic encephalopathy (E00–E90†)
- olivopontocerebellar atrophy (G11.22–G11.23†)
- toxic encephalopathy (G92.–†)

G26.–4* Tics in diseases classified elsewhere

G26.–5* Stereotypies in diseases classified elsewhere

Stereotypies in:
- autism (F84.0–F84.1†)
- mental retardation (F70–F79†)
- Rett's syndrome (F84.2†)

Other degenerative diseases of the nervous system (G30–G32)

G30 Alzheimer's disease

Includes: senile and presenile forms
Excludes: senile:
- degeneration of brain NEC (G31.1)
- dementia NOS (F03)

senility NOS (R54)

G30.0 Alzheimer's disease with early onset
Note: Onset usually before the age of 65 years.

G30.00 Alzheimer's disease with early onset, familial
G30.01 Alzheimer's disease with early onset, sporadic

G30.1 Alzheimer's disease with late onset
Note: Onset usually after the age of 65 years.

G30.10 Alzheimer's disease with late onset, familial
G30.11 Alzheimer's disease with late onset, sporadic

G30.8 Other Alzheimer's disease

G30.80 Guamanian-type Alzheimer's disease
Excludes: Guamanian-type parkinsonism–dementia complex (G23.84)

G30.9 Alzheimer's disease, unspecified

G31 Other degenerative diseases of nervous system, not elsewhere classified

Excludes: Reye's syndrome (G93.7)

G31.0 Circumscribed brain atrophy

G31.00 Pick's disease
G31.01 Progressive isolated aphasia [Mesulam]
G31.02 Frontal lobe dementia

G31.1 Senile degeneration of brain, not elsewhere classified
Excludes: Alzheimer's disease (G30.–)
senility NOS (R54)

G31.2 Degeneration of the nervous system due to alcohol

G31.20 Alcoholic cerebellar degeneration
Alcoholic cerebellar ataxia

G31.21 Alcoholic cerebral degeneration
Alcoholic encephalopathy
Excludes: central pontine myelinolysis (G37.2)
Korsakov's alcoholic amnestic syndrome (F10.6)
Wernicke's superior haemorrhagic polioencephalitis syndrome (E51.2)

G31.22 Alcoholic spinal cord degeneration

G31.23 Dysfunction of autonomic nervous system due to alcohol

G31.24 Morel's laminar sclerosis

G31.28 Other specified degeneration of nervous system due to alcohol

G31.8 Other specified degenerative diseases of nervous system

G31.80 Grey-matter degeneration [Alpers]

G31.81 Subacute necrotizing encephalopathy [Leigh]

G31.82 Neuroaxonal dystrophy [Seitelberger]

G31.83 Progressive subcortical gliosis

G31.84 Spongy degeneration of white matter in infancy [Canavan–van Bogaert–Bertrand]

G31.85 Diffuse Lewy body disease (dementia)

G31.9 Degenerative disease of the nervous system, unspecified

G32* Other degenerative disorders of the nervous system in diseases classified elsewhere

G32.0* Subacute combined degeneration of the spinal cord in diseases classified elsewhere

Subacute combined degeneration of the spinal cord in:
- thiamin deficiency (E51.–†)
- vitamin B_{12} deficiency (E53.80†)

G32.8* Other specified degenerative disorders of the nervous system in diseases classified elsewhere

Demyelinating diseases of the central nervous system (G35–G37)

G35 Multiple sclerosis

Includes: multiple sclerosis (of):
- NOS
- brain stem
- cord
- disseminated
- generalized

Excludes: concentric sclerosis [Baló] (G37.5)
neuromyelitis optica [Devic] (G36.0)

Note: These conditions are classified to other ICD-10 categories even if they are often considered as variants of multiple sclerosis.

G35.–0 Relapsing/remitting multiple sclerosis

G35.–1 Primary progressive multiple sclerosis
Chronic progressive multiple sclerosis, progressive from onset

G35.–2 Secondary progressive multiple sclerosis
Chronic progressive multiple sclerosis, after an initially relapsing/remitting course (includes remittent progressive)

G35.–8 Other symptomatic forms of multiple sclerosis

G36 Other acute disseminated demyelination

Excludes: postinfectious encephalitis and encephalomyelitis NOS (G04.8)

G36.0 Neuromyelitis optica [Devic]
Spinal cord demyelination in optic neuritis
Excludes: optic neuritis NOS (H46)

G36.1 Acute and subacute haemorrhagic leukoencephalitis [Hurst]

G36.8 Other specified acute disseminated demyelination

G36.9 Acute disseminated demyelination, unspecified

G37 Other demyelinating diseases of central nervous system

G37.0 Diffuse sclerosis
Periaxial encephalitis
Schilder's disease
Excludes: adrenoleukodystrophy [Addison–Schilder] (E71.330)

G37.1 Central demyelination of corpus callosum
Marchiafava–Bignami syndrome

Use additional code, if desired, to identify associated conditions(s) or cause.

G37.2 Central pontine myelinolysis
Use additional code, if desired, to identify associated conditions(s) or cause.

G37.3 Acute transverse myelitis in demyelinating disease of central nervous system
Acute transverse myelitis NOS

Use additional code, if desired, to identify associated condition(s) or cause.

Excludes: multiple sclerosis (G35.–)
neuromyelitis optica [Devic] (G36.0)

G37.4 Subacute necrotizing myelitis

G37.5 Concentric sclerosis [Baló]

G37.8 Other specified demyelinating diseases of the central nervous system
Use additional code, if desired, to identify associated condition(s) or cause.

G37.9 Demyelinating disease of the central nervous system, unspecified

Episodic and paroxysmal disorders (G40–G47)

G40 Epilepsy

Use additional code, if desired, to identify associated condition(s) or cause.

Excludes: convulsions of newborn (P90.–)
epileptic psychosis (F06.8)
febrile convulsions (R56.0)
isolated (first) seizure (R56.8)

Landau–Kleffner syndrome (F80.3)
seizure (convulsive) NOS (R56.8)
status epilepticus (G41.–)
Todd's paralysis (postepileptic) (G83.80)

G40.0 Localization-related (focal)(partial) idiopathic epilepsy and epileptic syndromes with seizures of localized onset

G40.00 Benign childhood epilepsy with centrotemporal EEG spikes
G40.01 Childhood epilepsy with occipital EEG paroxysms

G40.1 Localization-related (focal)(partial) symptomatic epilepsy and epileptic syndromes with simple partial seizures

G40.10 Simple partial seizures
Attacks without alteration of consciousness
G40.11 Simple partial seizures developing into complex partial seizures
G40.12 Simple partial seizures developing into secondarily generalized seizures

G40.2 Localization-related (focal)(partial) symptomatic epilepsy and epileptic syndromes with complex partial seizures
Includes: attacks with alteration of consciousness

G40.20 Complex partial seizures with only alteration of consciousness
G40.21 Complex partial seizures with alteration of consciousness and automatisms
G40.22 Complex partial seizures developing into secondarily generalized seizures

G40.3 Generalized idiopathic epilepsy and epileptic syndromes

G40.30 Benign myoclonic epilepsy in infancy
G40.31 Familial benign neonatal seizures
G40.32 Non-familial benign neonatal seizures
G40.33 Childhood absence epilepsy [pyknolepsy]
G40.34 Epilepsy with generalized tonic–clonic seizures on awakening
G40.35 Juvenile absence epilepsy
G40.36 Juvenile myoclonic epilepsy [impulsive petit mal]
G40.37 Baltic myoclonus [Unverricht–Lundborg]
G40.39 Unspecified generalized epileptic syndromes with atonic, clonic, myoclonic, tonic or tonic–clonic seizures

G40.4 Other generalized epilepsy and epileptic syndromes

G40.40 Infantile spasms [West]
Salaam attacks

G40.41 Early infantile epileptic encephalopathy with suppression burst EEG

G40.42 Epilepsy with myoclonic absences

G40.43 Epilepsy with myoclonic–astatic seizures

G40.44 Lennox–Gastaut syndrome

G40.45 Symptomatic early myoclonic encephalopathy

G40.46 Myoclonic epilepsy with ragged red fibres (MERRF)

G40.5 Special epileptic syndromes

G40.50 Epilepsia partialis continua [Kozhevnikof]

G40.51 Chronic progressive epilepsia partialis continua [Rasmussen]

G40.52 Epileptic seizures related to alcohol

G40.53 Epileptic seizures related to drugs
Use additional external cause code (Chapter XX), if desired, to identify drug.
Excludes: epileptic seizures related to psychoactive substance withdrawal (F1*x*.3 and F1*x*.4)

G40.54 Epileptic seizures related to hormonal changes
Use additional code, if desired, to identify cause.

G40.55 Epileptic seizures related to sleep deprivation

G40.56 Epileptic seizures related to stress

G40.57 Epilepsy with special mode of precipitation [reflex epilepsy]
Musicogenic epilepsy
Photosensitive epilepsy
Reading epilepsy

G40.58 Other situation-related epileptic seizures

G40.6 Grand mal seizures, unspecified (with or without petit mal)

Generalized tonic–clonic epileptic seizures (with or without seizures)

Note: This category should be used only for those conditions in which there is no additional information available that would allow appropriate classification in one of the categories G40.0–G40.5.

G40.7 Petit mal, unspecified, without grand mal seizures

Absence seizures

Note: Category G40.7 should be used only when there is insufficient information to allow the condition to be classified in G40.33 or G40.35.

G40.8 Other epilepsy

Excludes: acquired aphasia with epilepsy [Landau–Kleffner] (F80.3)
pseudoseizures (F44.5)

G40.80 Epilepsy with continuous EEG spike-waves during slow wave sleep
Electrical status epilepticus during sleep

G40.89 Epilepsies and epileptic syndromes, undetermined as to whether they are focal or generalized

G40.890 Severe myoclonic epilepsy in infancy

G40.9 Epilepsy, unspecified

Epileptic:
- convulsions NOS
- fits NOS
- seizures NOS

Postictal amnesia

G41 Status epilepticus

G41.0 Grand mal status epilepticus

Tonic–clonic status epilepticus
Excludes: epilepsia partialis continua [Kozhevnikof] (G40.50)

G41.1 Petit mal status epilepticus

Epileptic absence status
Nonconvulsive generalized status epilepticus

G41.2 Complex partial status epilepticus

G41.8 Other status epilepticus

G41.9 Status epilepticus, unspecified

G43 Migraine

Use additional external cause code (Chapter XX), if desired, to identify drug, if drug-induced.

Excludes: atypical facial pain (G50.1)
headache NOS (R51)

G43.0 Migraine without aura [common migraine]

G43.1 Migraine with aura [classical migraine]

G43.10 With typical aura
G43.11 With prolonged aura
G43.12 With acute onset aura

Use sixth character, if desired, to identify neurological symptoms:

G43.1*x*0 Hemianopic and other visual migraine
G43.1*x*1 Hemisensory migraine
G43.1*x*2 Migraine with aphasia
G43.1*x*3 Basilar migraine
G43.1*x*4 Migraine aura (all types) without headache
G43.1*x*5 Familial hemiplegic migraine
G43.1*x*7 Multiple types of aura
G43.1*x*8 Other specified migraine with aura

G43.2 Status migrainosus

G43.3 Complicated migraine

Migrainous cerebral infarction

G43.8 Other migraine

G43.80 Ophthalmoplegic migraine
G43.81 Retinal (monocular) migraine
G43.82 Childhood periodic migraine syndromes
G43.820 Abdominal migraine
G43.821 Benign paroxysmal vertigo of childhood
G43.822 Alternating hemiplegia of childhood
G43.83 Atypical migraine

G43.9 Migraine, unspecified

G44 Other headache syndromes

Excludes: atypical facial pain (G50.1)
glossopharyngeal neuralgia (G52.1)
headache NOS (R51)
other cranial neuralgia (G52.8)
post-lumbar-puncture headache (G97.1)
trigeminal neuralgia (G50.0)

G44.0 Cluster headache syndrome

G44.00 Cluster headache with periodicity undetermined
G44.01 Episodic cluster headache
G44.02 Chronic cluster headache
G44.03 Chronic paroxysmal hemicrania
G44.08 Other and atypical cluster headache

G44.1 Vascular headache, not elsewhere classified

G44.2 Tension-type headache

G44.20 Episodic tension-type headache associated with disorder of pericranial muscles

G44.21 Episodic tension-type headache without disorder of pericranial muscles

G44.22 Chronic tension-type headache with disorder of pericranial muscles

G44.23 Chronic tension-type headache without disorder of pericranial muscles

G44.28 Other tension-type headache
Atypical tension-type headache

G44.3 Chronic post-traumatic headache

G44.4 Drug-induced headache, not elsewhere classified
Use additional external cause code (Chapter XX), if desired, to identify drug.

Excludes: headache associated with psychoactive substance use (G44.83)

G44.8 Other specified headache syndromes

G44.80 Other headaches not associated with a structural lesion

G44.800 Idiopathic stabbing headache
Cephalgia fugax
Icepick headache

G44.801 External compression headache

G44.802 Cold stimulus headache

G44.803 Benign cough headache

G44.804 Benign exertional headache

G44.805 Headache associated with sexual activity
Coital (orgasmic) cephalalgia

G44.806 Idiopathic carotidynia

G44.81 Headaches associated with other vascular disorders
Use additional code (Chapter IX), if desired, to identify the vascular disorder.
Excludes: vascular headache NEC (G44.1)

G44.82 Headache associated with other intracranial disorders
Use additional code, if desired, to identify associated condition.

G44.83 Headache associated with psychoactive substance use
Use additional code, if desired, to identify substance (F10–F19) and associated condition (F1*x*.0–F1*x*.9), e.g.

harmful use (F1*x*.1), dependence (F1*x*.2), withdrawal (F1*x*.3 or F1*x*.4).

G44.84 Headache or facial pain associated with disorders of cranium, cranial and facial structures, cranial nerves, neck and spine
Use additional code, if desired, to identify associated condition(s) or cause.

G44.85 Other specified syndromes of facial and ocular pain
Excludes: atypical facial pain (G50.1)
ocular pain NOS (H57.1)

G44.850 Tolosa–Hunt syndrome

G44.851 Neck–tongue syndrome

G44.88 Headache associated with other specified disorders
Use additional code, if desired, to indicate associated condition.
Excludes: post-lumbar-puncture headache (G97.0)

G45 Transient cerebral ischaemic attacks and related syndromes

Excludes: neonatal cerebral ischaemia (P91.0)

Use additional fifth character, if desired, to indicate side of ischaemia:

G45.*x*0 Left
G45.*x*1 Right
G45.*x*2 Left and right (symmetrical)

G45.0 Vertebro-basilar artery syndrome
Subclavian steal syndrome

G45.1 Carotid artery syndrome (hemispheric)
Excludes: amaurosis fugax (G45.3)

G45.2 Multiple and bilateral precerebral artery syndromes
Bilateral episodes in non-symmetrical territories
Unilateral episodes in different territories (vertebro-basilar and carotid)
Excludes: symmetrical (G45.*x*2)

G45.3 Amaurosis fugax

G45.4 Transient global amnesia
Excludes: amnesia NOS (R41.3)

G45.8 Other transient cerebral ischaemic attacks and related syndromes

G45.9 Transient cerebral ischaemic attack, unspecified
Spasm of cerebral artery
Transient cerebral ischaemia NOS

G46* Vascular syndromes of brain in cerebrovascular diseases (I60–I67†)

Excludes: clinically silent cerebral infarction (R90.83)

Use additional sixth character, if desired, to indicate side of lesion:

G46.*xx*0 Left
G46.*xx*1 Right
G46.*xx*2 Left and right (symmetrical)

For multiple specified vascular syndromes of the brain, code each one separately.

G46.0* Middle cerebral artery syndrome (I66.0†)

G46.00* Superficial middle cerebral artery syndrome (cortical)
G46.01* Deep middle cerebral artery syndrome (lenticulostriate)
G46.02* Combined deep and superficial middle cerebral artery syndrome (total)

G46.1* Anterior cerebral artery syndrome (I66.1†)

G46.10* Superficial anterior cerebral artery syndrome (cortical)
G46.11* Deep anterior cerebral artery syndrome [Heubner]
G46.12* Combined deep and superficial anterior cerebral artery syndrome (total)

G46.2* Posterior cerebral artery syndrome (I66.2†)

G46.20* Superficial posterior cerebral artery syndrome (occipital syndrome)
G46.21* Deep posterior cerebral artery syndrome (thalamic syndrome)
G46.22* Combined deep and superficial posterior cerebral artery syndrome (total)

G46.3* Brain stem stroke syndrome (I60–I67†)

G46.30* Peduncular syndrome [Benedikt] [Claude] [peduncular-Foville] [Weber]
G46.31* Pontine syndrome [pontine-Foville] [Millard–Gubler]
G46.32* Medullary syndrome [Wallenberg]
G46.37* Multiple, overlapping or bilateral brain stem stroke syndrome
G46.38* Other specified brain stem stroke syndromes

G46.4* **Cerebellar stroke syndrome (I60–I67†)**

G46.40* Superior cerebellar artery syndrome
G46.41* Anterior–inferior cerebellar artery syndrome
G46.42* Posterior–inferior cerebellar artery syndrome
G46.43* Pseudo-tumoral cerebellar infarction syndrome
G46.47* Multiple, overlapping or bilateral cerebellar infarction syndrome

G46.5* **Pure motor lacunar syndrome (I60–I67†)**

G46.50* Proportional pure motor lacunar syndrome
G46.51* Partial pure motor lacunar syndrome
G46.52* "Pure" motor lacunar syndrome with accompanying symptoms other than sensory

G46.6* **Pure sensory lacunar syndrome (I60–I67†)**

G46.60* Pure paraesthetic sensory lacunar syndrome
G46.61* Pure sensory lacunar syndrome with objective sensory deficit
G46.62* Pure sensory lacunar syndrome with pain

G46.7* **Other lacunar syndromes (I60–I67†)**

G46.70* Sensory motor stroke
G46.71* Dysarthria–clumsy hand syndrome
G46.72* Crural hemiparesis with homolateral ataxia
G46.73* Pseudobulbar lacunar syndrome
G46.77* Multiple and bilateral lacunae (lacunar state)
Excludes: causing parkinsonism (G22.1)
causing vascular dementia (F01.2)

G46.8* **Other vascular syndromes of brain in cerebrovascular diseases (I60–I67†)**

G46.80* Anterior choroidal artery syndrome
G46.81* Anterior superficial junctional syndrome
G46.82* Posterior superficial junctional syndrome
G46.83* Subcortical junctional syndrome
G46.84* Tuberothalamic artery syndrome
G46.87* Multiple vascular syndromes of brain NOS

G47 Sleep disorders

Excludes: nocturnal myoclonus (G25.80)
nonorganic sleep disorders (F51.–)
sleep terrors (F51.4)
sleepwalking (F51.3)

G47.0 Disorders of initiating and maintaining sleep [insomnias]
Excludes: altitudinal insomnia (T70.2)

G47.1 Disorders of excessive somnolence [hypersomnias]
Idiopathic hypersomnia

G47.2 Disorders of the sleep–wake schedule
- G47.20 Transient sleep–wake schedule disorder
- G47.21 Advanced sleep phase disorder
- G47.22 Delayed sleep phase syndrome
- G47.23 Irregular sleep–wake pattern
- G47.24 Non-24-hour sleep–wake cycle
- G47.28 Other disorders of the sleep–wake schedule

G47.3 Sleep apnoea
Sleep-related respiratory failure [Ondine]
Excludes: pickwickian syndrome (E66.2)

- G47.30 Alveolar hypoventilation syndrome
- G47.31 Central sleep apnoea
- G47.32 Obstructive sleep apnoea
- G47.38 Other sleep apnoea

G47.4 Narcolepsy and cataplexy

- G47.40 Narcolepsy
- G47.41 Cataplexy
- G47.42 Sleep paralysis
- G47.43 Hypnogogic or hypnopompic hallucinations
- G47.44 Any combination of narcolepsy, cataplexy, hypnogogic or hypnopompic hallucinations and sleep paralysis
- G47.48 Other forms of narcolepsy and cataplexy

G47.8 Other sleep disorders
Excludes: other sudden death, cause unknown (R96.–)
sleep apnoea (G47.3)
• newborn (R96.–)
sudden infant death syndrome (R95)

- G47.80 Other REM-sleep-related parasomnias
  Excludes: nightmares (F51.5)
  sleep paralysis G47.42
  - G47.800 REM-sleep-related behaviour disorder [phantasmagorias]
  - G47.801 Impaired REM-sleep-related non-painful penile erections
  - G47.802 REM-sleep-related painful erections

G47.803 REM-sleep-related cardiac sinus arrest
G47.804 REM-sleep-related headache
Use additional code, if required, to indicate type of headache.

G47.81 Other non-REM-sleep-related parasomnias
Excludes: benign neonatal sleep myoclonus (G25.37)
snoring (R06.5)
G47.810 Sleep-related bruxism
G47.811 Sleep-related enuresis
G47.812 Non-REM-sleep-related abnormal swallowing syndrome
G47.813 Nocturnal paroxysmal dystonia

G47.82 Sleep arousal disorders
Confusional arousals
Sleep drunkenness

G47.83 Sleep–wake transition disorders
Excludes: nocturnal leg cramps (R25.20)
G47.830 Sleep-related rhythmic movement disorder
Head-banging [jactatio capitis nocturnus]
G47.831 Sleep starts
G47.832 Sleeptalking

G47.84 Kleine–Levin syndrome
Recurrent hypersomnia

G47.88 Other specified sleep disorders

G47.9 Sleep disorder, unspecified

Nerve, nerve root and plexus disorders (G50–G59)

Excludes: current traumatic nerve, nerve root and plexus disorders — see nerve injury by body region (S04.–, S14.–, S24.–, S34.–, S44.–, S54.–, S64.–, S74.–, S84.–, S94.–)
neuralgia } NOS (M79.2)
neuritis }
peripheral neuritis in pregnancy (O26.8)
radiculitis NOS (M54.1)

G50 Disorders of trigeminal nerve

Includes: disorders of 5th cranial nerv

G50.0 Trigeminal neuralgia
Includes: syndrome of paroxysmal facial pain
tic douloureux

Excludes: postherpetic trigeminal neuralgia (B02.2)
postzoster trigeminal neuralgia (B02.2)
trigeminal neuropathy:
• idiopathic (G50.80)
• secondary NOS (G50.81)

G50.00 Idiopathic trigeminal neuralgia
G50.09 Secondary trigeminal neuralgia, unspecified

G50.1 Atypical facial pain

G50.8 Other disorders of trigeminal nerve
Excludes: benign neoplasm of trigeminal nerve (D33.33)
malignant neoplasm of trigeminal nerve (C72.51)

G50.80 Idiopathic trigeminal neuropathy
G50.81 Secondary trigeminal neuropathy NOS

G50.9 Disorder of trigeminal nerve, unspecified

G51 Facial nerve disorders

Includes: disorders of 7th cranial nerve

G51.0 Bell's palsy
Includes: facial palsy
Excludes: facial hemiatrophy [Romberg] (Q67.4)

G51.00 Idiopathic acute facial nerve palsy
G51.01 Familial acute facial nerve palsy
G51.02 Familial recurrent facial nerve palsy
G51.08 Other specified facial nerve palsy

G51.1 Geniculate ganglionitis
Excludes: postherpetic geniculate ganglionitis (B02.2)

G51.2 Melkersson's syndrome
Melkersson–Rosenthal syndrome

G51.3 Clonic hemifacial spasm

G51.4 Facial myokymia

G51.8 Other disorders of facial nerve
Excludes: facial hemiatrophy [Romberg] (Q67.4)

G51.9 Disorder of facial nerve, unspecified

G52 Disorders of other cranial nerves

Excludes: disorders of:
- acoustic [8th] nerve (H93.3)
- oculomotor nerves (H49.0–H49.3)
- optic [2nd] nerve (H46, H47.0)

paralytic strabismus due to nerve palsy (H49.0–H49.2)

Use sixth character, if desired, to indicate:

G52.*xx*0 Unilateral
G52.*xx*1 Bilateral

G52.0 Disorders of olfactory nerve

Disorder of 1st cranial nerve

Excludes: idiopathic:
- anosmia (R43.0)
- parosmia (R43.1)

G52.1 Disorders of glossopharyngeal nerve

Includes: disorder of 9th cranial nerve
Excludes: oculopalatal myoclonus (G25.33)

G52.10 Idiopathic glossopharyngeal neuralgia
G52.18 Other specified disorders of glossopharyngeal nerve

G52.2 Disorders of vagus nerve

Includes: disorder of pneumogastric [10th] cranial nerve
Excludes: paralysis of vocal cords and larynx (J38.0)

G52.20 Superior laryngeal neuralgia
G52.28 Other specified disorders of vagus nerve

G52.3 Disorders of hypoglossal nerve

Includes: disorder of 12th cranial nerve

G52.30 Idiopathic hypoglossal neuropathy
G52.38 Other specified disorders of hypoglossal nerve

G52.7 Disorders of multiple cranial nerves

Polyneuritis cranialis

G52.8 Disorders of other specified cranial nerves

G52.80 Occipital neuralgia [Arnold]
G52.81 Disorders of accessory nerve
Disorders of 11th cranial nerve

G52.9 Cranial nerve disorder, unspecified

G53* Cranial nerve disorders in diseases classified elsewhere

G53.0* Postzoster neuralgia (B02.2†)

G53.00* Acute trigeminal herpes zoster neuropathy
G53.01* Postzoster trigeminal neuralgia
G53.02* Acute glossopharyngeal herpes zoster neuropathy
G53.03* Postzoster glossopharyngeal neuralgia
G53.04* Acute herpetic geniculate ganglionitis
G53.05* Postherpetic geniculate ganglionitis
G53.06* Ocular nerve palsy due to herpes zoster

G53.1* Multiple cranial nerve palsies in infectious and parasitic diseases classified elsewhere (A00–B99†)

G53.2* Multiple cranial nerve palsies in sarcoidosis (D86.8†)

G53.3* Multiple cranial nerve palsies in neoplastic disease (C00–D48†)

G53.8* Other cranial nerve disorders in other diseases classified elsewhere

G53.80* Other trigeminal (5th cranial) nerve disorder in other diseases classified elsewhere
G53.81* Facial (7th cranial) nerve disorder in other diseases classified elsewhere
G53.82* Olfactory (1st cranial) nerve disorder in other diseases classified elsewhere
G53.83* Glossopharyngeal (9th cranial) nerve disorder in other diseases classified elsewhere
G53.84* Vagus (10th cranial) nerve disorder in other diseases classified elsewhere
G53.85* Hypoglossal (12th cranial) nerve disorder in other diseases classified elsewhere
G53.87* Multiple cranial nerve disorder in other diseases classified elsewhere

G54 Nerve root and plexus disorders

Excludes: current traumatic nerve root and plexus disorders — see nerve injury by body region
intervertebral disc disorders (M50–M51)
neuralgia or neuritis NOS (M79.2)

neuritis or radiculitis:
- brachial NOS (M54.1)
- lumbar NOS (M54.1)
- lumbosacral NOS (M54.1)
- thoracic NOS (M54.1)

radiculitis NOS (M54.1)
radiculopathy NOS (M54.1)
spondylosis (M47.–)

G54.0 Brachial plexus disorders

Excludes: idiopathic brachial plexopathy [neuralgic amyotrophy] [Parsonage–Aldren–Turner] (G54.5)

G54.00 Post-radiation (radiation-induced) brachial plexopathy
G54.01 Thoracic outlet syndrome due to cervical rib
G54.02 Thoracic outlet syndrome due to other anatomical abnormality
G54.03 Brachial plexus lesion due to vasculitis
G54.04 Brachial plexus lesion due to diabetes mellitus
G54.05 Brachial plexus lesion due to inflammatory neuropathy
Classify under inflammatory polyneuropathy (G61.–) if there are other lesions in addition to brachial plexus.
G54.08 Other brachial plexus lesions

G54.1 Lumbosacral plexus disorders

G54.10 Postradiation (radiation-induced) lumbosacral plexopathy
G54.11 Inflammatory lumbosacral plexopathy
G54.12 Vasculitic lumbosacral plexopathy
G54.13 Lumbosacral plexopathy due to diabetes mellitus
G54.14 Idiopathic lumbosacral plexopathy
G54.18 Other lumbosacral plexus disorders

G54.2 Cervical root disorders, not elsewhere classified

G54.3 Thoracic root disorders, not elsewhere classified

G54.4 Lumbosacral root disorders, not elsewhere classified

G54.5 Neuralgic amyotrophy

Includes: idiopathic brachial plexopathy [Parsonage–Aldren–Turner]
shoulder-girdle neuritis

G54.50 Sporadic acute brachial plexopathy
G54.51 Familial acute or recurrent brachial plexopathy

G54.6 Phantom limb syndrome with pain

G54.7 Phantom limb syndrome without pain
Phantom limb syndrome NOS

G54.8 Other nerve root and plexus disorders

G54.80 Nerve root cysts
Perineural cysts
Tarlov cysts
G54.81 Nerve root avulsion
Use additional code (S14.2 and S24.2), if desired, to indicate injury.
G54.82 Radiculo-plexopathy
Use additional code, if desired, to indicate cause, e.g. cytomegalovirus (B25.–).
G54.83 Radiculo-myelopathy
Use additional code, if desired, to indicate cause, e.g. cytomegalovirus (B25.–).

G54.9 Nerve root and plexus disorder, unspecified

G54.90 Nerve root disorder NOS
G54.91 Nerve plexus disorder NOS

G55* Nerve root and plexus compressions in diseases classified elsewhere

Use additional fifth character, if desired, to define location:

G55.*x*0 Cervical root
G55.*x*1 Thoracic root
G55.*x*2 Lumbar root
G55.*x*3 Sacral root
G55.*x*4 Cervical plexus
G55.*x*5 Brachial plexus
G55.*x*6 Lumbar plexus
G55.*x*7 Sacral plexus
G55.*x*8 Splanchnic plexus
G55.*x*9 Presacral plexus

Use additional sixth character, if desired, to define root level. G55.*xx*0 to G55.*xx*8 may be used for appropriately numbered cervical, thoracic, lumbar, sacral and coccygeal roots, for instance:

G55.*x*10 First thoracic root
G55.*x*11 Second thoracic root
G55.*x*12 Third or fourth thoracic root
G55.*x*13 Fifth or sixth thoracic root
G55.*x*14 Seventh or eighth thoracic root
G55.*x*15 Ninth or tenth thoracic root
G55.*x*16 Eleventh thoracic root
G55.*x*17 Twelfth thoracic root
G55.*x*18 Multiple nerve roots

G55.0* Nerve root and plexus compressions in neoplastic disease (C00–D48†)

G55.1* Nerve root and plexus compressions in intervertebral disc disorders (M50–M51†)

G55.2* Nerve root and plexus compressions in spondylosis (M47.–†)

G55.3* Nerve root and plexus compressions in other dorsopathies (M45–M46†, M48.–†, M53–M54†)

G55.8* Nerve root and plexus compressions in other diseases classified elsewhere

G56 Mononeuropathies of upper limb

Excludes: current traumatic nerve disorder — see nerve injury by body region

G56.0 Carpal tunnel syndrome

G56.1 Other lesions of median nerve

G56.10 Lesion of median nerve in axilla
G56.11 Lesion of median nerve at ligament of Struthers
G56.12 Median nerve pronator syndrome
G56.13 Median nerve anterior interosseous syndrome

G56.2 Lesion of ulnar nerve

G56.20 Ulnar nerve lesion in axilla
G56.21 Tardy ulnar nerve palsy (post-humeral fracture)
G56.22 Ulnar nerve cubital tunnel syndrome
G56.23 Ulnar nerve lesion at wrist
Guyon's canal syndrome

G56.24 Ulnar nerve lesion in palm
Lesion of deep branch of ulnar nerve
G56.28 Other lesions of ulnar nerve

G56.3 Lesion of radial nerve

G56.30 Radial nerve lesion in axilla
G56.31 Radial nerve lesion in radial groove
G56.32 Radial nerve posterior interosseous syndrome
G56.33 Superficial radial nerve lesion
G56.38 Other lesions of radial nerve

G56.4 Causalgia

G56.8 Other mononeuropathies of upper limb

G56.80 Lesion of musculocutaneous nerve
G56.81 Interdigital neuroma of upper limb

G56.9 Mononeuropathy of upper limb, unspecified

G57 Mononeuropathies of lower limb

Excludes: current traumatic nerve disorder — see nerve injury by body region

G57.0 Lesion of sciatic nerve

Excludes: sciatica:
- NOS (M54.3)
- attributed to intervertebral disc disorder (M51.1)

G57.00 Lesion of gluteal nerve
G57.01 Sciatic nerve pyriformis syndrome
G57.02 Lesion of sciatic nerve in thigh
G57.08 Other lesions of sciatic nerve

G57.1 Meralgia paraesthetica

Lateral cutaneous nerve of thigh syndrome

G57.2 Lesion of femoral nerve

G57.20 Femoral nerve lesion in abdomen
G57.21 Femoral nerve lesion in thigh
G57.22 Lesion of saphenous nerve

G57.3 Lesion of lateral popliteal nerve

Includes: peroneal nerve palsy

G57.30 Lesion of superficial peroneal nerve
G57.31 Lesion of deep peroneal nerve

G57.4 Lesion of medial popliteal nerve

G57.40 Lesion of medial popliteal nerve at knee
G57.41 Lesion of medial popliteal nerve in calf
G57.42 Lesion of sural nerve

G57.5 Tarsal tunnel syndrome

G57.6 Lesion of plantar nerve

G57.60 Lesion of lateral plantar nerve
G57.61 Lesion of medial plantar nerve
G57.62 Morton's metatarsalgia

G57.8 Other mononeuropathies of lower limb

G57.80 Lesion of genitofemoral nerve
G57.81 Lesion of ilioinguinal nerve
G57.82 Lesion of pudendal nerve
G57.83 Interdigital neuroma of lower limb

G57.9 Mononeuropathy of lower limb, unspecified

G58 Other mononeuropathies

G58.0 Intercostal neuropathy

G58.7 Mononeuritis multiplex

G58.8 Other specified mononeuropathies

G58.80 Lesion of phrenic nerve
G58.81 Traumatic neuroma
Excludes: interdigital neuroma of:
- lower limb (G57.84)
- upper limb (G56.81)

neuroma of plantar nerve (G57.6)
G58.82 Lesion of suprascapular nerve
G58.83 Lesion of axillary nerve
G58.84 Lesion of long thoracic nerve

G58.9 Mononeuropathy, unspecified

G59* Mononeuropathy in diseases classified elsewhere

G59.0* Diabetic mononeuropathy (E10–E14† with common fourth character .4)

G59.8* Other mononeuropathies in diseases classified elsewhere
Mononeuropathy in (due to):
- leprosy (A30.–†)

- radiation (G97.80†)
- vasculitis (M30.–†, M31.–†)
- zoster (B02.2†)

Polyneuropathies and other disorders of the peripheral nervous system (G60–G64)

Excludes: acute poliomyelitis (A80.–)
neuralgia NOS (M79.2)
neuritis NOS (M79.2)
peripheral neuritis in pregnancy (O26.8)
radiculitis NOS (M54.1)

G60 Hereditary and idiopathic neuropathy

Excludes: neuropathic heredofamilial amyloidosis (E85.1)

Use sixth character for mode of inheritance when applicable:

G60.*xx*0 Autosomal dominant
G60.*xx*1 Autosomal recessive
G60.*xx*2 Sex-linked dominant
G60.*xx*3 Sex-linked recessive
G60.*xx*4 Maternal inheritance
G60.*xx*5 Familial with uncertain inheritance
G60.*xx*6 Non-familial
G60.*xx*8 Other specified mode of inheritance

G60.0 Hereditary motor and sensory neuropathy

Excludes: hereditary motor and sensory neuropathy, type IV [Refsum] (G60.1)

G60.00 Type I: Charcot–Marie–Tooth disease, hypertrophic demyelinative type
Peroneal muscular atrophy, hypertrophic type

G60.01 Type II: Charcot–Marie–Tooth disease, neuronal type
Peroneal muscular atrophy, axonal type

G60.02 Type III: hypertrophic demyelinative neuropathy of infancy [Déjerine–Sottas]

G60.03 Type V: hereditary spastic paraplegia with motor and sensory neuropathy

G60.04 Type VI: hereditary motor and sensory neuropathy with optic atrophy

G60.05 Type VII: hereditary motor and sensory neuropathy with retinitis pigmentosa

G60.06 Roussy–Lévy syndrome
G60.08 Other types of hereditary motor and sensory neuropathy

G60.1 Refsum's disease
Hereditary motor and sensory neuropathy, type IV
Hereditary phytanic acidaemia
Excludes: infantile Refsum's disease (E80.300)

G60.2 Neuropathy in association with hereditary ataxia

G60.3 Idiopathic progressive neuropathy

G60.30 Diffuse posterior root ganglion degeneration
G60.31 Segmental posterior root ganglion degeneration

G60.8 Other hereditary and idiopathic neuropathies
Excludes: familial dysautonomia [Riley–Day] (G90.1)

G60.80 Hereditary sensory and autonomic neuropathy, type I
G60.81 Hereditary sensory and autonomic neuropathy, type II
G60.82 Hereditary sensory and autonomic neuropathy, type III
G60.83 Hereditary sensory and autonomic neuropathy, type IV
Congenital insensitivity to pain, anhidrosis and mental retardation [Swanson]
G60.84 Hereditary sensory and autonomic neuropathy, type V
Congenital sensory neuropathy with selective loss of pain perception [Low]
G60.85 Familial giant axonal neuropathy
G60.86 Neuropathy associated with multiple endocrine neoplasia, type 2B
G60.87 Hereditary pressure-sensitive neuropathy
Inherited tendency to develop pressure palsies
Tomaculous neuropathy

G60.9 Hereditary and idiopathic neuropathy, unspecified

G61 Inflammatory polyneuropathy

G61.0 Guillain–Barré syndrome
Includes: acute (post-)infective polyneuritis

Use additional code, if desired, to identify cause.

G61.00 Predominantly motor Guillain–Barré syndrome
G61.01 Guillain–Barré syndrome with severe autonomic involvement
G61.02 Guillain–Barré syndrome with significant sensory involvement
G61.03 Guillain–Barré syndrome with ophthalmoplegia
Descending type with ophthalmoplegia and ataxia [Fisher]

G61.1 Serum neuropathy
Use additional external cause code (Chapter XX), if desired, to identify cause.

G61.8 Other inflammatory polyneuropathies
Excludes: acute pandysautonomia (G90.00)
progressive dorsal root degeneration (G60.3)

G61.80 Progressive chronic inflammatory demyelinating polyneuropathy
G61.81 Relapsing–remitting chronic inflammatory demyelinating polyneuropathy
G61.82 Sensory perineuritis
G61.83 Acute sensory polyneuropathy

G61.9 Inflammatory polyneuropathy, unspecified

G62 Other polyneuropathies

Excludes: neuropathic heredofamilial amyloidosis (E85.1)

G62.0 Drug-induced polyneuropathy
Use additional external cause code (Chapter XX), if desired, to identify drug.

G62.1 Alcoholic polyneuropathy

G62.2 Polyneuropathy due to other toxic agents
Use additional external cause code (Chapter XX), if desired, to identify toxic agent.

G62.8 Other specified polyneuropathies
Use additional external cause code (Chapter XX), if desired, to identify cause.

G62.80 Postradiation (radiation-induced) polyneuropathy
G62.81 Small fibre neuropathy NOS

G62.9 Polyneuropathy, unspecified
Neuropathy NOS

G63* Polyneuropathy in diseases classified elsewhere

G63.0* Polyneuropathy in infectious and parasitic diseases classified elsewhere
Polyneuropathy (in):
- diphtheria (A36.8†)
- hepatitis B infection (B16.–†, B18.–†)
- HIV disease (B23.8†)
- infectious mononucleosis (B27.–†)
- leprosy (A30.–†)
- Lyme disease (A69.2†)
- mumps (B26.8†)
- postherpetic (B02.2†)
- shigellosis (A03.–†)
- syphilis, late (A52.1†)
  - congenital (A50.4†)
- tuberculous (A17.8†)
- typhoid fever (A01.0†)
- zoster (B02.2†)

G63.1* Polyneuropathy in neoplastic disease (C00–D48†)

G63.2* Diabetic polyneuropathy (E10–E14† with common fourth character .4)

G63.3* Polyneuropathy in other endocrine and metabolic diseases (E00–E06†, E15–E16†, E20–E34†, E70–E89†)
Polyneuropathy in:
- amyloidosis (E85.1†)
- xanthoma tuberosum (E78.26†)

G63.4* Polyneuropathy in nutritional deficiency (E40–E64†)
Polyneuropathy in vitamin B_{12} deficiency (E53.80†)

G63.5* Polyneuropathy in systemic connective tissue disorders (M30–M35†)

G63.6* Polyneuropathy in other musculoskeletal disorders (M00–M25†, M40–M96†)
Polyneuropathy in rheumatoid arthritis (M05.3†)

G63.8* Polyneuropathy in other diseases classified elsewhere
Polyneuropathy in:
- chronic hepatic failure (K72.–†)

- ciguatera fish poisoning (T61.0†)
- critical illness, e.g. asphyxiation (R09.0†); cardiac arrest with successful rescuscitation (I46.0†); septic shock (A41.9†)
- sarcoidosis (D86.88†)
- uraemic neuropathy (N18.8†)

G64 Other disorders of peripheral nervous system

Includes: disorder of peripheral nervous system NOS

G64.–0 Generalized myokymia
G64.–1 Myokymia, hyperhidrosis, impaired muscle relaxation syndrome
G64.–2 Focal myokymia

Diseases of myoneural junction and muscle (G70–G73)

G70 Myasthenia gravis and other myoneural disorders

Excludes: botulism (A05.1)
transient neonatal myasthenia gravis (P94.0)

Use sixth character for topography, if desired:

G70.*xx*0 Ocular
G70.*xx*1 Bulbar
G70.*xx*2 Mild generalized
G70.*xx*3 Severe generalized

G70.0 Myasthenia gravis

G70.00 Acquired idiopathic autoimmune myasthenia gravis
G70.01 Myasthenia gravis associated with thymoma
G70.02 Myasthenia gravis associated with other autoimmune diseases
G70.03 Penicillamine-induced myasthenia gravis
G70.08 Other myasthenia gravis
Use additional external cause code (Chapter XX), if desired, to identify drug, if drug-induced.

G70.1 Toxic myoneural disorders

Use additional external cause code (Chapter XX), if desired, to identify toxic agent.

G70.2 Congenital and developmental myasthenia

G70.20 Congenital endplate acetylcholinesterase deficiency
G70.21 Congenital endplate acetylcholine receptor deficiency
G70.22 Congenital slow channel syndrome
G70.23 Congenital myasthenia with presynaptic defect
G70.24 Familial infantile myasthenia
G70.25 Limb-girdle myasthenia, familial
G70.26 Limb-girdle myasthenia, nonfamilial
G70.28 Other specified congenital or developmental myasthenia

G70.8 Other specified myoneural disorders

G70.80 Eaton–Lambert syndrome unassociated with neoplasm

G70.9 Myoneural disorder, unspecified

G71 Primary disorders of muscles

Excludes: arthrogryposis multiplex congenita (Q74.3)
dermatopolymyositis (M33.–)
metabolic disorders (E70–E90)
myositis (M60.–)

G71.0 Muscular dystrophy

Excludes: congenital myopathy:
- NOS (G71.2)
- with specific morphological abnormalities of the muscle fibre (G71.2)

G71.00 Benign dystrophin-deficient Becker-type muscular dystrophy
G71.01 Benign scapuloperoneal muscular dystrophy with early contractures [Emery–Dreifuss]
G71.02 Facioscapulohumeral muscular dystrophy [Landouzy–Déjerine]
G71.03 Limb-girdle muscular dystrophy [Erb]
G71.04 Ocular muscular dystrophy
G71.05 Oculopharyngeal muscular dystrophy
G71.06 Scapuloperoneal muscular dystrophy
G71.07 Severe dystrophin-deficient Duchenne-type muscular dystrophy
G71.08 Other muscular dystrophy
G71.080 Autosomal recessive muscular dystrophy, childhood type, resembling Duchenne/Becker

G71.081 Distal muscular dystrophy
Distal myopathy

G71.082 Humeroperoneal muscular dystrophy with early contractures

G71.083 Muscular dystrophy with excessive autophagy

G71.084 Congenital muscular dystrophy with central nervous system abnormalities [Fukuyama]

G71.085 Congenital muscular dystrophy without central nervous system abnormalities

G71.1 Myotonic disorders

G71.10 Chondrodystrophic myotonia [Schwartz–Jampel]

G71.11 Drug-induced myotonia
Use additional external cause code (Chapter XX), if desired, to identify drug.

G71.12 Dystrophia myotonica [Steinert]

G71.120 Neonatal dystrophia myotonica

G71.121 Juvenile onset dystrophia myotonica

G71.122 Adult onset dystrophia myotonica

G71.13 Myotonia congenita

G71.130 Myotonia congenita, dominant [Thomsen]

G71.131 Myotonia congenita, recessive [Becker]

G71.14 Neuromyotonia [Isaacs]

G71.15 Paramyotonia congenita

G71.16 Pseudomyotonia

G71.18 Other myotonic disorders
Symptomatic myotonia
Use additional code, if desired, to identify the primary cause.

G71.2 Congenital myopathies

G71.20 Central core disease

G71.21 Fibre-type disproportion

G71.22 Multicore (minicore) disease

G71.23 Centronuclear myopathy
Includes: myotubular myopathy

G71.230 Centronuclear myopathy with type I fibre hypotrophy

G71.24 Nemaline myopathy

G71.25 Myopathy with tubular aggregates

G71.26 Fingerprint body myopathy

G71.28 Other congenital myopathies

G71.280 Sarcotubular myopathy

G71.281 Reducing body myopathy

G71.3 Mitochondrial myopathy, not elsewhere classified

Excludes: defects of mitochondrial respiratory chain (E88.83)
Kearns–Sayre syndrome (H49.8)
myoclonic epilepsy with ragged red fibres (MERRF) (G40.46)

G71.30 Mitochondrial myopathy with cytochrome *c* oxidase deficiency
G71.31 Mitochondrial myopathy with coenzyme Q deficiency
G71.32 Mitochondrial myopathy with complex I deficiency
G71.33 Luft's disease
G71.34 Other ocular myopathy with mitochondrial abnormalities
G71.35 Mitochondrial encephalopathy with lactic acidosis and stroke-like episodes (MELAS)
G71.38 Other specified types of mitochondrial myopathy

G71.8 Other primary disorders of muscles

G71.80 Myopathies with specific structural abnormalities
Excludes: congenital myopathies (G71.2)
G71.800 Myopathy with cytoplasmic bodies
G71.801 Myopathy with cylindrical bodies
G71.802 Myopathy with zebra bodies
G71.803 Myopathy with rimmed vacuoles
G71.804 Myopathy with spheromembranous bodies
G71.805 Familial granulovacuolar myopathy with electrical myotonia
G71.806 Myosclerosis
G71.807 Type I muscle fibre atrophy
G71.808 Type II muscle fibre atrophy
G71.81 Ocular myopathy
Oculocraniosomatic myopathy
Excludes: ocular muscular dystrophy (G71.04)
ocular myopathy with mitochondrial abnormalities (G71.35)
oculopharyngeal muscular dystrophy (G71.05)
G71.82 Monomelic hypertrophic myopathy
G71.83 Hypertrophic brachial myopathy
G71.84 Malignant hyperthermia
Malignant hyperpyrexia
Excludes: malignant neuroleptic syndrome (G21.0)

G71.85 Myopathy with deficiency of sarcotubular calcium binding [Brodie]
G71.86 Quadriceps myopathy

G71.9 Primary disorder of muscle, unspecified
Hereditary myopathy NOS

G72 Other myopathies

Excludes: arthrogryposis multiplex congenita (Q74.3)
dermatopolymyositis (M33.–)
ischaemic infarction of muscle (M62.2)
myositis (M60.–)
polymyositis (M33.2)

G72.0 Drug-induced myopathy
Use additional external cause code (Chapter XX), if desired, to identify drug.

G72.1 Alcoholic myopathy

G72.10 Acute alcoholic myopathy
G72.11 Chronic alcoholic neuromyopathy

G72.2 Myopathy due to other toxic agents
Use additional external cause code (Chapter XX), if desired, to identify toxic agent.

G72.3 Periodic paralysis

G72.30 Familial hypokalaemic periodic paralysis
G72.31 Familial hyperkalaemic periodic paralysis
G72.32 Familial normokalaemic periodic paralysis
G72.33 Periodic paralysis associated with hyperthyroidism
G72.34 Secondary periodic paralysis due to hypokalaemia
G72.35 Secondary periodic paralysis due to hyperkalaemia
G72.36 Periodic paralysis with cardiac arrhythmias
G72.38 Other periodic paralysis

G72.4 Inflammatory myopathy, not elsewhere classified
Use additional code, if desired, to identify cause, e.g. HIV disease (B23.8).

G72.8 Other specified myopathies
Excludes: disorders of muscle tone of newborn (P94.–)
Volkmann's ischaemic contracture (T79.6)

G72.80 Secondary rhabdomyolysis [myoglobinuria]
Use additional code, if desired, to identify any associated condition, e.g. acute poliomyelitis (A80.–);

dermatomyositis (M33.0–M33.1); drug-induced myopathy (G72.0); metabolic diseases of muscle causing rhabdomyolysis (E70–E90); polymyositis (M33.2).

G72.81 Idiopathic rhabdomyolysis

G72.82 Delayed muscle maturation

G72.9 Myopathy, unspecified

G73* Disorders of myoneural junction and muscle in diseases classified elsewhere

G73.0* Myasthenic syndromes in endocrine diseases

Myasthenic syndromes in:

- diabetic amyotrophy (E10–E14† with common fourth character .4)
- thyrotoxicosis [hyperthyroidism] (E05.–†)

G73.1* Eaton–Lambert syndrome (C80†)

Excludes: Eaton–Lambert syndrome unassociated with neoplasm (G70.80)

G73.2* Other myasthenic syndromes in neoplastic disease (C00–D48†)

G73.3* Myasthenic syndromes in other diseases classified elsewhere

G73.4* Myopathy in infectious and parasitic diseases classified elsewhere

G73.5* Myopathy in endocrine diseases

Includes: myopathy (in) (due to):

- acromegaly (E22.0†)
- Cushing's syndrome (E24.–†)
- hyperparathyroidism (E21.–†)
- hyperthyroidism (E05.–†)
- hypoadrenalism (E27.1†, E27.3–E27.4†)
- hypoparathyroidism (E20.–†)
- hypothyroidism (E00–E03†)

Excludes: drug-induced corticosteroid myopathy (G72.0)

G73.50* Ocular myopathy in hyperthyroidism (E05.0†)
Dysthyroid ophthalmoplegia (orbitopathy)

G73.6* Myopathy in metabolic diseases

Myopathy in:

- carnitine deficiency (E71.32†)
- glycogen storage disease (E74.0†)

- hydroxymethylglutaryl-CoA lyase deficiency (E71.30†)
- isovaleryl-CoA dehydrogenase deficiency (E71.11†)
- lactate dehydrogenase deficiency (E74.86†)
- lipid storage disorders (E75.–†)
- mannose-6-phosphate isomerase deficiency (E74.83†)
- methylmalonyl-CoA mutase deficiency (E71.12†)
- multiple-chain acyl-CoA dehydrogenase deficiency (E88.820†)
- phosphoglycerate kinase deficiency (E74.85†)
- phosphoglycerate mutase deficiency (E74.84†)

G73.7* Myopathy in other diseases classified elsewhere

Includes: myopathy in:
- amyloidosis (E85.–†)
- carcinoid syndrome (E34.0†)
- intrauterine exposure to toxins (P04.–†)
- nutritional deficiencies (E40–E64†)
- osteomalacia (M83.–†)
- polyarteritis nodosa (M30.0†)
- rheumatoid arthritis (M05.3†)
- sarcoidosis (D86.88†)
- scleroderma (M34.8†)
- sicca syndrome [Sjögren] (M35.0†)
- syphilis (A51.4†, A52.7†)
- systemic lupus erythematosus (M32.1†)
- thalassemia (D56.–†)
- trauma and ischaemia (T79.6†)
- vitamin D deficiency (E55.–†)

G73.70* Muscle wasting in diseases classified elsewhere

Muscle wasting (in) (due to):
- cachexia NOS (R64†)
- disuse atrophy (M62.5†)
- immobility syndrome (M62.3†)
- malignant cachexia (C80†)

Cerebral palsy and other paralytic syndromes (G80–G83)

G80 Infantile cerebral palsy

Includes: Little's disease
Excludes: hereditary spastic paraplegia (G11.4)

G80.0 Spastic cerebral palsy
Congenital spastic paralysis (cerebral)

G80.1 Spastic diplegia

G80.2 Infantile hemiplegia

G80.3 Dyskinetic cerebral palsy
Athetoid cerebral palsy

G80.4 Ataxic cerebral palsy

G80.8 Other infantile cerebral palsy
Mixed cerebral palsy syndromes

G80.9 Infantile cerebral palsy, unspecified
Cerebral palsy NOS

G81 Hemiplegia

Note: For primary coding, this category is to be used only when hemiplegia (complete)(incomplete) is reported without further specification, or is stated to be old or longstanding but of unspecified cause. The category is also for use in multiple coding to identify these types of hemiplegia resulting from any cause.

Excludes: congenital and infantile cerebral palsy (G80.–)

G81.0 Flaccid hemiplegia

G81.1 Spastic hemiplegia

G81.9 Hemiplegia, unspecified

G82 Paraplegia and tetraplegia

Note: For primary coding, this category is to be used only when the listed conditions are reported without further specification, or are stated to be old or longstanding but of unspecified cause. The category is also for use in multiple coding to identify these conditions resulting from any cause.

Excludes: congenital and infantile cerebral palsy (G80.–)

G82.0 Flaccid paraplegia

G82.1 Spastic paraplegia
Excludes: tropical spastic paraplegia (G04.1)

G82.2 Paraplegia, unspecified
Paralysis of both lower limbs NOS
Paraplegia (lower) NOS

G82.3 Flaccid tetraplegia

G82.4 Spastic tetraplegia

G82.5 Tetraplegia, unspecified
Quadriplegia NOS

G83 Other paralytic syndromes

Note: For primary coding, this category is to be used only when the listed conditions are reported without further specification, or are stated to be old or longstanding but of unspecified cause. The category is also for use in multiple coding to identify these conditions resulting from any cause.

Includes: paralysis (complete)(incomplete), except as in G80–G82

G83.0 Diplegia of upper limbs
Diplegia (upper)
Paralysis of both upper limbs

G83.1 Monoplegia of lower limb
Paralysis of lower limb

G83.2 Monoplegia of upper limb
Paralysis of upper limb

G83.3 Monoplegia, unspecified

G83.4 Cauda equina syndrome
Excludes: cord bladder NOS (G95.84)

G83.40 Complete cauda equina syndrome
G83.41 Neurogenic bladder due to cauda equina syndrome
G83.42 Syndrome of intermittent claudication of cauda equina
G83.48 Other partial cauda equina syndrome

G83.8 Other specified paralytic syndromes

G83.80 Todd's paralysis (postepileptic)

G83.9 Paralytic syndrome, unspecified

Other disorders of the nervous system (G90–G99)

G90 Disorders of autonomic nervous system

Includes: disorders of (para)sympathetic nervous system

Excludes: dysfunction of autonomic nervous system due to alcohol (G31.2)
hereditary amyloid neuropathies (E85.1)
hereditary sensory and autonomic neuropathies (G60.80–G60.84)

G90.0 Idiopathic peripheral autonomic neuropathy

G90.00 Acute pandysautonomia
G90.01 Chronic pandysautonomia
G90.02 Carotid sinus syncope
G90.08 Other idiopathic peripheral autonomic neuropathy

G90.1 Familial dysautonomia [Riley–Day]

G90.10 Sympathetic dysfunction associated with dopamine β-hydroxylase deficiency
G90.18 Other familial dysautonomia

G90.2 Horner's syndrome

Bernard(–Horner) syndrome

G90.3 Multi-system degeneration

Includes: multi-system atrophy [MSA]

Excludes: corticobasal ganglionic degeneration (G23.81)
dentatorubral pallidoluysian degeneration (G23.83)
olivopontocerebellar degeneration (G11.22; G11.23)
orthostatic hypotension NOS (I95.1)
pallidopyramidal dentatoluysian degeneration (G23.82)

G90.30 Isolated neurogenic orthostatic hypotension
G90.31 Shy–Drager syndrome
G90.32 Other multi-system degeneration with dysautonomia

G90.8 Other disorders of autonomic nervous system

Excludes: causalgia (G56.4)

G90.80 Holmes–Adie syndrome
Excludes: Adie's (myotonic) pupil (H57.00)
G90.81 Cholinergic neuropathy
G90.82 Chronic idiopathic anhidrosis
G90.83 Sympathetic osteodystrophy
Reflex sympathetic dystrophy

G90.9 Disorder of autonomic nervous system, unspecified

G91 Hydrocephalus

Includes: acquired hydrocephalus
Excludes: hydrocephalus (in) (due to):
- congenital (Q03.–)
- congenital toxoplasmosis (P37.1)

G91.0 Communicating hydrocephalus

G91.1 Obstructive hydrocephalus

G91.2 Normal-pressure hydrocephalus

G91.3 Post-traumatic hydrocephalus, unspecified

G91.8 Other hydrocephalus

G91.9 Hydrocephalus, unspecified

G92 Toxic encephalopathy

Use additional external cause code (Chapter XX), if desired, to identify toxic agent, e.g. carbon monoxide (T58).

G92.–0 Early toxic encephalopathy
G92.–1 Delayed toxic encephalopathy

G93 Other disorders of brain

G93.0 Cerebral cysts

Excludes: acquired periventricular cysts of newborn (P91.1)
congenital cerebral cysts (Q04.6)

G93.00 Arachnoid cyst
G93.01 Porencephalic cyst, acquired

G93.1 Anoxic brain damage, not elsewhere classified

Use additional code, if desired, to identify the associated condition, e.g.

- amnesic syndrome (F04)
- cerebellar syndrome (G96.80)
- cognitive impairment (F06.7)
- cortical blindness (H47.6)
- parkinsonian syndrome (G21.8)
- persistent vegetative state (G96.81)
- prolonged coma (R40.2)

Excludes: anoxic brain damage with action myoclonus [Lance–Adams] (G25.38)
complicating:
- abortion, ectopic or molar pregnancy (O08.8)
- pregnancy, labour or delivery (O29.2, O74.3, O89.2)

complication of surgical and medical care (T80–T88)
neonatal anoxia (P21.9)

G93.2 Benign intracranial hypertension

Includes: pseudotumor cerebri
Excludes: hypertensive encephalopathy (I67.4)

G93.20 Idiopathic intracranial hypertension

G93.21 Intracranial hypertension secondary to obesity

G93.22 Intracranial hypertension secondary to toxic exposure
Use additional external cause code (Chapter XX), if desired, to identify toxic agent.

G93.23 Intracranial hypertension secondary to hormone abnormality
Use additional code, if desired, to identify hormone abnormality.

G93.24 Intracranial hypertension secondary to cerebral venous thrombosis

G93.28 Other secondary intracranial hypertension

G93.3 Postviral fatigue syndrome

Benign myalgic encephalomyelitis

G93.4 Encephalopathy, unspecified

Excludes: encephalopathy:
- alcoholic (G31.2)
- toxic (G92.–)

G93.5 Compression of brain

Includes: compression / herniation } of brain (stem)

Excludes: traumatic compression of brain (diffuse) (S06.2)
- focal (S06.3)

G93.50 Medial temporal transtentorial herniation
G93.51 Central transtentorial herniation
G93.52 Cerebellar tonsillar herniation
G93.53 Upwards transtentorial cerebellar herniation
G93.58 Other specified type of brain or brain stem compression

G93.6 Cerebral oedema

Excludes: cerebral oedema:
- due to birth injury (P11.0)
- traumatic (S06.1)

G93.7 Reye's syndrome

Use additional external cause code (Chapter XX), if desired, to identify cause.

G93.8 Other specified disorders of brain

Use additional external cause code (Chapter XX), if desired, to identify cause.

G93.80 Postradiation (radiation-induced) encephalopathy

G93.9 Disorder of brain, unspecified

G94* Other disorders of brain in diseases classified elsewhere

G94.0* Hydrocephalus in infectious and parasitic diseases classified elsewhere (A00–B99†)

G94.1* Hydrocephalus in neoplastic disease (C00–D48†)

G94.2* Hydrocephalus in other diseases classified elsewhere

G94.8* Other specified disorders of brain in diseases classified elsewhere

G94.80* Metabolic encephalopathy in diseases classified elsewhere

Metabolic encephalopathy in:
- hepatic failure (K70–K72†)
- hypercalcaemia (E83.5†)
- hypernatraemia (E87.0†)

- hyperparathyroidism (E21.–†)
- hyperthyroidism (E05.–†)
- hypocalcaemia (E58†, E83.5†)
- hyponatraemia (E87.1†)
- hypoparathyroidism (E20.–†)
- hypothyroidism (E00–E03†)
- uraemia (N17–N19†)

G94.81* Ischaemic and hypoxic encephalopathy in diseases classified elsewhere

Ischaemic and hypoxic encephalopathy in:
- chronic cardiac failure (I50†)
- respiratory failure (J00–J99†)
- severe anaemia (D50–D59†)
- sickle-cell anaemia with crisis (D57.0†)

G94.82* Encephalopathy due to nutritional deficiencies

Encephalopathy due to deficiency of:
- niacin (E52†)
- vitamin B_6 (E53.1†)
- vitamin B_{12} (E53.80†)

Excludes: Wernicke's encephalopathy due to thiamine deficiency (E51.2)

G95 Other diseases of spinal cord

Excludes: myelitis (G04.–)

G95.0 Syringomyelia and syringobulbia

Excludes: congenital hydromyelia (Q06.4)

Use sixth character, if desired, to indicate:

G95.0*x*0 Syringomyelia
G95.0*x*1 Syringobulbia
G95.0*x*2 Syringobulbia and syringomyelia
G95.0*x*3 Syringomesencephalia
G95.0*x*4 Hydromyelia

G95.00 Syringomyelia, hydromyelia and syringobulbia associated with Arnold–Chiari malformation

G95.01 Syringomyelia, hydromyelia and syringobulbia associated with Dandy–Walker syndrome

G95.02 Syringomyelia, hydromyelia and syringobulbia associated with spinal intramedullary neoplasm

G95.03 Syringomyelia, hydromyelia and syringobulbia associated with spinal intramedullary vascular malformation

G95.04 Syringomyelia, hydromyelia and syringobulbia associated with chronic traumatic myelopathy
G95.05 Syringomyelia, hydromyelia and syringobulbia following previous haematomyelia
G95.06 Syringomyelia, hydromyelia and syringobulbia associated with posterior fossa arachnoiditis
G95.08 Other specified causes of syringomyelia, hydromelia and syringobulbia

G95.1 Vascular myelopathies

Excludes: intraspinal phlebitis and thrombophlebitis, except nonpyogenic (G08.–)

G95.10 Acute arterial infarction of spinal cord (embolic) (nonembolic)
G95.11 Arterial thrombosis of spinal cord
G95.12 Haematomyelia
G95.13 Subacute necrotic myelopathy
G95.14 Acute venous infarction of spinal cord
G95.15 Chronic venous infarction of spinal cord
G95.16 Nonpyogenic intraspinal phlebitis and thrombophlebitis
G95.17 Oedema of spinal cord
G95.18 Other specified types of vascular myelopathy

G95.2 Cord compression, unspecified

G95.8 Other specified diseases of spinal cord

Excludes: neurogenic bladder:
- NOS (N31.9)
- due to cauda equina syndrome (G83.4)

neuromuscular dysfunction of bladder without mention of spinal cord lesion (N31.–)

G95.80 Drug-induced myelopathy
Use additional external cause code (Chapter XX), if desired, to identify drug.
G95.81 Toxin-induced myelopathy
Use additional external cause code (Chapter XX), if desired, to identify toxic agent.
G95.82 Postradiation (radiation-induced) myelopathy
G95.83 Myelopathy due to lathyrism
G95.84 Cord bladder NOS

G95.9 Disease of spinal cord, unspecified

Myelopathy NOS

G96 Other disorders of central nervous system

G96.0 Cerebrospinal fluid leak

Excludes: from spinal puncture (G97.0)

G96.00 Cerebrospinal fluid rhinorrhoea
G96.01 Cerebrospinal fluid otorrhoea

G96.1 Disorders of meninges, not elsewhere classified

Includes: chronic adhesive meningitis
meningeal adhesions (cerebral)(spinal)

Excludes: spinal arachnoiditis NOS (G03.9)

G96.10 Opto-chiasmatic arachnoiditis
G96.11 Cranial arachnoiditis NOS
G96.18 Other specified disorders of meninges, not elsewhere classified

G96.8 Other specified disorders of central nervous system

G96.80 Cerebellar syndrome
G96.81 Persistent vegetative state
G96.82 Locked-in syndrome
G96.83 Akinetic mutism

G96.9 Disorder of central nervous system, unspecified

G97 Postprocedural disorders of nervous system, not elsewhere classified

G97.0 Cerebrospinal fluid leak from spinal puncture

G97.1 Other reaction to spinal and lumbar puncture

Post-lumbar puncture headache

G97.2 Intracranial hypotension following ventricular shunting

G97.8 Other postprocedural disorders of nervous system

G97.80 Late effects of radiation not elsewhere classified

Excludes: postradiation (radiation-induced):
- brachial plexopathy (G54.00)
- encephalopathy (G93.8)
- lumbosacral plexopathy (G54.10)
- myelopathy (G95.82)
- polyneuropathy (G62.80)

G97.9 Postprocedural disorder of nervous system, unspecified

G98 Other disorders of nervous system, not elsewhere classified

Nervous system disorder NOS

G99* Other disorders of nervous system in diseases classified elsewhere

G99.0* Autonomic neuropathy in endocrine and metabolic diseases

Diabetic autonomic neuropathy (E10–E14† with common fourth character .4)

Neuropathic heredofamilial amyloidosis (E85.1†)

G99.1* Other disorders of the autonomic nervous system in other diseases classified elsewhere

Autonomic nervous system disorder in:

- Chagas' disease (B57.4†)
- diabetic neuropathy (E10–E14† with common fourth character .4)
- HIV disease (B23.8†)
- injury of sympathetic nerves and plexuses (S14.5†, S24.4†, S34.5†)
- leprosy (A30.–†)
- neuropathic heredofamilial amyloidosis (E85.1†)
- other degenerative diseases of the basal ganglia (G23.–†)
- Parkinson's disease (G20.–†)
- porphyric neuropathy (E80.–†)
- remote effect of neoplasia (C00–D48†)
- spinal cord injury (S14.0†, S24.0†, S34.0†)
- syringomyelia and syringobulbia (G95.0†)
- thiamine deficiency (E51.–†)

G99.2* Myelopathy in diseases classified elsewhere

Includes: myelopathy (in) (due to):

- anterior spinal and vertebral artery compression syndromes (M47.0†)
- HIV disease (vacuolar myelopathy) (B23.8†)
- intervertebral disc disorders (M50.0†, M51.0†)
- neoplastic disease (C00–D48†)
- spinal cord compression due to diseases classified elsewhere
- spondylosis (M47.–†)
- vitamin B_{12} deficiency (E53.80†)

Excludes: myelopathy due to spinal cord injury (S14.0, S24.0, S34.0)

Use fifth character, if desired, to specify spinal cord level:

G99.20 Cervical spinal cord

G99.21 Cervicothoracic spinal cord
G99.22 Thoracic spinal cord
G99.23 Thoracolumbar spinal cord
G99.24 Lumbosacral spinal cord
G99.25 Sacral spinal cord
G99.27 Multiple or overlapping

G99.8* Other specified disorders of the nervous system in diseases classified elsewhere

CHAPTER VII

Diseases of the eye and adnexa (H00–H59)

Disorders of eyelid, lacrimal system and orbit (H00–H06)

H02 Other disorders of eyelid

H02.4 Ptosis of eyelid

H05 Disorders of orbit

Excludes: congenital malformation of orbit (Q10.7)

H05.0 Acute inflammation of orbit

Abscess, Cellulitis, Osteomyelitis, Periostitis } of orbit

Tenonitis

H05.1 Chronic inflammatory disorders of orbit

Granuloma of orbit

H05.2 Exophthalmic conditions

H05.20 Haemorrhage of orbit

H05.21 Oedema of orbit

H05.22 Ophthalmic Graves' disease (euthyroid)

Excludes: hypothyroidism with exophthalmus (E05.0)

H05.28 Other exophthalmic conditions

H05.29 Displacement of globe, unspecified

H05.3 Deformity of orbit

Atrophy, Exostosis } of orbit

H05.4 Enophthalmos

H05.5 Retained (old) foreign body following penetrating wound of orbit

Retrobulbar foreign body

H05.8 Other disorders of orbit
Cyst of orbit
Excludes: dysthyroid ophthalmoplegia (orbitopathy) (G73.50)

H05.9 Disorder of orbit, unspecified

Disorders of sclera, cornea, iris and ciliary body (H15–H22)

H16.– Keratitis

H20 Iridocyclitis

H20.0 Acute and subacute iridocyclitis
Anterior uveitis, Cyclitis, Iritis } acute, recurrent or subacute

H20.1 Chronic iridocyclitis

H20.2 Lens-induced iridocyclitis

H20.8 Other iridocyclitis

H20.9 Iridocyclitis, unspecified

Disorders of lens (H25–H28)

H25.– Senile cataract

Excludes: capsular glaucoma with pseudoexfoliation of lens (H40.1)

H26 Other cataract

H26.0 Infantile, juvenile and presenile cataract

H26.1 Traumatic cataract
Use additional external cause code (Chapter XX), if desired, to identify cause.

H26.2 Complicated cataract
Cataract in chronic iridocyclitis
Cataract secondary to ocular disorders
Glaucomatous flecks (subcapsular)

H26.3 Drug-induced cataract
Use additional external cause code (Chapter XX), if desired, to identify drug.

H26.4 After-cataract
Secondary cataract
Soemmerring's ring

H26.8 Other specified cataract

H26.9 Cataract, unspecified

H28* Cataract and other disorders of lens in diseases classified elsewhere

H28.0* Diabetic cataract (E10–E14† with common fourth character .3)

H28.1* Cataract in other endocrine, nutritional and metabolic diseases
Cataract in hypoparathyroidism (E20.–†)
Malnutrition–dehydration cataract (E46†)

H28.2* Cataract in other diseases classified elsewhere
Myotonic cataract (G71.1†)

H28.8* Other disorders of lens in diseases classified elsewhere

Disorders of choroid and retina (H30–H36)

H30 Chorioretinal inflammation

H30.0 Focal chorioretinal inflammation
Focal:
- chorioretinitis
- choroiditis
- retinitis
- retinochoroiditis

H30.1 Disseminated chorioretinal inflammation
Disseminated:
- chorioretinitis
- choroiditis
- retinitis
- retinochoroiditis

Excludes: exudative retinopathy (H35.0)

H30.2 Posterior cyclitis
Pars planitis

H30.8 Other chorioretinal inflammations
Harada's disease [Vogt–Koyanagi–Harada]

H30.9 Chorioretinal inflammation, unspecified
Chorioretinitis NOS
Choroiditis NOS
Retinitis NOS
Retinochoroiditis NOS

H31 Other disorders of choroid

H31.0 Chorioretinal scars
Macula scars of posterior pole (postinflammatory) (post-traumatic)
Solar retinopathy

H31.1 Choroidal degeneration
Atrophy of choroid
Sclerosis of choroid
Excludes: angioid streaks (H35.3)

H31.2 Hereditary choroidal dystrophy
Choroideremia
Dystrophy, choroidal (central areolar)(generalized)(peripapillary)
Gyrate atrophy, choroid
Excludes: ornithinaemia (E72.4)

H31.3 Choroidal haemorrhage and rupture
Choroidal haemorrhage:
- NOS
- expulsive

H31.4 Choroidal detachment

H31.8 Other specified disorders of choroid

H31.9 Disorder of choroid, unspecified

H32* Chorioretinal disorders in diseases classified elsewhere

H32.0* Chorioretinal inflammation in infectious and parasitic diseases classified elsewhere
Chorioretinitis:
- syphilitic, late (A52.7†)

- toxoplasma (B58.0†)
- tuberculous (A18.5†)

H32.8* **Other chorioretinal disorders in diseases classified elsewhere**

H33 Retinal detachments and breaks

H33.0 **Retinal detachment with retinal break**
Rhegmatogenous retinal detachment

H33.4 **Traction detachment of retina**
Proliferative vitreo-retinopathy with retinal detachment

H34 Retinal vascular occlusions

Excludes: amaurosis fugax (G45.3)

H34.0 **Transient retinal artery occlusion**

H34.1 **Central retinal artery occlusion**

H34.2 **Other retinal artery occlusions**
Hollenhorst's plaque
Retinal:
- artery occlusion:
  - branch
  - partial
- microembolism

H34.8 **Other retinal vascular occlusions**
Retinal vein occlusion:
- central
- incipient
- partial
- tributary

H34.9 **Retinal vascular occlusion, unspecified**

H35 Other retinal disorders

H35.0 **Background retinopathy and retinal vascular changes**
Changes in retinal vascular appearance
Retinal:
- micro-aneurysms
- neovascularization
- perivasculitis
- varices

- vascular sheathing
- vasculitis

Retinopathy:
- NOS
- background NOS
- Coats'
- exudative
- hypertensive

H35.1 Retinopathy of prematurity
Retrolental fibroplasia

H35.2 Other proliferative retinopathy
Proliferative vitreo-retinopathy
Excludes: proliferative vitreo-retinopathy with retinal detachment (H33.4)

H35.3 Degeneration of macula and posterior pole
Angioid streaks, Cyst, Drusen (degenerative), Hole, Puckering } of macula
Kuhnt–Junius degeneration
Senile macular degeneration (atrophic)(exudative)
Toxic maculopathy

Use additional external cause code (Chapter XX), if desired, to identify drug, if drug-induced.

H35.4 Peripheral retinal degeneration
Degeneration, retina:
- NOS
- lattice
- microcystoid
- palisade
- paving stone
- reticular

H35.5 Hereditary retinal dystrophy
Dystrophy:
- retinal (albipunctate)(pigmentary)(vitelliform)
- tapetoretinal
- vitreoretinal

Retinitis pigmentosa
Stargardt's disease

H35.6 Retinal haemorrhage

H35.7 Separation of retinal layers
Central serous chorioretinopathy
Detachment of retinal pigment epithelium

H35.8 Other specified retinal disorders

H35.9 Retinal disorder, unspecified

H36* Retinal disorders in diseases classified elsewhere

H36.0* Diabetic retinopathy (E10–E14† with common fourth character .3)

H36.8* Other retinal disorders in diseases classified elsewhere
Atherosclerotic retinopathy (I70.80†)
Proliferative sickle-cell retinopathy (D57.–†)
Retinal dystrophy in lipid storage disorders (E75.–†)

Glaucoma (H40–H42)

H40 Glaucoma

Excludes: congenital glaucoma (Q15.0)

H40.0 Glaucoma suspect
Ocular hypertension

H40.1 Primary open-angle glaucoma
Glaucoma (primary)(residual stage):
- capsular with pseudoexfoliation of lens
- chronic simple
- low-tension
- pigmentary

H40.2 Primary angle-closure glaucoma
Angle-closure glaucoma (primary)(residual stage):
- acute
- chronic
- intermittent

H40.3 Glaucoma secondary to eye trauma
Use additional code, if desired, to identify cause.

H40.4 Glaucoma secondary to eye inflammation
Use additional code, if desired, to identify cause.

H40.5 Glaucoma secondary to other eye disorders
Use additional code, if desired, to identify cause.

H40.6 Glaucoma secondary to drugs
Use additional external cause code (Chapter XX), if desired, to identify drug.

H40.8 Other glaucoma

H40.9 Glaucoma, unspecified

H42.–* Glaucoma in diseases classified elsewhere

Disorders of vitreous body and globe (H43–H45)

H44 Disorders of globe

Includes: disorders affecting multiple structures of eye

H44.2 Degenerative myopia

H44.4 Hypotony of eye

H44.7 Retained (old) intraocular foreign body, nonmagnetic

Disorders of optic nerve and visual pathways (H46–H48)

H46 Optic neuritis

Optic:
- neuropathy, except ischaemic
- papillitis

Retrobulbar neuritis NOS

Excludes: ischaemic optic neuropathy (H47.02)
neuromyelitis optica [Devic] (G36.0)

H47 Other disorders of optic [2nd] nerve and visual pathways

H47.0 Disorders of optic nerve, not elsewhere classified

H47.00 Compression of optic nerve
H47.01 Haemorrhage in optic nerve sheath

H47.02 Ischaemic optic neuropathy
H47.03 Post-infection optic neuropathy
H47.08 Other disorders of optic nerve, not elsewhere classified

H47.1 Papilloedema, unspecified

H47.2 Optic atrophy
Includes: temporal pallor of optic disc

H47.20 Primary optic atrophy
H47.21 Leber's optic atrophy
H47.22 Dominantly inherited optic atrophy
H47.23 Recessively inherited optic atrophy
H47.24 Optic atrophy with the syndrome of diabetes insipidus, diabetes mellitus and deafness
H47.28 Other specified type of optic atrophy

H47.3 Other disorders of optic disc

H47.30 Drusen of optic disc
H47.31 Pseudopapilloedema

H47.4 Disorders of optic chiasm

H47.5 Disorders of other visual pathways

H47.50 Disorders of optic tracts
H47.51 Disorders of geniculate nuclei
H47.52 Disorders of optic radiations

H47.6 Disorders of visual cortex
Cortical blindness

H47.7 Disorder of visual pathways, unspecified

H48* Disorders of optic [2nd] nerve and visual pathways in diseases classified elsewhere

H48.0* Optic atrophy in diseases classified elsewhere
Optic atrophy in late syphilis (A52.1†)

H48.1* Retrobulbar neuritis in diseases classified elsewhere
Retrobulbar neuritis in:
- late syphilis (A52.1†)
- meningococcal infection (A39.8†)
- multiple sclerosis (G35.–†)

H48.8* **Other disorders of optic nerve and visual pathways in diseases classified elsewhere**

H48.80* Papilloedema in diseases classified elsewhere
Papilloedema in:
- decreased ocular pressure (H44.4†)
- pseudotumor cerebri (G93.2†)
- raised intracranial pressure (G91.–†, G94.1†, G94.2†)
- retinal lesion (H33–H36†)
- systemic hypertension (I10†)

H48.81* Disorders of optic nerve in diseases classified elsewhere

H48.82* Disorders of visual pathways in diseases classified elsewhere

Disorders of ocular muscles, binocular movement, accommodation and refraction (H49–H52)

Excludes: nystagmus and other irregular eye movements (H55.–)

H49 Paralytic strabismus

Excludes: ophthalmoplegia:
- internal (H52.50)
- internuclear (H51.2)
- progressive supranuclear (G23.1)

H49.0 **Third [oculomotor] nerve palsy**

H49.00 Third [oculomotor] nerve palsy, extrinsic and intrinsic
H49.01 Third [oculomotor] nerve palsy, extrinsic (sparing pupil)
H49.02 Third [oculomotor] nerve palsy, nuclear

H49.1 **Fourth [trochlear] nerve palsy**

H49.2 **Sixth [abducent] nerve palsy**

H49.20 Sixth [abducent] nerve palsy, peripheral
H49.21 Sixth [abducent] nerve palsy, nuclear

H49.3 **Total (external) ophthalmoplegia**

H49.4 **Progressive external ophthalmoplegia**

H49.8 **Other paralytic strabismus**
External ophthalmoplegia NOS
Kearns–Sayre syndrome

H49.9 Paralytic strabismus, unspecified

H50 Other strabismus

H50.0 Convergent concomitant strabismus
Esotropia (alternating)(monocular), except intermittent

H50.1 Divergent concomitant strabismus
Exotropia (alternating)(monocular), except intermittent

H50.2 Vertical strabismus

H50.3 Intermittent heterotropia
Intermittent:
- esotropia } (alternating)(monocular)
- exotropia }

H50.4 Other and unspecified heterotropia
Concomitant strabismus NOS
Cyclotropia
Hypertropia
Hypotropia
Microtropia
Monofixation syndrome

H50.5 Heterophoria
Alternating hyperphoria
Esophoria
Exophoria
Skew deviation

H50.6 Mechanical strabismus
Brown's sheath syndrome
Strabismus due to adhesions
Traumatic limitation of duction of eye muscle

H50.8 Other specified strabismus
Duane's syndrome

H50.9 Strabismus, unspecified

H51 Other disorders of binocular movement

H51.0 Palsy of conjugate gaze
Excludes: in brain stem syndromes (G46.3)

H51.00 Supranuclear lateral gaze palsy
H51.01 One-and-a-half syndrome
H51.08 Other palsy of conjugate gaze

H51.1 Convergence insufficiency and excess

H51.2 Internuclear ophthalmoplegia

H51.8 Other specified disorders of binocular movement

H51.80 Oculomotor apraxia
H51.81 Paralysis of upward gaze
H51.82 Paralysis of downward gaze
H51.83 Parinaud's syndrome

H51.9 Disorder of binocular movement, unspecified

H52 Disorders of refraction and accommodation

H52.0 Hypermetropia

H52.1 Myopia
Excludes: degenerative myopia (H44.2)

H52.2 Astigmatism

H52.3 Anisometropia and aniseikonia

H52.4 Presbyopia

H52.5 Disorders of accommodation

H52.50 Internal ophthalmoplegia (complete)(total)
H52.51 Paresis or spasm of accommodation
H52.52 Spasm of the near reflex
H52.58 Other disorders of accommodation

H52.6 Other disorders of refraction

H52.7 Disorder of refraction, unspecified

Visual disturbances and blindness (H53–H54)

H53 Visual disturbances

H53.0 Amblyopia ex anopsia
Amblyopia:
- anisometropic
- deprivation
- strabismic

H53.1 Subjective visual disturbances

Asthenopia
Day blindness
Hemeralopia
Metamorphopsia
Photophobia
Scintillating scotoma
Sudden visual loss
Visual halos
Excludes: visual hallucinations (R44.1)

H53.2 Diplopia

Includes: double vision

H53.20 Organic monocular diplopia
H53.21 Binocular diplopia

H53.3 Other disorders of binocular vision

Abnormal retinal correspondence
Fusion with defective stereopsis
Simultaneous visual perception without fusion
Suppression of binocular vision

H53.4 Visual field defects

Enlarged blind spot
Generalized contraction of visual field
Hemianop(s)ia (heteronymous)(homonymous)
Quadrant anop(s)ia
Scotoma:
- arcuate
- Bjerrum
- central
- ring

H53.5 Colour vision deficiencies

Achromatopsia
Acquired colour vision deficiency
Colour blindness
Deuteranomaly
Deuteranopia
Protanomaly
Protanopia
Tritanomaly
Tritanopia
Excludes: day blindness (H53.1)

H53.6 Night blindness
Excludes: due to vitamin A deficiency (E50.5)

H53.8 Other visual disturbances

H53.9 Visual disturbance, unspecified

H54 Blindness and low vision

Note: For definition of visual impairment categories see table on p. 246.

Excludes: amaurosis fugax (G45.3)

H54.0 Blindness, both eyes
Visual impairment categories 3, 4, 5 in both eyes.

H54.1 Blindness, one eye, low vision other eye
Visual impairment categories 3, 4, 5 in one eye, with category 1 or 2 in the other eye.

H54.2 Low vision, both eyes
Visual impairment category 1 or 2 in both eyes.

H54.3 Unqualified visual loss, both eyes
Visual impairment category 9 in both eyes.

H54.4 Blindness, one eye
Visual impairment categories 3, 4, 5 in one eye [normal vision in other eye].

H54.5 Low vision, one eye
Visual impairment category 1 or 2 in one eye [normal vision in other eye].

H54.6 Unqualified visual loss, one eye
Visual impairment category 9 in one eye [normal vision in other eye].

H54.7 Unspecified visual loss
Visual impairment category 9 NOS

Note: The table on p. 246 gives a classification of severity of visual impairment recommended by a WHO Study Group on the Prevention of Blindness, Geneva, 6–10 November 1972.[1]

The term "low vision" in category H54 comprises categories 1 and 2 of the table, the term "blindness" categories 3, 4 and 5 and the term "unqualified visual loss" category 9.

---

[1] WHO Technical Report Series, No. 518, 1973.

Category of visual impairment	Visual acuity with best possible correction	
	Maximum less than:	Minimum equal to or better than:
1	6/18 3/10 (0.3) 20/70	6/60 1/10 (0.1) 20/200
2	6/60 1/10 (0.1) 20/200	3/60 1/20 (0.05) 20/400
3	3/60 1/20 (0.05) 20/400	1/60 (finger counting at 1 metre) 1/50 (0.02) 5/300 (20/1200)
4	1/60 (finger counting at 1 metre) 1/50 (0.02) 5/300	Light perception
5	No light perception	
9	Undetermined or unspecified	

If the extent of the visual field is taken into account, patients with a field no greater than 10° but greater than 5° around central fixation should be placed in category 3 and patients with a field no greater than 5° around central fixation should be placed in category 4, even if the central acuity is not impaired.

Other disorders of eye and adnexa (H55–H59)

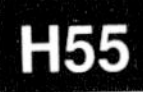 H55 Nystagmus and other irregular eye movements

Includes: nystagmus:
- NOS
- congenital
- deprivation
- dissociated
- latent

Excludes: idiopathic central positional nystagmus (H81.40)

H55.–0 Upbeat nystagmus
H55.–1 Downbeat nystagmus
H55.–2 Phasic lateral nystagmus
H55.–3 Rotatory (torsional) nystagmus
H55.–4 See-saw nystagmus
H55.–5 Nystagmus retractorius
H55.–6 Deficiencies of saccadic eye movements
H55.–7 Deficiencies of smooth pursuits
H55.–8 Other irregular eye movements

H57 Other disorders of eye and adnexa

H57.0 Anomalies of pupillary function

Excludes: Holmes–Adie syndrome (G90.80)

H57.00 Adi's (myotonic) pupil
H57.01 Paraneoplastic myotonic pupil
H57.02 Springing pupil
H57.03 Anisocoria NOS
H57.08 Other anomaly of pupillary function

H57.1 Ocular pain

H57.8 Other specified disorders of eye and adnexa

H57.9 Disorder of eye and adnexa, unspecified

H58* Other disorders of eye and adnexa in diseases classified elsewhere

H58.0* Anomalies of pupillary function in diseases classified elsewhere

Argyll Robertson phenomenon or pupil, syphilitic (A52.1†)

H58.1* Visual disturbances in diseases classified elsewhere

H58.8* Other specified disorders of eye and adnexa in diseases classified elsewhere

Syphilitic oculopathy NEC:
- congenital:
  - early (A50.0†)
  - late (A50.3†)
- early (secondary) (A51.4†)
- late (A52.7†)

H59 Postprocedural disorders of eye and adnexa, not elsewhere classified

H59.0 Vitreous syndrome following cataract surgery

H59.8 Other postprocedural disorders of eye and adnexa
Chorioretinal scars after surgery for detachment

H59.9 Postprocedural disorder of eye and adnexa, unspecified

CHAPTER VIII

Diseases of the ear and mastoid process (H60–H95)

Diseases of middle ear and mastoid (H65–H75)

H65 Nonsuppurative otitis media

Includes: with myringitis

H65.0 Acute serous otitis media

Acute and subacute secretory otitis media

H65.1 Other acute nonsuppurative otitis media

Otitis media, acute and subacute:
- allergic (mucoid)(sanguinous)(serous)
- mucoid
- nonsuppurative NOS
- sanguinous
- seromucinous

Excludes: otitic barotrauma (T70.0)
otitis media (acute) NOS (H66.9)

H65.2 Chronic serous otitis media

Chronic tubotympanal catarrh

H65.3 Chronic mucoid otitis media

Glue ear

Otitis media, chronic:
- mucinous
- secretory
- transudative

H65.4 Other chronic nonsuppurative otitis media

Otitis media, chronic:
- allergic
- exudative
- nonsuppurative NOS
- seromucinous
- with effusion (nonpurulent)

H65.9 Nonsuppurative otitis media, unspecified
Otitis media:
- allergic
- catarrhal
- exudative
- mucoid
- secretory
- seromucinous
- serous
- transudative
- with effusion (nonpurulent)

H66 Suppurative and unspecified otitis media
Includes: with myringitis

H66.0 Acute suppurative otitis media

H66.1 Chronic tubotympanic suppurative otitis media
Benign chronic suppurative otitis media
Chronic tubotympanic disease

H66.2 Chronic atticoantral suppurative otitis media
Chronic atticoantral disease

H66.3 Other chronic suppurative otitis media
Chronic suppurative otitis media NOS

H66.4 Suppurative otitis media, unspecified
Purulent otitis media NOS

H66.9 Otitis media, unspecified
Otitis media:
- NOS
- acute NOS
- chronic NOS

H70 Mastoiditis and related conditions

H70.0 Acute mastoiditis
Abscess } of mastoid
Empyema }

H70.1 Chronic mastoiditis
Caries } of mastoid
Fistula }

H70.2 Petrositis
Inflammation of petrous bone (acute)(chronic)

H70.8 Other mastoiditis and related conditions

H70.9 Mastoiditis, unspecified

H71 Cholesteatoma of middle ear

Cholesteatoma tympani

Excludes: recurrent cholesteatoma of postmastoidectomy cavity (H95.0)

H72.– Perforation of tympanic membrane

Includes: perforation of ear drum:
- persistent post-traumatic
- postinflammatory

Excludes: traumatic rupture of ear drum (S09.2)

H73.– Other disorders of tympanic membrane

Diseases of inner ear (H80–H83)

H81 Disorders of vestibular function

Excludes: vertigo:
- NOS (R42)
- epidemic (A88.1)

H81.0 Ménière's disease

Labyrinthine hydrops

Ménière's syndrome or vertigo

H81.1 Benign paroxysmal vertigo

H81.10 Idiopathic benign positional vertigo

H81.11 Post-traumatic benign positional vertigo

H81.18 Other benign paroxysmal vertigo

H81.2 Vestibular neuronitis

H81.3 Other peripheral vertigo

Includes: peripheral vertigo NOS

H81.30 Lermoyez' syndrome

H81.31 Aural vertigo

H81.32 Otogenic vertigo

H81.33 Drug-induced peripheral vertigo

Use additional code (Chapter XX), if desired, to identify drug.

H81.4 Vertigo of central origin

H81.40 Idiopathic central positional nystagmus

H81.41 Drug-induced vertigo of central origin
Use additional code (Chapter XX), if desired, to identify drug.

H81.48 Other vertigo of central origin

H81.8 Other disorders of vestibular function

H81.9 Disorder of vestibular function, unspecified
Includes: vertiginous syndrome NOS

H81.90 Drug-induced vertigo, unspecified as peripheral or central
Use additional code (Chapter XX), if desired, to identify drug.

H82* Vertiginous syndromes in diseases classified elsewhere

H83 Other diseases of inner ear

H83.0 Labyrinthitis

H83.1 Labyrinthine fistula

H83.2 Labyrinthine dysfunction
Hypersensitivity } of labyrinth
Hypofunction } of labyrinth
Loss of function } of labyrinth

H83.3 Noise effects on inner ear
Acoustic trauma
Noise-induced hearing loss

H83.8 Other specified diseases of inner ear

H83.9 Disease of inner ear, unspecified

Other disorders of ear (H90–H95)

H90 Conductive and sensorineural hearing loss

Includes: congenital deafness
Excludes: deaf mutism NEC (H91.3)
deafness NOS (H91.9)

hearing loss:
- NOS (H91.9)
- noise-induced (H83.3)
- ototoxic (H91.0)
- sudden (idiopathic) (H91.2)

H90.1 Conductive hearing loss, unilateral with unrestricted hearing on the contralateral side

H90.2 Conductive hearing loss, unspecified
Conductive deafness NOS

H90.3 Sensorineural hearing loss, bilateral

H90.4 Sensorineural hearing loss, unilateral with unrestricted hearing on the contralateral side

H90.5 Sensorineural hearing loss, unspecified
Hearing loss:
- central NOS
- neural NOS
- perceptive NOS
- sensory NOS

Sensorineural deafness NOS

H90.6 Mixed conductive and sensorineural hearing loss, bilateral

H90.7 Mixed conductive and sensorineural hearing loss, unilateral with unrestricted hearing on the contralateral side

H90.8 Mixed conductive and sensorineural hearing loss, unspecified

H91 Other hearing loss

Excludes: abnormal auditory perception (H93.2)
noise-induced hearing loss (H83.3)
psychogenic deafness (F44.6)
transient ischaemic deafness (H93.0)

H91.0 Ototoxic hearing loss
Use additional external cause code (Chapter XX), if desired, to identify toxic agent.

H91.1 Presbycusis
Presbyacusia

H91.2 Sudden idiopathic hearing loss
Sudden hearing loss NOS

H91.3 **Deaf mutism, not elsewhere classified**

H91.8 **Other specified hearing loss**

H91.9 **Hearing loss, unspecified**

Deafness:

- NOS
- high frequency
- low frequency

H92 Otalgia and effusion of ear

H92.0 **Otalgia**

H92.1 **Otorrhoea**

Excludes: leakage of cerebrospinal fluid through ear (G96.0)

H92.2 **Otorrhagia**

Excludes: traumatic otorrhagia — code by type of injury

H93 Other disorders of ear, not elsewhere classified

H93.0 **Degenerative and vascular disorders of ear**

Transient ischaemic deafness

Excludes: presbycusis (H91.1)

H93.1 **Tinnitus**

H93.2 **Other abnormal auditory perceptions**

Auditory recruitment

Diplacusis

Hyperacusis

Temporary auditory threshold shift

Excludes: auditory hallucinations (R44.0)

H93.3 **Disorders of acoustic nerve**

Includes: disorder of 8th cranial nerve

H93.30 Schwannoma [neurinoma] [neurilemmoma] of acoustic nerve

H93.31 Compression of acoustic nerve in tumours of cerebello-pontine angle

Use morphology code, if desired, to identify the tumour.

H93.32 Acoustic nerve damage due to meningitis

H93.33 Acoustic nerve damage due to vascular diseases

H93.38 Other specified disorders of acoustic nerve

H93.8 **Other specified disorders of ear**

H93.9 Disorder of ear, unspecified

H94* Other disorders of ear in diseases classified elsewhere

H94.0* Acoustic neuritis in infectious and parasitic diseases classified elsewhere

Acoustic neuritis in syphilis (A52.1†)

H94.8* Other specified disorders of ear in diseases classified elsewhere

H95 Postprocedural disorders of ear and mastoid process, not elsewhere classified

H95.0 Recurrent cholesteatoma of postmastoidectomy cavity

CHAPTER IX

Diseases of the circulatory system (I00–I99)

Excludes: transient cerebral ischaemic attacks and related syndromes (G45.–)

Acute rheumatic fever (I00–I02)

I00 Rheumatic fever without mention of heart involvement

Arthritis, rheumatic, acute or subacute

I01 Rheumatic fever with heart involvement

Excludes: chronic diseases of rheumatic origin (I05–I09)

I01.1 Acute rheumatic endocarditis

Acute rheumatic valvulitis

Any condition in I00 with endocarditis or valvulitis

I01.9 Acute rheumatic heart disease, unspecified

Any condition in I00 with unspecified type of heart involvement

Rheumatic:
- carditis, acute
- heart disease, active or acute

I02 Rheumatic chorea

Includes: Sydenham's chorea

Excludes: chorea:
- NOS (G25.5)
- Huntington (G10.–)

I02.0 Rheumatic chorea with heart involvement

Chorea NOS with heart involvement

Rheumatic chorea with heart involvement of any type classifiable under I01.–

I02.9 Rheumatic chorea without heart involvement

Rheumatic chorea NOS

Chronic rheumatic heart diseases (I05–I09)

I05 Rheumatic mitral valve diseases

Excludes: when specified as nonrheumatic (I34.–)

I05.0 Mitral stenosis

Mitral (valve) obstruction (rheumatic)

I05.1 Rheumatic mitral insufficiency

Rheumatic mitral:
- incompetence
- regurgitation

I05.2 Mitral stenosis with insufficiency

Mitral stenosis with incompetence or regurgitation

I06.– Rheumatic aortic valve diseases

Excludes: when not specified as rheumatic (I35.–)

I07.– Rheumatic tricuspid valve diseases

Includes: whether specified as rheumatic or not
Excludes: when specified as nonrheumatic (I36.–)

I08 Multiple valve diseases

Includes: whether specified as rheumatic or not
Excludes: endocarditis, valve unspecified (I38)
rheumatic disease of endocardium, valve unspecified (I09.1)

I08.0 Disorders of mitral and aortic valves

Involvement of both mitral and aortic valves whether specified as rheumatic or not

I09 Other rheumatic heart diseases

I09.1 Rheumatic diseases of endocardium, valve unspecified

Rheumatic:
- endocarditis (chronic)
- valvulitis (chronic)

Excludes: endocarditis, valve unspecified (I38)

I09.8 Other specified rheumatic heart diseases

Rheumatic disease of pulmonary valve

I09.9 Rheumatic heart disease, unspecified

Rheumatic:
- carditis
- heart failure

Excludes: rheumatoid carditis (M05.3)

Hypertensive diseases (I10–I15)

I10 Essential (primary) hypertension

High blood pressure

Hypertension (arterial)(benign)(essential)(malignant)(primary)(systemic)

Excludes: involving vessels of:
- brain (I60–I69)
- eye (H35.0)

I11.– Hypertensive heart disease

Includes: any condition in I50.– due to hypertension

I12.– Hypertensive renal disease

Includes: any condition in N18.– or N19 with any condition in I10
arteriosclerosis of kidney
arteriosclerotic nephritis (chronic)(interstitial)
hypertensive nephropathy
nephrosclerosis

Excludes: secondary hypertension (I15.–)

I13.– Hypertensive heart and renal disease

Includes: any condition in I11.– with any condition in I12.–
disease:
- cardiorenal
- cardiovascular renal

I15.– Secondary hypertension

Excludes: involving vessels of:
- brain (I60–I69)
- eye (H35.0)

Ischaemic heart disease (I20–I25)

Note: For morbidity, duration as used in categories I21–I25 refers to the interval elapsing between onset of the ischaemic episode and admission to care. For mortality, duration refers to the interval elapsing between onset and death.

Includes: with mention of hypertension (I10–I15)

Use additional code, if desired, to identify presence of hypertension.

I20.– Angina pectoris

I21.– Acute myocardial infarction

Includes: myocardial infarction specified as acute or with a stated duration of 4 weeks (28 days) or less from onset

Excludes: myocardial infarction:
- old (I25.2)
- specified as chronic or with a stated duration of more than 4 weeks (more than 28 days) from onset (I25.8)
- subsequent (I22.–)

I22.– Subsequent myocardial infarction

Includes: recurrent myocardial infarction

Excludes: specified as chronic or with a stated duration of more than 4 weeks (more than 28 days) from onset (I25.8)

I24.– Other acute ischaemic heart diseases

Excludes: angina pectoris (I20.–)

I25 Chronic ischaemic heart disease

I25.0 Atherosclerotic cardiovascular disease, so described

I25.1 Atherosclerotic heart disease

Coronary (artery):
- atheroma
- atherosclerosis
- disease
- sclerosis

I25.2 Old myocardial infarction

Healed myocardial infarction

Past myocardial infarction diagnosed by ECG or other special investigation, but currently presenting no symptoms

I25.3 Aneurysm of heart
Aneurysm:
- mural
- ventricular

I25.5 Ischaemic cardiomyopathy

I25.8 Other forms of chronic ischaemic heart disease
Any condition in I21–I22 and I24.– specified as chronic or with a stated duration of more than 4 weeks (more than 28 days) from onset

I25.9 Chronic ischaemic heart disease, unspecified
Ischaemic heart disease (chronic) NOS

Other forms of heart disease (I30–I52)

I34.– Nonrheumatic mitral valve disorders

Excludes: when of unspecified cause but with mention of:
- diseases of aortic valve (I08.0)
- mitral stenosis or obstruction (I05.0)

when specified as rheumatic (I05.–)

I35.– Nonrheumatic aortic valve disorders

Excludes: when of unspecified cause but with mention of diseases of mitral valve (I08.0)
when specified as rheumatic (I06.–)

I36.– Nonrheumatic tricuspid valve disorders

Excludes: when of unspecified cause (I07.–)
when specified as rheumatic (I07.–)

I37.– Pulmonary valve disorders

Excludes: when specified as rheumatic (I09.8)

I38 Endocarditis, valve unspecified

Endocarditis (chronic) NOS
Valvular:
- incompetence
- insufficiency
- regurgitation
- stenosis

Valvulitis (chronic)

} of unspecified valve { NOS or of specified cause, except rheumatic

Excludes: when specified as rheumatic (I09.1)

I39*.– Endocarditis and heart valve disorders in diseases classified elsewhere

Includes: endocardial involvement in:
- gonococcal infection (A54.8†)
- Libman–Sacks disease (M32.1†)
- meningococcal infection (A39.5†)
- rheumatoid arthritis (M05.3†)
- syphilis (A52.0†)
- typhoid fever (A01.–†)

I41* Myocarditis in diseases classified elsewhere

I41.0* Myocarditis in bacterial diseases classified elsewhere

I41.1* Myocarditis in viral diseases classified elsewhere

I41.2* Myocarditis in other infectious and parasitic diseases classified elsewhere

Myocarditis in:
- Chagas' disease (chronic) (B57.2†)
  - acute (B57.0†)
- toxoplasmosis (B58.8†)

I41.8* Myocarditis in other diseases classified elsewhere

Rheumatoid myocarditis (M05.3†)

I42.– Cardiomyopathy

Excludes: ischaemic cardiomyopathy (I25.5)

I43.*– Cardiomyopathy in diseases classified elsewhere

I44 Atrioventricular and left bundle-branch block

I44.0 Atrioventricular block, first degree

I44.1 Atrioventricular block, second degree

Atrioventricular block, type I and II
Möbitz block, type I and II
Second-degree block, type I and II
Wenckebach's block

I44.2 Atrioventricular block, complete

Complete heart block NOS
Third-degree block

I44.3 Other and unspecified atrioventricular block

Atrioventricular block NOS

I44.4 **Left anterior fascicular block**

I44.5 **Left posterior fascicular block**

I44.6 **Other and unspecified fascicular block**
Left bundle-branch hemiblock NOS

I44.7 **Left bundle-branch block, unspecified**

I45 Other conduction disorders

I45.0 **Right fascicular block**

I45.1 **Other and unspecified right bundle-branch block**
Right bundle-branch block NOS

I45.2 **Bifascicular block**

I45.3 **Trifascicular block**

I45.4 **Nonspecific intraventricular block**
Bundle-branch block NOS

I45.5 **Other specified heart block**
Sinoatrial block
Sinoauricular block
Excludes: heart block NOS (I45.9)

I45.9 **Conduction disorder, unspecified**
Heart block NOS
Stokes–Adams syndrome

I46 Cardiac arrest

Excludes: cardiogenic shock (R57.0)

I46.0 **Cardiac arrest with successful resuscitation**

I47 Paroxysmal tachycardia

I47.0 **Re-entry ventricular arrhythmia**

I47.1 **Supraventricular tachycardia**
Paroxysmal tachycardia:
- atrial
- atrioventricular [AV]
- junctional
- nodal

I47.2 **Ventricular tachycardia**

I47.9 **Paroxysmal tachycardia, unspecified**
Bouveret(–Hoffman) syndrome

I48 Atrial fibrillation and flutter

I49 Other cardiac arrhythmias

I49.0 Ventricular fibrillation and flutter

I49.1 Atrial premature depolarization
Atrial premature beats

I49.2 Junctional premature depolarization

I49.3 Ventricular premature depolarization

I49.4 Other and unspecified premature depolarization
Ectopic beats
Extrasystoles
Extrasystolic arrhythmias
Premature:
• beats NOS
• contractions

I49.5 Sick sinus syndrome
Tachycardia–bradycardia syndrome

I49.8 Other specified cardiac arrhythmias
Rhythm disorder:
• coronary sinus
• ectopic
• nodal

I49.9 Cardiac arrhythmia, unspecified
Arrhythmia (cardiac) NOS

I50.– Heart failure

Excludes: due to hypertension (I11.–)
• with renal disease (I13.–)

Cerebrovascular diseases (I60–I69)

Includes: with mention of hypertension (conditions in I10 and I15.–)

Use additional code, if desired, to identify presence of hypertension.

Excludes: transient cerebral ischaemic attacks and related syndromes (G45.–)
traumatic intracranial haemorrhage (S06.–)
vascular dementia (F01.–)

I60 Subarachnoid haemorrhage

Includes: ruptured cerebral aneurysm

In case of multiple intracranial aneurysms, use additional code(s) (I67.1*xxx*), if desired, to identify the unruptured aneurysm(s).

Excludes: sequelae of subarachnoid haemorrhage (I69.0)
traumatic subarachnoid haemorrhage (S06.6)

For I60.0–I60.6: use additional sixth character, if desired, to indicate side:

I60.*xx*0 Left
I60.*xx*1 Right
I60.*xx*2 Bilateral

I60.0 Subarachnoid haemorrhage from carotid siphon and bifurcation

I60.00 Aneurysm at origin of ophthalmic artery
I60.01 Aneurysm at origin of anterior choroidal artery
I60.02 Aneurysm at origin of posterior communicating artery
I60.03 Aneurysm at bifurcation of internal carotid artery
I60.04 Carotido-cavernous aneurysm

I60.1 Subarachnoid haemorrhage from middle cerebral artery

Use additional code (I60.83), if desired, in case of mycotic aneurysm.

I60.10 Proximal (M1-horizontal segment) middle cerebral artery aneurysm
I60.11 Aneurysm at major bi- or trifurcation of middle cerebral artery
I60.12 Distal middle cerebral artery aneurysm

I60.2 Subarachnoid haemorrhage from anterior communicating artery

Use additional code (I60.83), if desired, in case of mycotic aneurysm.

I60.20 Anterior communicating artery aneurysm
I60.21 Proximal (A1-horizontal segment) anterior cerebral artery aneurysm

I60.22 Distal (A2-vertical segment) anterior cerebral artery aneurysm
I60.23 Pericallosal bifurcation artery aneurysm

I60.3 Subarachnoid haemorrhage from posterior communicating artery
Distal posterior communicating artery aneurysm

I60.4 Subarachnoid haemorrhage from basilar artery
Use additional code (I60.85), if desired, in case of dissecting aneurysm.

I60.40 Proximal basilar artery (vertebral artery confluence) aneurysm
I60.41 Midbasilar artery aneurysm
I60.42 Top of basilar artery aneurysm
I60.43 Bifid basilar artery aneurysm
I60.44 Aneurysm at origin of superior cerebellar artery
I60.45 Aneurysm at origin of anterior inferior cerebellar artery

I60.5 Subarachnoid haemorrhage from vertebral artery
Includes: intracranial vertebral artery aneurysm
Use additional code (I60.85), if desired, in case of dissecting aneurysm.

I60.50 Aneurysm at origin of posterior inferior cerebellar artery
I60.51 Subarachnoid haemorrhage from ruptured spinal artery aneurysm

I60.6 Subarachnoid haemorrhage from other intracranial arteries

I60.60 Distal superior cerebellar artery aneurysm
I60.61 Distal anterior inferior cerebellar artery aneurysm
I60.62 Distal posterior inferior cerebellar artery aneurysm
I60.63 Internal auditory artery aneurysm
I60.64 Proximal posterior cerebral artery aneurysm
I60.65 Distal posterior cerebral artery aneurysm
I60.67 Ruptured aneurysms of several intracranial arteries
I60.68 Aneurysm of other specified intracranial arteries

I60.7 Subarachnoid haemorrhage from intracranial artery, unspecified
Ruptured (congenital) berry aneurysm NOS
Subarachnoid haemorrhage from:
- cerebral artery NOS
- communicating artery NOS
- multiple cerebral arteries NOS

I60.8 Other subarachnoid haemorrhage

Includes: meningeal haemorrhage

I60.80 Rupture of specified arteriovenous malformation

Excludes: nonruptured arteriovenous malformation of cerebral vessels (Q28.2)

I60.800 Ruptured arteriovenous malformation in hemisphere, cortical

I60.8000 Frontal

I60.8001 Temporal

I60.8002 Parietal

I60.8003 Occipital

I60.8007 Involving more than one lobe

I60.801 Ruptured arteriovenous malformation in hemisphere, subcortical

I60.8010 Basal ganglia

I60.8011 Internal capsule

I60.8012 Thalamus

I60.8013 Hypothalamus

I60.8014 Corpus callosum

I60.8017 Involving more than one subcortical structure

I60.802 Ruptured arteriovenous malformation in hemisphere, unspecified

I60.803 Ruptured arteriovenous malformation in brain stem

I60.8030 Midbrain

I60.8031 Pons

I60.8032 Medulla

I60.8037 Involving more than one subdivision of brain stem

I60.804 Ruptured arteriovenous malformation in cerebellum

I60.805 Ruptured arteriovenous malformation in choroid plexus

I60.8050 Choroid plexus in lateral ventricle

I60.8051 Choroid plexus in third ventricle

I60.8052 Choroid plexus in fourth ventricle

I60.8057 Multiple locations in choroid plexus

I60.806 Ruptured arteriovenous malformation in spinal cord

I60.8060 Cervical spinal cord

I60.8061 Thoracic spinal cord

I60.8062 Lumbosacral spinal cord

I60.8067 More than one subdivision of spinal cord

I60.807 Multiple or widespread ruptured arteriovenous malformation

I60.81 Subarachnoid haemorrhage from coagulation disorder classified elsewhere
Use additional code, if desired, to indicate associated disorder.

I60.82 Subarachnoid haemorrhage from primary intracerebral haemorrhage classified elsewhere
Use additional code (I61), if desired, to indicate the type of haemorrhage.

I60.83 Subarachnoid haemorrhage from ruptured mycotic aneurysm

I60.84 Subarachnoid haemorrhage from intracranial artery dissection (dissecting aneurysm)

I60.85 Subarachnoid haemorrhage due to tumour
Use additional code, if desired, to identify tumour.

I60.9 Subarachnoid haemorrhage, unspecified

I60.90 Ruptured (congenital) cerebral aneurysm NOS

I60.91 Primary subarachnoid haemorrhage (without aneurysm, arteriovenous malformation or other cause)

I61 Intracerebral haemorrhage

Use additional code, if desired, to identify cause.

Excludes: sequelae of intracerebral haemorrhage (I69.1)
traumatic intracerebral haemorrhage (S06.3)

Use additional sixth character, if desired, to indicate side:

I61.*xx*0 Left
I61.*xx*1 Right
I61.*xx*2 Bilateral

I61.0 Intracerebral haemorrhage in hemisphere, subcortical

Includes: deep intracerebral haemorrhage

I61.00 Basal ganglia
I61.01 Thalamus
I61.02 Internal capsule
I61.03 Hypothalamus
I61.04 Corpus callosum
I61.07 Involving more than one subcortical structure

I61.1 Intracerebral haemorrhage in hemisphere, cortical

Includes: cerebral lobe haemorrhage
superficial intracerebral haemorrhage

I61.10 Frontal
I61.11 Temporal
I61.12 Parietal
I61.13 Occipital
I61.17 Involving more than one lobe

I61.2 Intracerebral haemorrhage in hemisphere, unspecified

I61.3 Intracerebral haemorrhage in brain stem

I61.30 Midbrain
I61.31 Pons
I61.32 Medulla
I61.37 Involving more than one subdivision of brain stem

I61.4 Intracerebral haemorrhage in cerebellum

I61.40 Cerebellar hemisphere
I61.41 Cerebellar tonsil
I61.42 Vermis
I61.47 Involving more than one subdivision of cerebellum

I61.5 Intracerebral haemorrhage, intraventricular

I61.50 Lateral ventricle
I61.51 Third ventricle
I61.52 Fourth ventricle
I61.57 Multiple ventricles

I61.6 Intracerebral haemorrhage, multiple localized

I61.8 Other intracerebral haemorrhage

I61.9 Intracerebral haemorrhage, unspecified

I62 Other nontraumatic intracranial haemorrhage

Excludes: sequelae of intracranial haemorrhage (I69.2)

I62.0 Subdural haemorrhage (acute)(nontraumatic)

Excludes: traumatic subdural haematoma (S06.5)

Use additional sixth character, if desired, to indicate side:

I62.0*x*0 Left
I62.0*x*1 Right
I62.0*x*2 Bilateral

I62.00 Acute nontraumatic subdural haemorrhage (haematoma)
I62.01 Subacute nontraumatic subdural haemorrhage (haematoma)

I62.02 Chronic nontraumatic subdural haemorrhage (haematoma)

I62.1 Nontraumatic extradural haemorrhage

Includes: nontraumatic epidural haemorrhage
Excludes: traumatic extradural haematoma (S06.4)

I62.10 Acute nontraumatic extradural haemorrhage (haematoma)
I62.11 Subacute nontraumatic extradural haemorrhage (haematoma)
I62.12 Chronic nontraumatic extradural haemorrhage (haematoma)

I62.9 Intracranial haemorrhage (nontraumatic), unspecified

I63 Cerebral infarction

Excludes: sequelae of cerebral infarction (I69.3)

Use additional sixth character, if desired, to indicate side:

I63.*xx*0 Left
I63.*xx*1 Right
I63.*xx*2 Bilateral

I63.0 Cerebral infarction due to thrombosis of precerebral arteries

Use additional code, if desired, to identify etiology of thrombosis.

I63.00 Internal carotid artery
I63.01 Common carotid artery
I63.02 Innominate artery
I63.03 Vertebral artery
I63.04 Basilar artery
I63.05 Subclavian artery
I63.06 External carotid artery
I63.07 Multiple or bilateral precerebral arteries

I63.1 Cerebral infarction due to embolism of precerebral arteries

Use additional code, if desired, to identify source of embolus, for example:

- atrial fibrillation (I48)
- cardiac intraventricular clot due to myocardial infarction (I21.–)
- congenital heart valve disease (I38)
- endocarditis in diseases classified elsewhere (I39.–*)
- rheumatic heart valve disease (I05–I09)

I63.10 Internal carotid artery
I63.11 Common carotid artery

I63.12	Innominate artery
I63.13	Vertebral artery
I63.14	Basilar artery
I63.15	Subclavian artery
I63.16	External carotid artery
I63.17	Multiple or bilateral precerebral arteries

I63.2 Cerebral infarction due to unspecified occlusion or stenosis of precerebral arteries

Use additional code, if desired, to indicate etiology of occlusion or stenosis.

I63.20	Internal carotid artery
I63.21	Common carotid artery
I63.22	Innominate artery
I63.23	Vertebral artery
I63.24	Basilar artery
I63.25	Subclavian artery
I63.26	External carotid artery
I63.27	Multiple or bilateral precerebral arteries

I63.3 Cerebral infarction due to thrombosis of cerebral arteries

Use additional code, if desired, to indicate etiology of thrombosis.

I63.30	Middle cerebral artery
I63.31	Anterior cerebral artery
I63.32	Posterior cerebral artery
I63.33	Superior cerebellar artery
I63.34	Anterior inferior cerebellar artery
I63.35	Posterior inferior cerebellar artery
I63.36	Lenticulo-striate arteries
I63.37	Anterior choroidal artery
I63.38	Posterior communicating artery
I63.39	Multiple or bilateral arteries

I63.4 Cerebral infarction due to embolism of cerebral arteries

Use additional code, if desired, to identify source of embolus, for example:

- atrial fibrillation (I48)
- cardiac intraventricular clot due to myocardial infarction (I21.–)
- congenital heart valve disease (I38)
- endocarditis in diseases classified elsewhere (I39.–*)
- rheumatic heart valve disease (I05–I09)

I63.40 Middle cerebral artery
I63.41 Anterior cerebral artery
I63.42 Posterior cerebral artery
I63.43 Superior cerebellar artery
I63.44 Anterior inferior cerebellar artery
I63.45 Posterior inferior cerebellar artery
I63.46 Lenticulo-striate arteries
I63.47 Anterior choroidal artery
I63.48 Posterior communicating artery
I63.49 Multiple or bilateral arteries

I63.5 Cerebral infarction due to unspecified occlusion or stenosis of cerebral arteries

I63.50 Middle cerebral artery
I63.51 Anterior cerebral artery
I63.52 Posterior cerebral artery
I63.53 Superior cerebellar artery
I63.54 Anterior inferior cerebellar artery
I63.55 Posterior inferior cerebellar artery
I63.56 Lenticulo-striate arteries
I63.57 Anterior choroidal artery
I63.58 Posterior communicating artery
I63.59 Multiple or bilateral arteries

I63.6 Cerebral infarction due to cerebral venous thrombosis, nonpyogenic

I63.60 Cerebral cortical vein
I63.61 Sagittal sinus
I63.62 Great cerebral vein (Galen)
I63.63 Straight sinus
I63.64 Sigmoid sinus
I63.65 Jugular vein
I63.66 Cavernous sinus
I63.67 Multiple or bilateral veins or sinus

I63.8 Other cerebral infarction

I63.9 Cerebral infarction, unspecified

I64 Stroke, not specified as haemorrhage or infarction

Cerebrovascular accident NOS

Excludes: sequelae of stroke (I69.4)

I65 Occlusion and stenosis of precerebral arteries, not resulting in cerebral infarction

Includes: embolism, narrowing, obstruction (complete) (partial), thrombosis } of basilar, carotid and vertebral arteries, not resulting in cerebral infarction

Excludes: atherosclerosis of ophthalmic artery (I70.81)
when causing cerebral infarction (I63.–)

Use additional sixth character, if desired, to indicate side:

I65.*xx*0 Left
I65.*xx*1 Right
I65.*xx*2 Bilateral

I65.0 Occlusion and stenosis of vertebral artery

I65.00 Plaque on vertebral artery
I65.01 Non-obstructive stenosis of vertebral artery
I65.02 Obstructive (>70%) stenosis of vertebral artery
I65.03 Occlusion of vertebral artery

I65.1 Occlusion and stenosis of basilar artery

I65.10 Plaque on basilar artery
I65.11 Non-obstructive stenosis of basilar artery
I65.12 Obstructive (>70%) stenosis of basilar artery
I65.13 Occlusion of basilar artery

I65.2 Occlusion and stenosis of carotid artery

I65.20 Plaque on internal carotid artery
I65.21 Non-obstructive stenosis of internal carotid artery
I65.22 Obstructive (>70%) stenosis of internal carotid artery
I65.23 Occlusion of internal carotid artery
I65.24 Plaque on common carotid artery
I65.25 Non-obstructive stenosis of common carotid artery
I65.26 Obstructive (>70%) stenosis of common carotid artery
I65.27 Occlusion of common carotid artery
I65.28 Stenosis of external carotid artery
I65.29 Occlusion of external carotid artery

I65.3 Occlusion and stenosis of multiple and bilateral precerebral arteries

I65.8 Occlusion and stenosis of other precerebral arteries

I65.80 Plaque on innominate artery
I65.81 Non-obstructive stenosis of innominate artery

I65.82 Obstructive (>70%) stenosis of innominate artery
I65.83 Occlusion of innominate artery
I65.84 Plaque on subclavian artery
I65.85 Non-obstructive stenosis of subclavian artery
I65.86 Obstructive (>70%) stenosis of subclavian artery
I65.87 Occlusion of subclavian artery

I65.9 Occlusion and stenosis of unspecified precerebral artery
Precerebral artery NOS

I66 Occlusion and stenosis of cerebral arteries, not resulting in cerebral infarction

Includes: embolism, narrowing, obstruction (complete) (partial), thrombosis — of middle, anterior and posterior cerebral arteries, and cerebellar arteries, not resulting in cerebral infarction

Excludes: when causing cerebral infarction (I63.–)

Use additional sixth character, if desired, to indicate side:

I66.*xx*0 Left
I66.*xx*1 Right
I66.*xx*2 Bilateral

I66.0 Occlusion and stenosis of middle cerebral artery

I66.00 Plaque on middle cerebral artery
I66.01 Non-obstructive stenosis of middle cerebral artery
I66.02 Obstructive (>70%) stenosis of middle cerebral artery
I66.03 Occlusion of middle cerebral artery

I66.1 Occlusion and stenosis of anterior cerebral artery

I66.10 Plaque on anterior cerebral artery
I66.11 Non-obstructive stenosis of anterior cerebral artery
I66.12 Obstructive (>70%) stenosis of anterior cerebral artery
I66.13 Occlusion of anterior cerebral artery

I66.2 Occlusion and stenosis of posterior cerebral artery

I66.20 Plaque on posterior cerebral artery
I66.21 Non-obstructive stenosis of posterior cerebral artery
I66.22 Obstructive (>70%) stenosis of posterior cerebral artery
I66.23 Occlusion of posterior cerebral artery

I66.3 Occlusion and stenosis of cerebellar arteries

I66.30 Plaque on cerebellar arteries
I66.31 Non-obstructive stenosis of cerebellar arteries
I66.32 Obstructive (>70%) stenosis of cerebellar arteries
I66.33 Occlusion of cerebellar arteries

I66.4 Occlusion and stenosis of multiple and bilateral cerebral arteries

I66.8 Occlusion and stenosis of other cerebral arteries

I66.80 Occlusion and stenosis of perforating arteries
I66.81 Occlusion and stenosis of anterior communicating artery
I66.82 Occlusion and stenosis of posterior communicating artery
I66.83 Occlusion and stenosis of aberrant cerebral artery

I66.9 Occlusion and stenosis of unspecified cerebral artery

I67 Other cerebrovascular diseases

Excludes: sequelae of the listed conditions (I69.8)

I67.0 Dissection of cerebral arteries, nonruptured

Includes: precerebral arteries, nonruptured
Excludes: ruptured cerebral arteries (I60.7)

Use additional sixth character, if desired, to indicate side:

I67.0*x*0 Left
I67.0*x*1 Right
I67.0*x*2 Bilateral

I67.00 Dissection of common carotid artery
I67.01 Dissection of extracranial internal carotid artery
I67.02 Dissection of intracranial internal carotid artery
I67.03 Dissection of extracranial vertebral artery
I67.04 Dissection of intracranial vertebral artery
I67.05 Dissection of basilar artery
I67.06 Dissection of middle cerebral artery
I67.07 Dissection of anterior cerebral artery
I67.08 Dissection of posterior cerebral artery
I67.09 Dissection of other specified cerebral or precerebral artery

I67.1 Cerebral aneurysm, nonruptured

Includes: cerebral:
- aneurysm NOS
- arteriovenous fistula, acquired

Excludes: congenital cerebral aneurysm, nonruptured (Q28.-)
ruptured cerebral aneurysm NOS (I60.9)

Use additional seventh character, if desired, to indicate side:

I67.1xx0 Left
I67.1xx1 Right
I67.1xx2 Bilateral

For multiple specified nonruptured cerebral aneurysms, code each one separately.

I67.10 Carotid siphon and internal carotid artery bifurcation
- I67.100 Aneurysm at origin of ophthalmic artery
- I67.101 Aneurysm at origin of anterior choroidal artery
- I67.102 Aneurysm at origin of posterior communicating artery
- I67.103 Aneurysm at bifurcation of internal carotid artery
- I67.104 Carotido-cavernous aneurysm

I67.11 Middle cerebral artery
- I67.110 Proximal (M1-horizontal segment) middle cerebral artery aneurysm
- I67.111 Aneurysm at major bi- or trifurcation of middle cerebral artery
- I67.112 Distal middle cerebral artery aneurysm
  Use additional code (I60.83), if desired, in case of mycotic aneurysm.

I67.12 Anterior cerebral and communicating artery
- I67.120 Anterior communicating artery aneurysm
- I67.121 Proximal (A1-horizontal segment) anterior cerebral artery aneurysm
- I67.122 Distal (A2-vertical segment) anterior cerebral artery aneurysm
- I67.123 Pericallosal artery aneurysm
  Use additional code (I60.83), if desired, in case of mycotic aneurysm.

I67.13 Posterior communicating artery
Distal posterior communicating artery aneurysm

I67.14 Basilar artery
- I67.140 Proximal basilar artery (vertebral artery confluence) aneurysm
- I67.141 Midbasilar artery aneurysm

I67.142 Top of basilar artery aneurysm
I67.143 Bifid basilar artery aneurysm
I67.144 Aneurysm at origin of superior cerebellar artery
I67.145 Aneurysm at origin of anterior inferior cerebellar artery

I67.15 Vertebral artery
Includes: intracranial vertebral artery aneurysm
I67.150 Aneurysm at origin of posterior inferior cerebellar artery

I67.17 Multiple intracranial aneurysms, unspecified
I67.18 Other intracranial arteries
I67.180 Distal superior cerebellar artery
I67.181 Distal anterior inferior cerebellar artery
I67.182 Distal posterior inferior cerebellar artery
I67.183 Internal auditory artery
I67.184 Proximal posterior cerebral artery
I67.185 Distal posterior cerebral artery

I67.2 Cerebral atherosclerosis

Atheroma of cerebral arteries

I67.3 Progressive vascular leukoencephalopathy

Binswanger's disease

Use additional code (F01.2), if appropriate, to indicate the presence of a vascular dementia syndrome.

I67.4 Hypertensive encephalopathy

I67.5 Moyamoya disease

I67.50 Primary moyamoya disease
Idiopathic occlusion of basal arteries with rete mirabilis

I67.51 Secondary moyamoya disease
Use additional code, if desired, to identify the cause of basal artery occlusion.

I67.6 Nonpyogenic thrombosis of intracranial venous system

Includes: nonpyogenic thrombosis of:
- cerebral vein
- intracranial venous sinus

Excludes: when causing infarction (I63.6)

I67.60 Cerebral cortical vein
I67.61 Sagittal sinus
I67.62 Great cerebral artery (Galen)
I67.63 Straight sinus
I67.64 Sigmoid sinus

I67.65 Jugular vein
I67.66 Cavernous sinus
I67.67 Multiple cerebral vein(s) and sinus(es)
I67.68 Other cerebral vein or sinus

I67.7 Cerebral arteritis, not elsewhere classified

I67.70 Primary cerebral angiitis
Granulomatous angiitis of the nervous system
I67.78 Other cerebral arteritis, not elsewhere classified

I67.8 Other specified cerebrovascular diseases
Excludes: cerebral arteriovenous fistula, acquired (I67.1)

I67.9 Cerebrovascular disease, unspecified

I68* Cerebrovascular disorders in diseases classified elsewhere

I68.0* Cerebral amyloid angiopathy (E85.–†)
Includes: congophilic angiopathy

I68.00* Familial
I68.01* Nonfamilial

I68.1* Cerebral arteritis in infectious and parasitic diseases
Cerebral arteritis:
- listerial (A32.8†)
- syphilitic (A52.0†)
- tuberculous (A18.8†)

I68.2* Cerebral arteritis in other diseases classified elsewhere
Cerebral arteritis in systemic lupus erythematosus (M32.1†)

I68.8* Other cerebrovascular disorders in diseases classified elsewhere

I69 Sequelae of cerebrovascular disease

Note: This category is to be used to indicate conditions in I60–I67 as the cause of sequelae, themselves classified elsewhere. The "sequelae" include conditions specified as such or as late effects, or those present one year or more after onset of the causal condition (see also Section II, note 1.5, coding of late effects).

I69.0 Sequelae of subarachnoid haemorrhage

I69.1 Sequelae of intracerebral haemorrhage

I69.2 Sequelae of other nontraumatic intracranial haemorrhage

I69.3 Sequelae of cerebral infarction

I69.4 Sequelae of stroke, not specified as haemorrhage or infarction

I69.8 Sequelae of other and unspecified cerebrovascular diseases

Diseases of arteries, arterioles and capillaries (I70–I79)

I70 Atherosclerosis

Includes: arteriolosclerosis
arteriosclerosis
arteriosclerotic vascular disease
atheroma
degeneration:
- arterial
- arteriovascular
- vascular

endarteritis deformans or obliterans
senile:
- arteritis
- endarteritis

Excludes: cerebral (I67.2)
coronary (I25.1)

I70.0 Atherosclerosis of aorta

I70.1 Atherosclerosis of renal artery

Goldblatt's kidney
Excludes: atherosclerosis of renal arterioles (I12.–)

I70.2 Atherosclerosis of arteries of extremities

Atherosclerotic gangrene
Mönckeberg's (medial) sclerosis

I70.8 Atherosclerosis of other arteries

I70.80† Atherosclerotic retinopathy (H36.8*)
I70.81 Atherosclerosis of ophthalmic artery

I70.9 Generalized and unspecified atherosclerosis

I71 Aortic aneurysm and dissection

I71.0 Dissection of aorta [any part]

Dissecting aneurysm of aorta (ruptured) [any part]

I71.9 Aortic aneurysm of unspecified site, without mention of rupture

Aneurysm, Dilatation, Hyaline necrosis } of aorta

I72 Other aneurysms

Includes: aneurysm (cirsoid)(false)(ruptured)

Excludes: aneurysm (of):
- aorta (I71.–)
- arteriovenous, acquired (I77.0)
- cerebral (nonruptured) (I67.1)
  - ruptured (I60.–)
- heart (I25.3)
- retinal (H35.0)
- varicose (I77.0)

I72.0 Aneurysm of carotid artery

Excludes: carotid siphon and internal carotid artery bifurcation (I60.0, I67.10)

I72.1 Aneurysm of artery of upper extremity

I72.2 Aneurysm of renal artery

I72.3 Aneurysm of iliac artery

I72.4 Aneurysm of artery of lower extremity

I72.8 Aneurysm of other specified arteries

I72.9 Aneurysm of unspecified site

I73 Other peripheral vascular diseases

Excludes: spasm of cerebral artery (G45.9)

I73.0 Raynaud's syndrome

Raynaud's:
- disease
- gangrene
- phenomenon (secondary)

I73.1 Thromboangiitis obliterans [Buerger]

I73.8 Other specified peripheral vascular diseases

Acrocyanosis
Acroparaesthesia:
- simple [Schultze's type]
- vasomotor [Nothnagel's type]

Erythrocyanosis
Erythromelalgia

I73.9 Peripheral vascular disease, unspecified

Intermittent claudication
Spasm of artery

I74 Arterial embolism and thrombosis

Includes: infarction:
- embolic
- thrombotic

occlusion:
- embolic
- thrombotic

Excludes: embolism and thrombosis:
- basilar (I63.0–I63.2, I65.1)
- carotid (I63.0–I63.2, I65.2)
- cerebral (I63.3–I63.5, I66.9)
- complicating:
  - abortion or ectopic or molar pregnancy (O08.2)
  - pregnancy, childbirth and the puerperium (O88.–)
- coronary (I21–I25)
- precerebral (I63.0–I63.2, I65.9)
- retinal (H34.–)
- vertebral (I63.0–I63.2, I65.0)

I74.0 Embolism and thrombosis of abdominal aorta

Aortic bifurcation syndrome
Leriche's syndrome

I74.1 Embolism and thrombosis of other and unspecified parts of aorta

I74.2 Embolism and thrombosis of arteries of upper extremities

I74.3 Embolism and thrombosis of arteries of lower extremities

I74.4 Embolism and thrombosis of arteries of extremities, unspecified

Peripheral arterial embolism

I74.5 Embolism and thrombosis of iliac artery

I74.8 Embolism and thrombosis of other arteries

I74.9 Embolism and thrombosis of unspecified artery

I77 Other disorders of arteries and arterioles

Excludes: collagen (vascular) diseases (M30–M36)
hypersensitivity angiitis (M31.0)

I77.0 Arteriovenous fistula, acquired

Aneurysmal varix
Arteriovenous aneurysm, acquired
Excludes: cerebral (I67.1)
traumatic — see injury of blood vessel by body region

I77.1 Stricture of artery

I77.2 Rupture of artery

Erosion } of artery
Fistula } of artery
Ulcer } of artery

Excludes: traumatic rupture of artery — see injury of blood vessel by body region

I77.3 Arterial fibromuscular dysplasia

I77.30 Arterial fibromuscular dysplasia of (pre)cerebral arteries

I77.300 Internal carotid artery
I77.301 Common carotid artery
I77.302 Innominate artery
I77.303 Vertebral artery
I77.304 Basilar artery
I77.305 Middle cerebral artery
I77.306 Anterior cerebral artery
I77.307 Posterior cerebral artery
I77.308 Other cerebral artery

I77.4 Coeliac artery compression syndrome

I77.5 Necrosis of artery

I77.6 Arteritis, unspecified

Aortitis NOS
Endarteritis NOS
Excludes: arteritis or endarteritis:
- aortic arch [Takayasu] (M31.4)
- cerebral NEC (I67.7)
- coronary (I25.8)

- deformans (I70.–)
- giant cell (M31.5–M31.6)
- obliterans (I70.–)
- senile (I70.–)

I77.8 Other specified disorders of arteries and arterioles

I78 Diseases of capillaries

I78.0 Hereditary haemorrhagic telangiectasia
Rendu–Osler–Weber disease

I79* Disorders of arteries, arterioles and capillaries in diseases classified elsewhere

I79.0* Aneurysm of aorta in diseases classified elsewhere
Syphilitic aneurysm of aorta (A52.0†)

I79.1* Aortitis in diseases classified elsewhere
Syphilitic aortitis (A52.0†)

Diseases of veins, lymphatic vessels and lymph nodes, not elsewhere classified (I80–I89)

I80.– Phlebitis and thrombophlebitis

Includes: endophlebitis
inflammation, vein
periphlebitis
suppurative phlebitis

Use additional external cause code (Chapter XX), if desired, to identify drug, if drug-induced.

Other and unspecified disorders of the circulatory system (I95–I99)

I95 Hypotension

Excludes: cardiovascular collapse (R57.9)

I95.0 Idiopathic hypotension

I95.1 Orthostatic hypotension

Hypotension, postural

Excludes: neurogenic orthostatic hypotension (G90.30)
Shy–Drager syndrome (G90.31)

I95.2 Hypotension due to drugs

Use additional external cause code (Chapter XX), if desired, to identify drug.

I95.8 Other hypotension

Chronic hypotension

I95.9 Hypotension, unspecified

I97.– Postprocedural disorders of circulatory system, not elsewhere classified

I98* Other disorders of circulatory system in diseases classified elsewhere

I98.0* Cardiovascular syphilis

Cardiovascular syphilis:
- NOS (A52.0†)
- congenital, late (A50.5†)

I98.1* Cardiovascular disorders in other infectious and parasitic diseases classified elsewhere

Cardiovascular involvement NEC in Chagas' disease (chronic) (B57.2†)

CHAPTER X

Diseases of the respiratory system (J00–J99)

Acute upper respiratory infections (J00–J06)

J01 Acute sinusitis

Includes: abscess, empyema, infection, inflammation, suppuration } acute, of sinus (accessory)(nasal)

Use additional code (B95–B97), if desired, to identify infectious agent.

Excludes: sinusitis, chronic or NOS (J32.–)

J01.0 Acute maxillary sinusitis
Acute antritis

J01.1 Acute frontal sinusitis

J01.2 Acute ethmoidal sinusitis

J01.3 Acute sphenoidal sinusitis

J01.4 Acute pansinusitis

J01.8 Other acute sinusitis
Acute sinusitis involving more than one sinus but not pansinusitis

J01.9 Acute sinusitis, unspecified

Influenza and pneumonia (J10–J18)

J10 Influenza due to identified influenza virus

Excludes: *Haemophilus influenzae* [*H. influenzae*] meningitis (G00.0)

J10.0 Influenza with pneumonia, influenza virus identified

J10.8 Influenza with other manifestations, influenza virus identified

Encephalopathy due to influenza
Influenzal:
- gastroenteritis
- myocarditis (acute)

} influenza virus identified

J11 Influenza, virus not identified

J11.0 Influenza with pneumonia, virus not identified

J11.8 Influenza with other manifestations, virus not identified

Encephalopathy due to influenza
Influenzal:
- gastroenteritis
- myocarditis (acute)

} unspecified or specific virus not identified

J13 Pneumonia due to *Streptococcus pneumoniae*

Bronchopneumonia due to *S. pneumoniae*

J14 Pneumonia due to *Haemophilus influenzae*

Bronchopneumonia due to *H. influenzae*

J15.– Bacterial pneumonia, not elsewhere classified

Includes: bronchopneumonia due to bacteria other than *S. pneumoniae* and *H. influenzae*

J16.– Pneumonia due to other infectious organisms, not elsewhere classified

J17* Pneumonia in diseases classified elsewhere

J17.0* Pneumonia in bacterial diseases classified elsewhere

J18.– Pneumonia, organism unspecified

Excludes: aspiration pneumonia (due to):
- NOS (J69.0)
- newborn (P24.–)
- solids and liquids (J69.–)

Other diseases of upper respiratory tract (J30–J39)

J32 Chronic sinusitis

Includes: abscess, empyema, infection, suppuration } (chronic) of sinus (accessory)(nasal)

Use additional code (B95–B97), if desired, to identify infectious agent.

Excludes: acute sinusitis (J01.–)

J32.0 Chronic maxillary sinusitis

Antritis (chronic)

J32.1 Chronic frontal sinusitis

J32.2 Chronic ethmoidal sinusitis

J32.3 Chronic sphenoidal sinusitis

J32.4 Chronic pansinusitis

J32.8 Other chronic sinusitis

Sinusitis (chronic) involving more than one sinus but not pansinusitis

J32.9 Chronic sinusitis, unspecified

J38 Diseases of vocal cords and larynx, not elsewhere classified

J38.0 Paralysis of vocal cords and larynx

Laryngoplegia

Paralysis of glottis

Chronic lower respiratory diseases (J40–J47)

Excludes: cystic fibrosis (E84.–)

J40 Bronchitis, not specified as acute or chronic

Bronchitis:
- NOS
- catarrhal
- with tracheitis NOS

Tracheobronchitis NOS

J42 Unspecified chronic bronchitis

Chronic:
- bronchitis NOS
- tracheitis
- tracheobronchitis

J43.– Emphysema

J45.– Asthma

Excludes: acute severe asthma (J46)
status asthmaticus (J46)

J46 Status asthmaticus

Acute severe asthma

J47 Bronchiectasis

Bronchiolectasis

Lung diseases due to external agents (J60–J70)

J69 Pneumonitis due to solids and liquids

Use additional external cause code (Chapter XX), if desired, to identify cause.

Excludes: neonatal aspiration syndromes (P24.–)

J69.0 Pneumonitis due to food and vomit

Aspiration pneumonia (due to):
- NOS
- food (regurgitated)
- gastric secretions
- milk
- vomit

Other respiratory diseases principally affecting the interstitium (J80–J84)

J81 Pulmonary oedema

Acute oedema of lung
Pulmonary congestion (passive)

Suppurative and necrotic conditions of lower respiratory tract (J85–J86)

J85.– Abscess of lung and mediastinum

Other diseases of pleura (J90–J94)

J90 Pleural effusion, not elsewhere classified

Pleurisy with effusion

J93.– Pneumothorax

Other diseases of the respiratory system (J95–J99)

J95 Postprocedural respiratory disorders, not elsewhere classified

J95.0 Tracheostomy malfunction

Haemorrhage from tracheostomy stoma
Obstruction of tracheostomy airway
Sepsis of tracheostomy stoma
Tracheo-oesophageal fistula following tracheostomy

J98 Other respiratory disorders

Excludes: apnoea NOS (R06.8)
sleep apnoea (G47.3)

J98.6 Disorders of diaphragm

Diaphragmatitis
Paralysis of diaphragm
Relaxation of diaphragm

CHAPTER XI

Diseases of the digestive system (K00–K93)

Diseases of oral cavity, salivary glands and jaws (K00–K14)

K04.– Diseases of pulp and periapical tissues

K07 Dentofacial anomalies [including malocclusion]

Excludes: hemifacial atrophy or hypertrophy (Q67.4)

K07.0 Major anomalies of jaw size

Hyperplasia, hypoplasia:
- mandibular
- maxillary

Macrognathism (mandibular)(maxillary)
Micrognathism (mandibular)(maxillary)
Excludes: acromegaly (E22.0)
Robin's syndrome (Q87.07)

K07.1 Anomalies of jaw–cranial base relationship

Asymmetry of jaw
Prognathism (mandibular)(maxillary)
Retrognathism (mandibular)(maxillary)

K07.2 Anomalies of dental arch relationship

Crossbite (anterior)(posterior)
Disto-occlusion
Mesio-occlusion
Midline deviation of dental arch
Openbite (anterior)(posterior)
Overbite (excessive):
- deep
- horizontal
- vertical

Overjet
Posterior lingual occlusion of mandibular teeth

K07.3 Anomalies of tooth position

Crowding, Diastema, Displacement, Rotation, Spacing, abnormal, Transposition } of tooth or teeth

Impacted or embedded teeth with abnormal position of such teeth or adjacent teeth

K07.4 Malocclusion, unspecified

K07.5 Dentofacial functional abnormalities

Abnormal jaw closure

Malocclusion due to:
- abnormal swallowing
- mouth breathing
- tongue, lip or finger habits

K07.6 Temporomandibular joint disorders

Costen's complex or syndrome

Derangement of temporomandibular joint

Snapping jaw

Temporomandibular joint-pain-dysfunction syndrome

Excludes: current temporomandibular joint:
- dislocation (S03.0)
- strain (S03.4)

K07.8 Other dentofacial anomalies

K07.9 Dentofacial anomaly, unspecified

K12 Stomatitis and related lesions

K12.0 Recurrent oral aphthae

Aphthous stomatitis (major)(minor)

Bednar's aphthae

Periadenitis mucosa necrotica recurrens

Recurrent aphthous ulcer

Stomatitis herpetiformis

Diseases of oesophagus, stomach and duodenum (K20–K31)

K20 Oesophagitis

Abscess of oesophagus
Oesophagitis:
- NOS
- chemical
- peptic

Use additional external cause code (Chapter XX), if desired, to identify cause.

Excludes: erosion of oesophagus (K22.1)

K22 Other diseases of oesophagus

K22.1 Ulcer of oesophagus

Erosion of oesophagus
Ulcer of oesophagus:
- NOS
- due to ingestion of:
  - chemicals
  - drugs and medicaments
- fungal
- peptic

Use additional external cause code (Chapter XX), if desired, to identify cause.

The following fourth-character subdivisions are for use with categories K25–K28:

K2x.0 Acute with haemorrhage

K2x.1 Acute with perforation

K2x.2 Acute with both haemorrhage and perforation

K2x.3 Acute without haemorrhage or perforation

K2x.4 Chronic or unspecified with haemorrhage

K2x.5 Chronic or unspecified with perforation

K2x.6 Chronic or unspecified with both haemorrhage and perforation

K2x.7 Chronic without haemorrhage or perforation

K2x.9 Unspecified as acute or chronic, without haemorrhage or perforation

K25 Gastric ulcer

[See pages 291–292 for subdivisions]

Includes: erosion (acute) of stomach
ulcer (peptic):
- pylorus
- stomach

Use additional external cause code (Chapter XX), if desired, to identify drug, if drug-induced.

K26 Duodenal ulcer

[See pages 291–292 for subdivisions]

Includes: erosion (acute) of duodenum
ulcer (peptic):
- duodenal
- postpyloric

Use additional external cause code (Chapter XX), if desired, to identify drug, if drug-induced.

Excludes: peptic ulcer NOS (K27.–)

K27 Peptic ulcer, site unspecified

[See pages 291–292 for subdivisions]

Includes: gastroduodenal ulcer NOS
peptic ulcer NOS

K28 Gastrojejunal ulcer

[See pages 291–292 for subdivisions]

Includes: ulcer (peptic) or erosion:
- anastomotic
- gastrocolic
- gastrointestinal
- gastrojejunal
- jejunal
- marginal
- stomal

K29 Gastritis and duodenitis

Excludes: Zollinger–Ellison syndrome (E16.8)

K29.2 Alcoholic gastritis

K29.8 Duodenitis

K29.9 Gastroduodenitis, unspecified

K30 Dyspepsia

Indigestion

Excludes: dyspepsia:
- nervous (F45.3)
- neurotic (F45.3)
- psychogenic (F45.3)

K31 Other diseases of stomach and duodenum

Excludes: gastrointestinal haemorrhage (K92.0–K92.2)

K31.3 Pylorospasm, not elsewhere classified

Excludes: pylorospasm:
- neurotic (F45.3)
- psychogenic (F45.3)

Noninfective enteritis and colitis (K50–K52)

Includes: noninfective inflammatory bowel disease

K50.– Crohn's disease [regional enteritis]

Includes: granulomatous enteritis

K51.– Ulcerative colitis

Other diseases of intestines (K55–K63)

K58 Irritable bowel syndrome

Includes: irritable colon

K58.0 Irritable bowel syndrome with diarrhoea

K58.9 Irritable bowel syndrome without diarrhoea

K59 Other functional intestinal disorders

Excludes: intestinal malabsorption (K90.–)
psychogenic intestinal disorders (F45.3)

K59.0 **Constipation**

K59.1 **Functional diarrhoea**

K59.2 **Neurogenic bowel, not elsewhere classified**

K59.4 **Anal spasm**
Proctalgia fugax

Diseases of peritoneum (K65–K67)

K65 Peritonitis

Diseases of liver (K70–K77)

Excludes: haemochromatosis (E83.10)
Reye's syndrome (G93.7)
viral hepatitis (B15–B19)
Wilson's disease (E83.01)

K70 Alcoholic liver disease

K70.0 **Alcoholic fatty liver**

K70.1 **Alcoholic hepatitis**

K70.2 **Alcoholic fibrosis and sclerosis of liver**

K70.3 **Alcoholic cirrhosis of liver**

K70.4 **Alcoholic hepatic failure**
Alcoholic hepatic failure:
- NOS
- acute
- chronic
- subacute
- with or without hepatic coma

K70.9 **Alcoholic liver disease, unspecified**

K71 Toxic liver disease

Includes: drug-induced:
- idiosyncratic (unpredictable) liver disease
- toxic (predictable) liver disease

Use additional external cause code (Chapter XX), if desired, to identify toxic agent.

Excludes: alcoholic liver disease (K70.–)

K71.0 Toxic liver disease with cholestasis
Cholestasis with hepatocyte injury
"Pure" cholestasis

K71.1 Toxic liver disease with hepatic necrosis
Hepatic failure (acute)(chronic) due to drugs

K72.– Hepatic failure, not elsewhere classified

Includes: hepatic:
- coma NOS
- encephalopathy NOS

hepatitis:
- acute
- fulminant
- malignant

} NEC, with hepatic failure

liver (cell) necrosis with hepatic failure
yellow liver atrophy or dystrophy

Excludes: alcoholic hepatic failure (K70.4)
viral hepatitis (B15–B19)
with toxic liver disease (K71.1)

Disorders of gallbladder, biliary tract and pancreas (K80–K87)

K85 Acute pancreatitis

Abscess of pancreas
Necrosis of pancreas:
- acute
- infective

Pancreatitis:
- NOS
- acute (recurrent)
- haemorrhagic
- subacute
- suppurative

K86 Other diseases of pancreas

K86.0 Alcohol-induced chronic pancreatitis

K86.1 Other chronic pancreatitis
Chronic pancreatitis:
- NOS
- infectious
- recurrent
- relapsing

Other diseases of the digestive system (K90–K93)

K90 Intestinal malabsorption

K90.8 Other intestinal malabsorption
Whipple's disease† (M14.8*)

K92 Other diseases of digestive system

K92.0 Haematemesis

K92.1 Melaena

K92.2 Gastrointestinal haemorrhage, unspecified
Haemorrhage:
- gastric NOS
- intestinal NOS

CHAPTER XII

Diseases of the skin and subcutaneous tissue (L00–L99)

Urticaria and erythema (L50–L54)

L51.– Erythema multiforme

L52 Erythema nodosum

Other disorders of the skin and subcutaneous tissue (L80–L99)

L89 Decubitus ulcer

Bed sore
Plaster ulcer
Pressure ulcer

L99* Other disorders of skin and subcutaneous tissue in diseases classified elsewhere

L99.0* Amyloidosis of skin (E85.–†)

L99.8* Other specified disorders of skin and subcutaneous tissue in diseases classified elsewhere

Syphilitic:
- alopecia (A51.3†)
- leukoderma (A51.3†, A52.7†)

Diseases of the musculoskeletal system and connective tissue (M00–M99)

Excludes: compartment syndrome (T79.6)
endocrine, nutritional and metabolic disorders (E00–E90)

Site of musculoskeletal involvement

The following subclassification to indicate the site of involvement is provided for optional use with appropriate categories in Chapter XIII. As local extensions or specialty adaptations may vary in the number of characters used, it is suggested that the supplementary site subclassification be placed in an identifiably separate position (e.g. in an additional box). Different subclassifications for use with dorsopathies are given on page 304.

0	Multiple sites		
1	Shoulder region	clavicle scapula	acromioclavicular, glenohumeral, sternoclavicular joints
2	Upper arm	humerus	elbow joint
3	Forearm	radius ulna	wrist joint
4	Hand	carpus fingers metacarpus	joints between these bones
5	Pelvic region and thigh	buttock femur pelvis	hip (joint) sacroiliac joint
6	Lower leg	fibula tibia	knee joint
7	Ankle and foot	metatarsus tarsus toes	ankle joint other joints in foot

8	Other	head neck ribs skull trunk vertebral column
9	Site unspecified	

Arthropathies (M00–M25)

Disorders affecting predominantly peripheral (limb) joints

M03* Postinfective and reactive arthropathies in diseases classified elsewhere

[See site code pages 298–299]

M03.0* Postmeningococcal arthritis (A39.8†)

M03.1* Postinfective arthropathy in syphilis
Clutton's joints (A50.5†)

M05 Seropositive rheumatoid arthritis

[See site code pages 298–299]

Excludes: rheumatic fever (I00)
rheumatoid arthritis of spine (M45.–)

M05.3† Rheumatoid arthritis with involvement of other organs and systems
Rheumatoid:
- endocarditis (I39.–*)
- myocarditis (I41.8*)
- myopathy (G73.7*)
- polyneuropathy (G63.6*)

M10.– Gout

[See site code pages 298–299]

M11.– Other crystal arthropathies

[See site code pages 298–299]

M14* Arthropathies in other diseases classified elsewhere

M14.0* Gouty arthropathy due to enzyme defects and other inherited disorders

Gouty arthropathy in:
- Lesch–Nyhan syndrome (E79.1†)
- sickle-cell disorders (D57.–†)

M14.1* Crystal arthropathy in other metabolic disorders

Crystal arthropathy in hyperparathyroidism (E21.–†)

M14.2* Diabetic arthropathy (E10–E14† with common fourth character .6)

M14.6* Neuropathic arthropathy

Charcot's or tabetic arthropathy (A52.1†)

Diabetic neuropathic arthropathy (E10–E14† with common fourth character .6)

M14.8* Arthropathies in other specified diseases classified elsewhere

Arthropathy in:
- erythema:
  - multiforme (L51.–†)
  - nodosum (L52†)
- sarcoidosis (D86.8†)
- Whipple's disease (K90.8†)

Systemic connective tissue disorders (M30–M36)

Includes: autoimmune disease:
- NOS
- systemic

collagen (vascular) disease:
- NOS
- systemic

Excludes: autoimmune disease, single organ or single cell-type (code to relevant condition category)

M30 Polyarteritis nodosa and related conditions

M30.0 Polyarteritis nodosa

M30.1 Polyarteritis with lung involvement [Churg–Strauss]
Allergic granulomatous angiitis

M30.2 Juvenile polyarteritis

M30.3 Mucocutaneous lymph node syndrome [Kawasaki]

M30.8 Other conditions related to polyarteritis nodosa
Polyangiitis overlap syndrome

M31 Other necrotizing vasculopathies

M31.0 Hypersensitivity angiitis
Goodpasture's syndrome

M31.1 Thrombotic microangiopathy
Thrombotic thrombocytopenic purpura

M31.2 Lethal midline granuloma

M31.3 Wegener's granulomatosis
Necrotizing respiratory granulomatosis

M31.4 Aortic arch syndrome [Takayasu]

M31.5 Giant cell arteritis with polymyalgia rheumatica

M31.6 Other giant cell arteritis

M31.8 Other specified necrotizing vasculopathies
Hypocomplementaemic vasculitis

M31.9 Necrotizing vasculopathy, unspecified

M32 Systemic lupus erythematosus

M32.0 Drug-induced systemic lupus erythematosus
Use additional external cause code (Chapter XX), if desired, to identify drug.

M32.1† Systemic lupus erythematosus with organ or system involvement
Libman–Sacks disease (I39*)

M32.8 Other forms of systemic lupus erythematosus

M32.9 Systemic lupus erythematosus, unspecified

M33 Dermatopolymyositis

M33.0 Juvenile dermatomyositis
Childhood dermatomyositis

M33.1 Other dermatomyositis

M33.10 Adult idiopathic dermatomyositis

M33.2 Polymyositis

M33.20 Juvenile polymyositis
Childhood polymyositis
M33.21 Adult idiopathic polymyositis
M33.22 Other secondary polymyositis
Use additional code, if desired, to identify cause, e.g. HIV disease (B23.8); sarcoidosis (D86.–).
M33.23 Eosinophilic polymyositis
M33.24 Perimyositis
M33.25 Eosinophilic perimyositis
M33.26 Inclusion body myositis
M33.28 Other specified dermatopolymyositis

M33.9 Dermatopolymyositis, unspecified

M34 Systemic sclerosis

Includes: scleroderma

M34.0 Progressive systemic sclerosis

M34.1 CR(E)ST syndrome

Combination of calcinosis, Raynaud's phenomenon, (o)esophageal dysfunction, sclerodactyly, telangiectasia.

M34.2 Systemic sclerosis induced by drugs and chemicals

Use additional external cause code (Chapter XX), if desired, to identify cause.

M34.8 Other forms of systemic sclerosis

Systemic sclerosis with myopathy† (G73.7*)

M34.9 Systemic sclerosis, unspecified

M35 Other systemic involvement of connective tissue

M35.0 Sicca syndrome [Sjögren]

Sjögren's syndrome with myopathy† (G73.7*)

M35.1 Other overlap syndromes

Mixed connective tissue disease
Excludes: polyangiitis overlap syndrome (M30.8)

M35.2 Behçet's disease

M35.3 Polymyalgia rheumatica
Excludes: polymyalgia rheumatica with giant cell arteritis (M31.5)

M35.4 Diffuse (eosinophilic) fasciitis

M35.5 Multifocal fibrosclerosis

M35.6 Relapsing panniculitis [Weber–Christian]

M35.7 Hypermobility syndrome
Familial ligamentous laxity
Excludes: Ehlers–Danlos syndrome (Q79.6)

M35.8 Other specified systemic involvement of connective tissue

M35.9 Systemic involvement of connective tissue, unspecified
Autoimmune disease (systemic) NOS
Collagen (vascular) disease NOS

M36* Systemic disorders of connective tissues in diseases classified elsewhere

M36.0* Dermato(poly)myositis in neoplastic disease (C00–D48†)

M36.00* Paraneoplastic dermatomyositis
M36.01* Paraneoplastic polymyositis

M36.1* Arthropathy in neoplastic disease (C00–D48†)
Arthropathy in:
- leukaemia (C91–C95†)
- malignant histiocytosis (C96.1†)
- multiple myeloma (C90.0†)

M36.2* Haemophilic arthropathy (D66–D68†)

M36.3* Arthropathy in other blood disorders (D50–D76†)

M36.4* Arthropathy in hypersensitivity reactions classified elsewhere
Arthropathy in Henoch(–Schönlein) purpura (D69.0†)

M36.8* Systemic disorders of connective tissue in other diseases classified elsewhere
Systemic disorders of connective tissue in ochronosis (E70.2†)

Dorsopathies (M40–M54)

The following supplementary subclassification to indicate the site of involvement is recommended for optional use with appropriate categories in the section on dorsopathies other than categories M50 and M51; see also note on page 298.

0 Multiple sites in spine
1 Occipito-atlanto-axial region
2 Cervical region
3 Cervicothoracic region
4 Thoracic region
5 Thoracolumbar region
6 Lumbar region
7 Lumbosacral region
8 Sacral and sacrococcygeal region
9 Site unspecified

M40 Kyphosis and lordosis

[See site code above]

Excludes: congenital:
- kyphosis (Q76.42)
- lordosis (Q76.43)

kyphoscoliosis (M41.–)

M40.0 Postural kyphosis
Excludes: osteochondrosis of spine (M42.–)

M40.1 Other secondary kyphosis

M40.2 Other and unspecified kyphosis

M40.3 Flatback syndrome

M40.4 Other lordosis
Lordosis:
- acquired
- postural

M40.5 Lordosis, unspecified

M41 Scoliosis

[See site code above]

Includes: kyphoscoliosis
Excludes: congenital scoliosis due to bony malformations (Q76.3)

M41.0 Infantile idiopathic scoliosis

M41.1 Juvenile idiopathic scoliosis
Adolescent scoliosis

M41.2 Other idiopathic scoliosis

M41.3 Thoracogenic scoliosis

M41.4 Neuromuscular scoliosis
Scoliosis secondary to cerebral palsy, Friedreich's ataxia, poliomyelitis, and other neuromuscular disorders.

M41.5 Other secondary scoliosis

M41.8 Other forms of scoliosis

M41.9 Scoliosis, unspecified

M42 Spinal osteochondrosis

[See site code page 304]

M42.0 Juvenile osteochondrosis of spine
Calvé's disease
Scheuermann's disease
Excludes: postural kyphosis (M40.0)

M42.1 Adult osteochondrosis of spine

M42.9 Spinal osteochondrosis, unspecified

M43 Other deforming dorsopathies

[See site code page 304]

Excludes: congenital malformations of the spine and bony thorax (Q76.–)
spinal curvature in:
- osteoporosis (M80–M81)
- Paget's disease of bone [osteitis deformans] (M88.–)

M43.0 Spondylolysis

M43.1 Spondylolisthesis

M43.2 Other fusion of spine
Ankylosis of spinal joint
Excludes: ankylosing spondylitis (M45)

M43.3 Recurrent atlantoaxial subluxation with myelopathy

M43.4 Other recurrent atlantoaxial subluxation

M43.5 Other recurrent vertebral subluxation

M43.6 Torticollis

Excludes: torticollis:
- congenital (sternomastoid) (Q68.0)
- current injury — see injury of spine by body region
- psychogenic (F45.8)
- spasmodic (G24.3)

M43.8 Other specified deforming dorsopathies

Excludes: kyphosis and lordosis (M40.–)
scoliosis (M41.–)

M43.9 Deforming dorsopathy, unspecified

Curvature of spine NOS

M45 Ankylosing spondylitis

[See site code page 304]

Excludes: Behçet's disease (M35.2)

M46 Other inflammatory spondylopathies

[See site code page 304]

M46.0 Spinal enthesopathy

Disorder of ligamentous or muscular attachments of spine

M46.1 Sacroiliitis, not elsewhere classified

M46.2 Osteomyelitis of vertebra

M46.3 Infection of intervertebral disc (pyogenic)

Use additional code (B95–B97), if desired, to identify infectious agent.

M46.4 Discitis, unspecified

M46.5 Other infective spondylopathies

M46.8 Other specified inflammatory spondylopathies

M46.9 Inflammatory spondylopathy, unspecified

M47 Spondylosis

[See site code page 304]

Includes: arthrosis or osteoarthritis of spine
degeneration of facet joints

M47.0† Anterior spinal or vertebral artery compression syndromes (G99.2*)

M47.1 Other spondylosis with myelopathy
Spondylogenic compression of spinal cord† (G99.2*)
Excludes: vertebral subluxation (M43.3–M43.5)

M47.2 Other spondylosis with radiculopathy

M47.8 Other spondylosis
Cervical spondylosis } without myelopathy or radiculopathy
Lumbosacral spondylosis } without myelopathy or radiculopathy
Thoracic spondylosis } without myelopathy or radiculopathy

M47.9 Spondylosis, unspecified

M48 Other spondylopathies

[See site code page 304]

M48.0 Spinal stenosis
Caudal stenosis

M48.1 Ankylosing hyperostosis [Forestier]
Diffuse idiopathic skeletal hyperostosis [DISH]

M48.2 Kissing spine

M48.3 Traumatic spondylopathy

M48.4 Fatigue fracture of vertebra
Stress fracture of vertebra

M48.5 Collapsed vertebra, not elsewhere classified
Collapsed vertebra NOS
Wedging of vertebra NOS
Excludes: collapsed vertebra in osteoporosis (M80.–)
current injury — see injury of spine by body region

M48.8 Other specified spondylopathies
Ossification of posterior longitudinal ligament

M48.9 Spondylopathy, unspecified

M49* Spondylopathies in diseases classified elsewhere

[See site code page 304]

M49.0* Tuberculosis of spine (A18.0†)
Pott's curvature

M49.1* Brucella spondylitis (A23.–†)

M49.2* Enterobacterial spondylitis (A01–A04†)

M49.3* **Spondylopathy in other infectious and parasitic diseases classified elsewhere**

M49.4* **Neuropathic spondylopathy**
Neuropathic spondylopathy in:
- syringomyelia and syringobulbia (G95.0†)
- tabes dorsalis (A52.1†)

M49.5* **Collapsed vertebra in diseases classified elsewhere**
Metastatic fracture of vertebra (C79.5†)

M49.8* **Spondylopathy in other diseases classified elsewhere**

M50 Cervical disc disorders

Includes: cervical disc disorders with cervicalgia
cervicothoracic disc disorders

M50.0† **Cervical disc disorder with myelopathy (G99.2*)**

M50.1 **Cervical disc disorder with radiculopathy**
Excludes: brachial radiculitis NOS (M54.1)

M50.2 **Other cervical disc displacement**

M50.3 **Other cervical disc degeneration**

M50.8 **Other cervical disc disorders**

M50.9 **Cervical disc disorder, unspecified**

M51 Other intervertebral disc disorders

Includes: thoracic, thoracolumbar and lumbosacral disc disorders

M51.0† **Lumbar and other intervertebral disc disorders with myelopathy (G99.2*)**

M51.1 **Lumbar and other intervertebral disc disorders with radiculopathy**
Excludes: lumbar radiculitis NOS (M54.1)

M51.10 Sciatica due to intervertebral disc disorder, L4/L5 (sciatica L5)
M51.11 Sciatica due to intervertebral disc disorder, L5/S1 (sciatica S1)
M51.12 Sciatica due to intervertebral disc disorder, combined
M51.13 Anterior thigh pain due to intervertebral disc disorder, L2/L3 (cruralgia L3)

M51.14 Anterior thigh pain due to intervertebral disc disorder, L3/L4 (cruralgia L4)

M51.17 Multiple radicular involvement

M51.2 Other specified intervertebral disc displacement
Lumbago due to displacement of intervertebral disc

M51.3 Other specified intervertebral disc degeneration

M51.4 Schmorl's nodes

M51.8 Other specified intervertebral disc disorders

M51.9 Intervertebral disc disorder, unspecified

M53 Other dorsopathies, not elsewhere classified

[See site code page 304]

M53.0 Cervicocranial syndrome
Posterior cervical sympathetic syndrome

M53.1 Cervicobrachial syndrome
Excludes: cervical disc disorder (M50.–)
thoracic outlet syndrome (G54.0)

M53.2 Spinal instabilities

M53.3 Sacrococcygeal disorders, not elsewhere classified
Coccygodynia

M53.8 Other specified dorsopathies

M53.9 Dorsopathy, unspecified

M54 Dorsalgia

[See site code page 304]

M54.0 Panniculitis affecting regions of neck or back
Excludes: relapsing panniculitis [Weber–Christian] (M35.6)

M54.1 Radiculopathy
Includes: neuritis or radiculitis:
- brachial NOS
- lumbar NOS
- lumbosacral NOS
- thoracic NOS

radiculitis NOS

Excludes: neuralgia and neuritis NOS (M79.2)
radiculopathy with:
- cervical disc disorder (M50.1)

- lumbar and other intervertebral disc disorder (M51.1)
- spondylosis (M47.2)

M54.10 Cervical radiculopathy, unspecified
M54.11 Thoracic radiculopathy, unspecified
M54.12 Lumbar radiculopathy, unspecified
M54.13 Lumbosacral radiculopathy, unspecified
M54.14 Sacral radiculopathy, unspecified

M54.2 Cervicalgia
Excludes: cervicalgia due to intervertebral disc disorder (M50.–)

M54.3 Sciatica
Excludes: lesion of sciatic nerve (G57.0)
sciatica:
- due to intervertebral disc lesion (M51.1)
- with lumbago (M54.4)

M54.4 Lumbago with sciatica
Excludes: that due to intervertebral disc disorder (M51.1)

M54.5 Low back pain
Loin pain
Low back strain
Lumbago NOS
Excludes: lumbago:
- due to intervertebral disc displacement (M51.2)
- with sciatica (M54.4)

M54.6 Pain in thoracic spine
Excludes: pain due to intervertebral disc disorder (M51.–)

M54.8 Other dorsalgia

M54.9 Dorsalgia, unspecified
Backache NOS

Soft tissue disorders (M60–M79)

Excludes: dermatopolymyositis (M33.–)
muscular dystrophies and other myopathies (G71–G72)
myopathy in:
- amyloidosis (E85.–)
- polyarteritis nodosa (M30.0)
- rheumatoid arthritis (M05.3)
- scleroderma (M34.–)

- Sjögren's syndrome (M35.0)
- systemic lupus erythematosus (M32.–)

M60 Myositis

[See site code pages 298–299]

Excludes: dermatomyositis (M33.–)

M60.0 Infective myositis

Tropical pyomyositis

Use additional code (B95–B97), if desired, to identify infectious agent.

M60.1 Interstitial myositis

M60.2 Foreign body granuloma in soft tissue, not elsewhere classified

M60.8 Other myositis

M60.80 Focal nodular myositis
Focal proliferative myositis
M60.81 Without other organ involvement
M60.82 With linear scleroderma
M60.83 Localized eosinophilic myositis

M60.9 Myositis, unspecified

M61 Calcification and ossification of muscle

[See site code pages 298–299]

M61.0 Myositis ossificans traumatica

M61.1 Myositis ossificans progressiva

Fibrodysplasia ossificans progressiva

M61.2 Paralytic calcification and ossification of muscle

Myositis ossificans associated with quadriplegia or paraplegia

M61.3 Calcification and ossification of muscles associated with burns

Myositis ossificans associated with burns

M61.4 Other calcification of muscle

M61.5 Other ossification of muscle

M61.9 Calcification and ossification of muscle, unspecified

M62 Other disorders of muscle

[See site code pages 298–299]

Excludes: cramp and spasm (R25.2)
myalgia (M79.1)
myopathy:
- alcoholic (G72.1)
- drug-induced (G72.0)

stiff-man syndrome (G25.84)

M62.0 Diastasis of muscle

M62.1 Other rupture of muscle (nontraumatic)

M62.2 Ischaemic infarction of muscle
Excludes: compartment syndrome (T79.6)
traumatic ischaemia of muscle (T79.6)
Volkmann's ischaemic contracture (T79.6)

M62.3 Immobility syndrome (paraplegic)

M62.4 Contracture of muscle

M62.5 Muscle wasting and atrophy, not elsewhere classified
Disuse atrophy NEC

M62.6 Muscle strain

M62.8 Other specified disorders of muscle

M62.80 Muscle (sheath) hernia
M62.81 Muscle hypertrophy
M62.82 Rigid spine syndrome due to muscle disorder

M63* Disorders of muscle in diseases classified elsewhere

M63.0* Myositis in bacterial diseases classified elsewhere
Myositis in:
- leprosy [Hansen's disease] (A30.–†)
- syphilis (A51.4†, A52.7†)

Excludes: pyomyositis (M60.0)

M63.1* Myositis in protozoal and parasitic infections classified elsewhere
Myositis in:
- cysticercosis (B69.8†)
- schistosomiasis [bilharziasis] (B65.–†)
- trichinellosis (B75†)

M63.2* **Myositis in other infectious diseases classified elsewhere**
Myositis in mycosis (B35–B49†)

M63.3* **Myositis in sarcoidosis (D86.8†)**

M63.8* **Other disorders of muscle in diseases classified elsewhere**

M79 Other soft tissue disorders, not elsewhere classified

[See site code pages 298–299]

Excludes: soft tissue pain, psychogenic (F45.4)

M79.0 **Rheumatism, unspecified**
Fibromyalgia
Fibrositis

M79.1 **Myalgia**
Excludes: myositis (M60.–)

M79.2 **Neuralgia and neuritis, unspecified**
Excludes: mononeuropathies (G56–G58)
radiculitis:
- NOS (M54.1)
- brachial (M54.1)
- lumbosacral (M54.1)

sciatica (M54.3–M54.4)

Osteopathies and chondropathies (M80–M94)

M80.– Osteoporosis with pathological fracture

[See site code pages 298–299]

Excludes: collapsed vertebra NOS (M48.5)
wedging of vertebra NOS (M48.5)

M81.– Osteoporosis without pathological fracture

[See site code pages 298–299]

M83.– Adult osteomalacia

[See site code pages 298–299]

Excludes: vitamin D-resistant osteomalacia (E83.33)

M85 Other disorders of bone density and structure

[See site code pages 298–299]

Excludes: osteogenesis imperfecta (Q78.0)
osteopetrosis (Q78.2)
osteopoikilosis (Q78.8)
polyostotic fibrous dysplasia (Q78.1)

M85.2 Hyperostosis of skull

M85.3 Osteitis condensans

M88 Paget's disease of bone [osteitis deformans]

[See site code pages 298–299]

M88.0 Paget's disease of skull

M88.8 Paget's disease of other bones

M89 Other disorders of bone

[See site code pages 298–299]

M89.0 Algoneurodystrophy
Shoulder–hand syndrome
Sudeck's atrophy
Sympathetic reflex dystrophy

M89.6 Osteopathy after poliomyelitis
Use additional code (B91), if desired, to identify previous poliomyelitis.

M89.8 Other specified disorders of bone
Infantile cortical hyperostoses
Post-traumatic subperiosteal ossification

Other disorders of the musculoskeletal system and connective tissue (M95–M99)

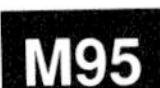

M95 Other acquired deformities of musculoskeletal system and connective tissue

Excludes: congenital malformations and deformations of the musculoskeletal system (Q65–Q79)
deforming dorsopathies (M40–M43)
dentofacial anomalies [including malocclusion] (K07.–)

M95.2 Other acquired deformity of head

M95.3 Acquired deformity of neck

M99 Biomechanical lesions, not elsewhere classified

Note: This category should not be used if the condition can be classified elsewhere.

The following supplementary subclassification to indicate the site of lesions is provided for optional use with appropriate subcategories in M99.–; see also note on page 298.

0	Head region	occipitocervical
1	Cervical region	cervicothoracic
2	Thoracic region	thoracolumbar
3	Lumbar region	lumbosacral
4	Sacral region	sacrococcygeal, sacroiliac
5	Pelvic region	hip, pubic
6	Lower extremity	
7	Upper extremity	acromioclavicular, sternoclavicular
8	Rib cage	costochondral, costovertebral, sternochondral
9	Abdomen and other	

M99.0 Segmental and somatic dysfunction

M99.1 Subluxation complex (vertebral)

M99.2 Subluxation stenosis of neural canal

M99.3 Osseous stenosis of neural canal

M99.4 Connective tissue stenosis of neural canal

M99.5 Intervertebral disc stenosis of neural canal

M99.6 Osseous and subluxation stenosis of intervertebral foramina

M99.7 Connective tissue and disc stenosis of intervertebral foramina

M99.8 Other biomechanical lesions

M99.9 Biomechanical lesion, unspecified

CHAPTER XIV

Diseases of the genitourinary system (N00–N99)

Glomerular diseases (N00–N08)

N00 **Acute nephritic syndrome**

N03 **Chronic nephritic syndrome**

N04 **Nephrotic syndrome**
Congenital nephrotic syndrome
Lipoid nephrosis

N05 **Unspecified nephritic syndrome**
Glomerular disease NOS
Glomerulonephritis NOS
Nephritis NOS
Nephropathy NOS

Renal failure (N17–N19)

Use additional external cause code (Chapter XX), if desired, to identify external agent.

N17.– **Acute renal failure**

N18 **Chronic renal failure**
Includes: chronic uraemia
diffuse sclerosing glomerulonephritis
Excludes: chronic renal failure with hypertension (I12.–)

N18.8 **Other chronic renal failure**
Uraemic neuropathy† (G63.8*)

N19 **Unspecified renal failure**
Uraemia NOS
Excludes: renal failure with hypertension (I12.–)

Other disorders of kidney and ureter (N25–N29)

N25 Disorders resulting from impaired renal tubular function

Excludes: metabolic disorders classifiable to E70–E90

N25.0 Renal osteodystrophy

Azotaemic osteodystrophy
Phosphate-losing tubular disorders
Renal:
- rickets
- short stature

N25.1 Nephrogenic diabetes insipidus

N25.8 Other disorders resulting from impaired renal tubular function

Lightwood–Albright syndrome
Renal tubular acidosis NOS
Secondary hyperparathyroidism of renal origin

Other diseases of the urinary system (N30–N39)

N31 Neuromuscular dysfunction of bladder, not elsewhere classified

Excludes: cord bladder NOS (G95.84)
due to spinal cord lesion (G95.8)
neurogenic bladder due to cauda equina syndrome (G83.41)
urinary incontinence NOS (R32)

N31.0 Uninhibited neuropathic bladder, not elsewhere classified

N31.1 Reflex neuropathic bladder, not elsewhere classified

N31.2 Flaccid neuropathic bladder, not elsewhere classified

Neuropathic bladder:
- atonic (motor)(sensory)
- autonomous
- nonreflex

N31.8 Other neuromuscular dysfunction of bladder

N31.9 Neuromuscular dysfunction of bladder, unspecified
Neurogenic bladder dysfunction NOS

Diseases of male genital organs (N40–N51)

N46 Male infertility

N48 Other disorders of penis

N48.3 Priapism
Painful erection
Excludes: sleep-related painful erections (G47.83)

N48.4 Impotence of organic origin
Use additional code, if desired, to identify cause.

Disorders of breast (N60–N64)

N64 Other disorders of breast

N64.3 Galactorrhoea not associated with childbirth

Noninflammatory disorders of female genital tract (N80–N98)

N91 Absent, scanty and rare menstruation

Excludes: ovarian dysfunction (E28.–)

N91.0 Primary amenorrhoea
Failure to start menstruation at puberty.

N91.1 Secondary amenorrhoea
Absence of menstruation in a woman who had previously menstruated.

N91.2 Amenorrhoea, unspecified
Absence of menstruation NOS

N91.3 Primary oligomenorrhoea
Menstruation which is scanty or rare from the start.

N91.4 Secondary oligomenorrhoea
Scanty and rare menstruation in a woman with previously normal periods.

N91.5 Oligomenorrhoea, unspecified
Hypomenorrhoea NOS

N94 Pain and other conditions associated with female genital organs and menstrual cycle

N94.0 Mittelschmerz

N94.1 Dyspareunia

N94.2 Vaginismus

N94.3 Premenstrual tension syndrome

N94.4 Primary dysmenorrhoea

N94.5 Secondary dysmenorrhoea

N94.6 Dysmenorrhoea, unspecified

N94.8 Other specified conditions associated with female genital organs and menstrual cycle

N94.9 Unspecified condition associated with female genital organs and menstrual cycle

N95 Menopausal and other perimenopausal disorders

Excludes: (postmenopausal) osteoporosis (M81.–)
• with pathological fracture (M80.–)

N95.0 Postmenopausal bleeding
Excludes: that associated with artificial menopause (N95.3)

N95.1 Menopausal and female climacteric states
Symptoms such as flushing, sleeplessness, headache, lack of concentration, associated with menopause
Excludes: that associated with artificial menopause (N95.3)

N95.2 Postmenopausal atrophic vaginitis
Senile (atrophic) vaginitis
Excludes: that associated with artificial menopause (N95.3)

N95.3 States associated with artificial menopause
Post-artificial-menopause syndrome

N97 Female infertility

Includes: inability to achieve a pregnancy
sterility, female NOS

N97.0 Female infertility associated with anovulation

CHAPTER XV

Pregnancy, childbirth and the puerperium (O00–O99)

Excludes: obstetrical tetanus (A34)
postpartum necrosis of pituitary gland (E23. 01)

Pregnancy with abortive outcome (O00–O08)

O08 Complications following abortion and ectopic and molar pregnancy

Note: This code is provided primarily for morbidity coding. For use of this category reference should be made to the morbidity coding rules and guidelines in Volume 2 of ICD-10.

O08.2 Embolism following abortion and ectopic and molar pregnancy

O08.3 Shock following abortion and ectopic and molar pregnancy

O08.4 Renal failure following abortion and ectopic and molar pregnancy

O08.5 Metabolic disorders following abortion and ectopic and molar pregnancy

O08.7 Other venous complications following abortion and ectopic and molar pregnancy

O08.8 Other complications following abortion and ectopic and molar pregnancy
Anoxic brain damage complicating abortion and ectopic and molar pregnancy

Oedema, proteinuria and hypertensive disorders in pregnancy, childbirth and the puerperium (O10–O16)

O10.– Pre-existing hypertension complicating pregnancy, childbirth and the puerperium

Includes: any condition in I10–I15 with pre-existing proteinuria

O12.– Gestational [pregnancy-induced] oedema and proteinuria without hypertension

O13 Gestational [pregnancy-induced] hypertension without significant proteinuria

Mild pre-eclampsia

O14 Gestational [pregnancy-induced] hypertension with significant proteinuria

O14.0 Moderate pre-eclampsia

O14.1 Severe pre-eclampsia

O14.9 Pre-eclampsia, unspecified

O15 Eclampsia

Includes: convulsions following conditions in O10, O12–O14 and O16
eclampsia with pregnancy-induced or pre-existing hypertension

O15.0 Eclampsia in pregnancy

O15.1 Eclampsia in labour

O15.2 Eclampsia in the puerperium

O15.9 Eclampsia, unspecified as to time period

Eclampsia NOS

O16 Unspecified maternal hypertension

Transient hypertension of pregnancy

Other maternal disorders predominantly related to pregnancy (O20–O29)

O21 Excessive vomiting in pregnancy

O21.0 **Mild hyperemesis gravidarum**
Hyperemesis gravidarum, mild or unspecified, starting before the end of the 22nd week of gestation

O21.1 **Hyperemesis gravidarum with metabolic disturbance**
Hyperemesis gravidarum, starting before the end of the 22nd week of gestation, with metabolic disturbance such as:
- carbohydrate depletion
- dehydration
- electrolyte imbalance

O21.2 **Late vomiting of pregnancy**
Excessive vomiting starting after 22 completed weeks of gestation

O21.8 **Other vomiting complicating pregnancy**
Vomiting due to diseases classified elsewhere, complicating pregnancy
Use additional code, if desired, to identify cause.

O21.9 **Vomiting of pregnancy, unspecified**

O22 Venous complications in pregnancy

O22.0 **Varicose veins of lower extremity in pregnancy**

O22.5 **Cerebral venous thrombosis in pregnancy**
Cerebrovenous sinus thrombosis in pregnancy

O26 Maternal care for other conditions predominantly related to pregnancy

O26.8 **Other specified pregnancy-related conditions**
Pregnancy-related peripheral neuritis

O29 Complications of anaesthesia during pregnancy

O29.2 **Central nervous system complications of anaesthesia during pregnancy**
Cerebral anoxia due to anaesthesia during pregnancy

Maternal care related to the fetus and amniotic cavity and possible delivery problems (O30–O48)

O35 Maternal care for known or suspected fetal abnormality and damage

Includes: the listed conditions in the fetus as a reason for observation, hospitalization or other obstetric care of the mother, or for termination of pregnancy

O35.0 Maternal care for (suspected) central nervous system malformation in fetus

Maternal care for (suspected) fetal:
- anencephaly
- spina bifida

Excludes: chromosomal abnormality in fetus (O35.1)

O35.1 Maternal care for (suspected) chromosomal abnormality in fetus

O35.2 Maternal care for (suspected) hereditary disease in fetus

Excludes: chromosomal abnormality in fetus (O35.1)

O35.3 Maternal care for (suspected) damage to fetus from viral disease in mother

Maternal care for (suspected) damage to fetus from maternal:
- cytomegalovirus infection
- rubella

O35.4 Maternal care for (suspected) damage to fetus from alcohol

O35.5 Maternal care for (suspected) damage to fetus by drugs

Maternal care for (suspected) damage to fetus from drug addiction

O35.6 Maternal care for (suspected) damage to fetus by radiation

O36 Maternal care for other known or suspected fetal problems

Includes: the listed conditions in the fetus as a reason for observation, hospitalization or other obstetric care of the mother, or for termination of pregnancy

O36.3 Maternal care for signs of fetal hypoxia

Complications of labour and delivery (O60–O75)

O74 Complications of anaesthesia during labour and delivery

Includes: maternal complications arising from the administration of a general or local anaesthetic, analgesic or other sedation during labour and delivery

O74.0 Aspiration pneumonitis due to anaesthesia during labour and delivery

Inhalation of stomach contents or secretions NOS } due to anaesthesia during labour and delivery
Mendelson's syndrome } due to anaesthesia during labour and delivery

O74.1 Other pulmonary complications of anaesthesia during labour and delivery

Pressure collapse of lung due to anaesthesia during labour and delivery

O74.2 Cardiac complications of anaesthesia during labour and delivery

Cardiac:
- arrest } due to anaesthesia during labour and delivery
- failure } due to anaesthesia during labour and delivery

O74.3 Central nervous system complications of anaesthesia during labour and delivery

Cerebral anoxia due to anaesthesia during labour and delivery

O74.4 Toxic reaction to local anaesthesia during labour and delivery

O74.5 Spinal and epidural anaesthesia-induced headache during labour and delivery

O74.6 Other complications of spinal and epidural anaesthesia during labour and delivery

O74.7 Failed or difficult intubation during labour and delivery

O74.8 Other complications of anaesthesia during labour and delivery

O74.9 Complication of anaesthesia during labour and delivery, unspecified

O75 Other complications of labour and delivery, not elsewhere classified

O75.0 Maternal distress during labour and delivery

O75.1 Shock during or following labour and delivery
Obstetric shock

O75.2 Pyrexia during labour, not elsewhere classified

O75.3 Other infection during labour
Septicaemia during labour

O75.4 Other complications of obstetric surgery and procedures
Cardiac:
- arrest
- failure

Cerebral anoxia

} following caesarean or other obstetric surgery or procedures, including delivery NOS

Complications predominantly related to the puerperium (O85–O92)

O87 Venous complications in the puerperium

Includes: in labour, delivery and the puerperium
Excludes: obstetric embolism (O88.–)
venous complications in pregnancy (O22.–)

O87.3 Cerebral venous thrombosis in the puerperium
Cerebrovenous sinus thrombosis in the puerperium

O87.8 Other venous complications in the puerperium

O87.9 Venous complication in the puerperium, unspecified
Puerperal:
- phlebitis NOS
- phlebopathy NOS
- thrombosis NOS

O88 Obstetric embolism

Includes: pulmonary emboli in pregnancy, childbirth or the puerperium
Excludes: embolism complicating abortion or ectopic or molar pregnancy (O08.2)

O88.0 Obstetric air embolism

O88.1 Amniotic fluid embolism

O88.2 Obstetric blood-clot embolism

O88.3 Obstetric pyaemic and septic embolism

O88.8 Other obstetric embolism
Obstetric fat embolism

O89 Complications of anaesthesia during the puerperium

O89.2 Central nervous system complications of anaesthesia during the puerperium
Cerebral anoxia due to anaesthesia during the puerperium

O89.3 Toxic reaction to local anaesthesia during the puerperium

O89.4 Spinal and epidural anaesthesia-induced headache during the puerperium

O89.5 Other complications of spinal and epidural anaesthesia during the puerperium

O99 Other maternal diseases classifiable elsewhere but complicating pregnancy, childbirth and the puerperium

Use additional code, if desired, to identify specific condition.

O99.3 Mental disorders and diseases of the nervous system complicating pregnancy, childbirth and the puerperium
Conditions in F00–F99 and G00–G99
Excludes: pregnancy-related peripheral neuritis (O26.8)

CHAPTER XVI

Certain conditions originating in the perinatal period (P00–P99)

Includes: conditions that have their origin in the perinatal period even though death or morbidity occurs later

Excludes: congenital malformations, deformations and chromosomal abnormalities (Q00–Q99)
endocrine, nutritional and metabolic diseases (E00–E90)
injury, poisoning and certain consequences of external causes (S00–T98)
neoplasms (C00–D48)
tetanus neonatorum (A33)

Fetus and newborn affected by maternal factors and by complications of pregnancy, labour and delivery (P00–P04)

Includes: the listed maternal conditions only when specified as a cause of mortality and morbidity in fetus or newborn

P00 Fetus and newborn affected by maternal conditions that may be unrelated to present pregnancy

P00.4 Fetus and newborn affected by maternal nutritional disorders

Fetus or newborn affected by maternal disorders classifiable to E40–E64
Maternal malnutrition NOS

P00.5 Fetus and newborn affected by maternal injury

Fetus or newborn affected by maternal conditions classifiable to S00–T79

P00.6 Fetus and newborn affected by surgical procedure on mother

Excludes: caesarean section for present delivery (P03.4)
previous surgery to uterus or pelvic organs (P03.8)

P00.7 Fetus and newborn affected by other medical procedures on mother, not elsewhere classified

Fetus or newborn affected by radiology

P01.– Fetus and newborn affected by maternal complications of pregnancy

P02.– Fetus and newborn affected by complications of placenta, cord and membranes

P03 Fetus and newborn affected by other complications of labour and delivery

P03.0 Fetus and newborn affected by breech delivery and extraction

P03.1 Fetus and newborn affected by other malpresentation, malposition and disproportion during labour and delivery

Contracted pelvis
Persistent occipitoposterior
Transverse lie

P03.2 Fetus and newborn affected by forceps delivery

P03.3 Fetus and newborn affected by delivery by vacuum extractor [ventouse]

P03.4 Fetus and newborn affected by caesarean delivery

P03.5 Fetus and newborn affected by precipitate delivery

Rapid second stage

P03.6 Fetus and newborn affected by abnormal uterine contractions

Hypertonic labour
Uterine inertia

P03.8 Fetus and newborn affected by other specified complications of labour and delivery

Abnormality of maternal soft tissues
Destructive operation to facilitate delivery
Fetus or newborn affected by other conditions classifiable to O60–O75 and by procedures used in labour and delivery not included in P02.– and P03.0–P03.6
Induction of labour

P03.9 Fetus and newborn affected by complication of labour and delivery, unspecified

P04 Fetus and newborn affected by noxious influences transmitted via placenta or breast milk

Excludes: congenital malformations (Q00–Q99)
neonatal jaundice from other excessive haemolysis due to drugs or toxins transmitted from mother (P58.–)

P04.0 Fetus and newborn affected by maternal anaesthesia and analgesia in pregnancy, labour and delivery

Reactions and intoxications from maternal opiates and tranquillizers administered during labour and delivery

P04.1 Fetus and newborn affected by other maternal medication

Cancer chemotherapy
Cytotoxic drugs

Excludes: dysmorphism due to warfarin (Q86.2)
fetal hydantoin syndrome (Q86.1)
maternal use of drugs of addiction (P04.4)

P04.2 Fetus and newborn affected by maternal use of tobacco

P04.3 Fetus and newborn affected by maternal use of alcohol

Excludes: fetal alcohol syndrome (Q86.0)

P04.4 Fetus and newborn affected by maternal use of drugs of addiction

Excludes: withdrawal symptoms from maternal use of drugs of addiction (P96.1)

P04.5 Fetus and newborn affected by maternal use of nutritional chemical substances

P04.6 Fetus and newborn affected by maternal exposure to environmental chemical substances

P04.8 Fetus and newborn affected by other maternal noxious influences

P04.9 Fetus and newborn affected by maternal noxious influence, unspecified

Disorders related to length of gestation and fetal growth (P05–P08)

P05 Slow fetal growth and fetal malnutrition

P05.0 **Light for gestational age**
Usually referred to as weight below but length above 10th centile for gestational age.

Light-for-dates

P05.1 **Small for gestational age**
Usually referred to as weight and length below 10th centile for gestational age.

Small-for-dates

P05.2 **Fetal malnutrition without mention of light or small for gestational age**
Infant, not light or small for gestational age, showing signs of fetal malnutrition, such as dry, peeling skin and loss of subcutaneous tissue.

P05.9 **Slow fetal growth, unspecified**
Fetal growth retardation NOS

P07.– Disorders related to short gestation and low birth weight, not elsewhere classified

Note: When both birth weight and gestational age are available, priority of assignment should be given to birth weight.

Includes: the listed conditions, without further specification, as causes of mortality, morbidity or additional care, in newborn

P08.– Disorders related to long gestation and high birth weight

Note: When both birth weight and gestational age are available, priority of assignment should be given to birth weight.

Includes: the listed conditions, without further specification, as causes of mortality, morbidity or additional care, in fetus or newborn

Birth trauma (P10–P15)

P10 Intracranial laceration and haemorrhage due to birth injury

Excludes: intracranial haemorrhage of fetus or newborn:
- NOS (P52.9)
- due to anoxia or hypoxia (P52.–)

P10.0 Subdural haemorrhage due to birth injury
Subdural haematoma (localized) due to birth injury
Excludes: subdural haemorrhage accompanying tentorial tear (P10.4)

P10.1 Cerebral haemorrhage due to birth injury

P10.2 Intraventricular haemorrhage due to birth injury

P10.3 Subarachnoid haemorrhage due to birth injury

P10.4 Tentorial tear due to birth injury

P10.8 Other intracranial lacerations and haemorrhages due to birth injury

P10.9 Unspecified intracranial laceration and haemorrhage due to birth injury

P11 Other birth injury to central nervous system

P11.0 Cerebral oedema due to birth injury

P11.1 Other specified brain damage due to birth injury

P11.2 Unspecified brain damage due to birth injury

P11.3 Birth injury to facial nerve
Facial palsy due to birth injury

P11.4 Birth injury to other cranial nerves

P11.5 Birth injury to spine and spinal cord
Fracture of spine due to birth injury

P11.9 Birth injury to central nervous system, unspecified

P14 Birth injury to peripheral nervous system

P14.0 Erb's paralysis due to birth injury

P14.1 Klumpke's paralysis due to birth injury

P14.2 **Phrenic nerve paralysis due to birth injury**

P14.3 **Other brachial plexus birth injuries**

P14.8 **Birth injuries to other parts of peripheral nervous system**

P14.9 **Birth injury to peripheral nervous system, unspecified**

Respiratory and cardiovascular disorders specific to the perinatal period (P20–P29)

P20 Intrauterine hypoxia

Includes: abnormal fetal heart rate
fetal or intrauterine:
- acidosis
- anoxia
- asphyxia
- distress
- hypoxia

meconium in liquor
passage of meconium

Excludes: intracranial haemorrhage due to anoxia or hypoxia (P52.–)

P20.0 **Intrauterine hypoxia first noted before onset of labour**

P20.1 **Intrauterine hypoxia first noted during labour and delivery**

P20.9 **Intrauterine hypoxia, unspecified**

P21 Birth asphyxia

P21.0 **Severe birth asphyxia**

Pulse less than 100 per minute at birth and falling or steady, respiration absent or gasping, colour poor, muscle tone absent.

Asphyxia with 1-minute Apgar score 0–3
White asphyxia

P21.1 **Mild and moderate birth asphyxia**

Normal respiration not established within one minute, but heart rate 100 or above, some muscle tone present, some response to stimulation.

Asphyxia with 1-minute Apgar score 4–7
Blue asphyxia

P21.9 Birth asphyxia, unspecified
Anoxia, Asphyxia, Hypoxia } NOS

P22 Respiratory distress of newborn

P22.0 Respiratory distress syndrome of newborn
Hyaline membrane disease

P22.1 Transient tachypnoea of newborn

P22.8 Other respiratory distress of newborn

P22.9 Respiratory distress of newborn, unspecified

P23.– Congenital pneumonia

Includes: infective pneumonia acquired in utero or during birth

P24.– Neonatal aspiration syndromes

Includes: neonatal pneumonia resulting from aspiration

Infections specific to the perinatal period (P35–P39)

Includes: infections acquired in utero or during birth
Excludes: asymptomatic human immunodeficiency virus [HIV] infection status (Z21)
congenital:
- gonococcal infection (A54.–)
- pneumonia (P23.–)
- syphilis (A50.–)

human immunodeficiency virus [HIV] disease (B20–B24)
infectious diseases acquired after birth (A00–B99, J10–J11)
laboratory evidence of human immunodeficiency virus [HIV] (R75)
tetanus neonatorum (A33)

P35 Congenital viral diseases

P35.0 Congenital rubella syndrome
Congenital rubella pneumonitis

P35.1 Congenital cytomegalovirus infection

P35.2 Congenital herpesviral [herpes simplex] infection

P35.3 Congenital viral hepatitis

P35.8 Other congenital viral diseases
Congenital varicella [chickenpox]

P35.9 Congenital viral disease, unspecified

P37 Other congenital infectious and parasitic diseases

Excludes: congenital syphilis (A50.–)
tetanus neonatorum (A33)

P37.0 Congenital tuberculosis

P37.1 Congenital toxoplasmosis
Hydrocephalus due to congenital toxoplasmosis

P37.2 Neonatal (disseminated) listeriosis

P37.3 Congenital falciparum malaria

P37.4 Other congenital malaria

P37.5 Neonatal candidiasis

P38 Omphalitis of newborn with or without mild haemorrhage

P39.– Other infections specific to the perinatal period

Haemorrhagic and haematological disorders of fetus and newborn (P50–P61)

P52 Intracranial nontraumatic haemorrhage of fetus and newborn

Includes: intracranial haemorrhage due to anoxia or hypoxia
Excludes: intracranial haemorrhage due to injury:
- birth (P10.–)
- maternal (P00.5)
- other (S06.–)

P52.0 Intraventricular (nontraumatic) haemorrhage, grade 1, of fetus and newborn
Subependymal haemorrhage (without intraventricular extension)

P52.1 Intraventricular (nontraumatic) haemorrhage, grade 2, of fetus and newborn
Subependymal haemorrhage with intraventricular extension

P52.2 Intraventricular (nontraumatic) haemorrhage, grade 3, of fetus and newborn
Subependymal haemorrhage with both intraventricular and intracerebral extension

P52.3 Unspecified intraventricular (nontraumatic) haemorrhage of fetus and newborn

P52.4 Intracerebral (nontraumatic) haemorrhage of fetus and newborn

P52.5 Subarachnoid (nontraumatic) haemorrhage of fetus and newborn

P52.6 Cerebellar (nontraumatic) and posterior fossa haemorrhage of fetus and newborn

P52.8 Other intracranial (nontraumatic) haemorrhages of fetus and newborn

P52.9 Intracranial (nontraumatic) haemorrhage of fetus and newborn, unspecified

P53 Haemorrhagic disease of fetus and newborn

Vitamin K deficiency of newborn

P57 Kernicterus

P57.0 Kernicterus due to isoimmunization

P57.8 Other specified kernicterus
Excludes: Crigler–Najjar syndrome (E80.5)

P57.9 Kernicterus, unspecified

P58.– Neonatal jaundice due to other excessive haemolysis

P59.– Neonatal jaundice from other and unspecified causes

Excludes: due to inborn errors of metabolism (E70–E90)
kernicterus (P57.–)

Transitory endocrine and metabolic disorders specific to fetus and newborn (P70–P74)

Includes: transitory endocrine and metabolic disturbances caused by the infant's response to maternal endocrine and metabolic factors, or its adjustment to extrauterine existence

P70 Transitory disorders of carbohydrate metabolism specific to fetus and newborn

P70.0 Syndrome of infant of mother with gestational diabetes

P70.1 Syndrome of infant of a diabetic mother
Maternal diabetes mellitus (pre-existing) affecting fetus or newborn (with hypoglycaemia)

P70.2 Neonatal diabetes mellitus

P70.3 Iatrogenic neonatal hypoglycaemia

P70.4 Other neonatal hypoglycaemia
Transitory neonatal hypoglycaemia

P71 Transitory neonatal disorders of calcium and magnesium metabolism

P71.0 Cow's milk hypocalcaemia in newborn

P71.1 Other neonatal hypocalcaemia
Excludes: neonatal hypoparathyroidism (P71.4)

P71.2 Neonatal hypomagnesaemia

P71.3 Neonatal tetany without calcium or magnesium deficiency
Neonatal tetany NOS

P71.4 Transitory neonatal hypoparathyroidism

P72 Other transitory neonatal endocrine disorders

Excludes: congenital hypothyroidism with or without goitre (E03.0–E03.1)

P72.1 Transitory neonatal hyperthyroidism
Neonatal thyrotoxicosis

P72.2 Other transitory neonatal disorders of thyroid function, not elsewhere classified
Transitory neonatal hypothyroidism

P74 Other transitory neonatal electrolyte and metabolic disturbances

P74.0 Late metabolic acidosis of newborn

P74.1 Dehydration of newborn

P74.2 Disturbances of sodium balance of newborn

P74.3 Disturbances of potassium balance of newborn

P74.5 Transitory tyrosinaemia of newborn

Other disorders originating in the perinatal period (P90–P96)

P90 Convulsions of newborn

Excludes: benign neonatal convulsions (familial) (G40.31)

Use an additional fifth character to indicate the type of convulsion:

P90.–0 Clonic
P90.–1 Tonic
P90.–2 Myoclonic
P90.–3 Other, including subtle

Use an additional sixth character to further specify the type of convulsion:

P90.–*x*0 Focal
P90.–*x*1 Multifocal
P90.–*x*2 Generalized

Use an additional code, if desired, to identify associated condition(s) or cause, such as birth injury (P10.–, P11.–), birth asphyxia (P21.–), infectious diseases (P35.–, P37.–), haemorrhagic disorders (P52.–, P53, P57.–), metabolic disorders (P70.–, P71.–, P74.–), withdrawal symptoms from maternal use of drugs of addiction (P96.1).

P91 Other disturbances of cerebral status of newborn

P91.0 Neonatal cerebral ischaemia

P91.1 Acquired periventricular cysts of newborn

P91.2 Neonatal cerebral leukomalacia

P91.3 Neonatal cerebral irritability

P91.4 Neonatal cerebral depression

P91.5 **Neonatal coma**

P91.8 **Other specified disturbances of cerebral status of newborn**

P91.9 **Disturbance of cerebral status of newborn, unspecified**

P94 Disorders of muscle tone of newborn

P94.0 **Transient neonatal myasthenia gravis**
Excludes: myasthenia gravis (G70.0)

P94.1 **Congenital hypertonia**

P94.2 **Congenital hypotonia**
Nonspecific floppy baby syndrome

P94.8 **Other disorders of muscle tone of newborn**

P94.9 **Disorder of muscle tone of newborn, unspecified**

P96 Other conditions originating in the perinatal period

P96.0 **Congenital renal failure**
Uraemia of newborn

P96.1 **Neonatal withdrawal symptoms from maternal use of drugs of addiction**
Drug withdrawal syndrome in infant of dependent mother
Excludes: reactions and intoxications from maternal opiates and tranquillizers administered during labour and delivery (P04.0)

P96.2 **Withdrawal symptoms from therapeutic use of drugs in newborn**

P96.3 **Wide cranial sutures of newborn**
Neonatal craniotabes

CHAPTER XVII

Congenital malformations, deformations and chromosomal abnormalities (Q00–Q99)

Excludes: inborn errors of metabolism (E70–E90)

Congenital malformations of the nervous system (Q00–Q07)

Q00 Anencephaly and similar malformations

Q00.0 Anencephaly

Q00.00 Acrania
Q00.01 Acephaly
Q00.02 Atelencephaly clausa
Q00.03 Atelencephaly aperta
Q00.04 Hemicephaly
Q00.05 Hemianencephaly
Q00.06 Amyelencephaly
Q00.07 Hydranencephaly
Q00.08 Other anencephaly

Q00.1 Craniorachischisis

Q00.2 Iniencephaly

Q00.20 Iniencephaly clausa
Q00.21 Iniencephaly aperta

Q01 Encephalocele

Use additional sixth character, if desired, to indicate:

Q01.*xx*0 Encephalomyelocele
Q01.*xx*1 Hydroencephalocele
Q01.*xx*2 Hydromeningocele, cranial
Q01.*xx*3 Meningocele, cerebral
Q01.*xx*4 Meningoencephalocele

Q01.0 **Frontal encephalocele**

Q01.1 **Nasofrontal encephalocele**

Q01.2 **Occipital encephalocele**

Q01.8 **Encephalocele of other sites**

Q01.80 Parietal encephalocele
Q01.81 Nasopharyngeal encephalocele
Q01.82 Temporal encephalocele
Q01.83 Orbital encephalocele

Q01.9 **Encephalocele, unspecified**

Q02 Microcephaly

Q02.–0 Hydromicrocephaly
Q02.–1 Micrencephalon

Q03 Congenital hydrocephalus

Includes: hydrocephalus in newborn
Excludes: Arnold–Chiari syndrome (Q07.0)
hydrocephalus:
- acquired (G91.–)
- due to congenital toxoplasmosis (P37.1)
- with spina bifida (Q05.0–Q05.4)

Q03.0 **Malformations of aqueduct of Sylvius**

Aqueduct of Sylvius:
- anomaly
- obstruction, congenital
- stenosis

Q03.1 **Atresia of foramina of Magendie and Luschka**

Dandy–Walker syndrome

Q03.8 **Other congenital hydrocephalus**

Q03.80 Congenital hydrocephalus in malformations classified elsewhere

Q03.9 **Congenital hydrocephalus, unspecified**

Q04 Other congenital malformations of brain

Excludes: cyclopia (Q87.02)
macrocephaly (Q75.3)

Q04.0 **Congenital malformations of corpus callosum**

Q04.00 Total agenesis of corpus callosum
Q04.01 Partial agenesis of corpus callosum
Q04.02 Agenesis with lipoma of corpus callosum
Q04.08 Other congenital malformations of corpus callosum

Q04.1 Arhinencephaly

Q04.2 Holoprosencephaly

Q04.3 Other reduction deformities of brain
Excludes: congenital malformation of corpus callosum (Q04.0)

Q04.30 Agyria
Q04.31 Lissencephaly
Q04.32 Microgyria
Q04.33 Pachygyria
Q04.34 Agenesis of part of brain, unspecified
Includes: absence, aplasia, hypoplasia } of part of brain, unspecified

Use additional sixth character, if desired and appropriate, to indicate location:

Q04.3*x*0 Frontal
Q04.3*x*1 Temporal
Q04.3*x*2 Parietal
Q04.3*x*3 Occipital
Q04.3*x*4 Brain stem
Q04.3*x*5 Cerebellum hemispheres
Q04.3*x*6 Cerebellar vermis
Q04.3*x*7 Optic nerves
Q04.3*x*8 Thalamus or basal ganglia
Q04.3*x*9 Hypothalamus

Q04.4 Septo-optic dysplasia

Q04.5 Megalencephaly

Q04.50 Symmetrical megalencephaly

Q04.6 Congenital cerebral cysts
Excludes: acquired porencephalic cyst (G93.01)

Q04.60 Porencephaly
Q04.61 Schizencephaly
Q04.62 Multicystic encephalomalacia
Q04.63 Congenital leptomeningeal cyst

Q04.8 Other specified congenital malformations of brain

Q04.80 Macrogyria
Q04.81 Ulegyria
Q04.82 Agenesis of septum pellucidum
Q04.83 Copocephaly
Q04.84 Disorders of neuronal migration
  Q04.840 Cortical lamination abnormality
  Q04.841 Neuronal heterotopia

Q04.9 Congenital malformation of brain, unspecified

Congenital:
- anomaly
- deformity
- disease or lesion
- multiple anomalies

} NOS of brain

Q05 Spina bifida

For spina bifida associated with other congenital abnormalities, use additional codes, if desired, to identify each condition.

Excludes: Arnold–Chiari syndrome (Q07.0)
spina bifida occulta (Q76.0)

Use additional fifth character, if desired, to indicate:
Q05.*x*0 Hydromeningocele, spinal
Q05.*x*1 Lipomeningocele
Q05.*x*2 Meningomyelocele
Q05.*x*3 Myelocele
Q05.*x*4 Myelomeningocele
Q05.*x*5 Rachischisis
Q05.*x*6 Spina bifida (aperta)(cystica)
Q05.*x*7 Syringomyelocele

Q05.0 Cervical spina bifida with hydrocephalus

Q05.1 Thoracic spina bifida with hydrocephalus

Spina bifida:
- dorsal
- thoracolumbar

} with hydrocephalus

Q05.2 Lumbar spina bifida with hydrocephalus

Lumbosacral spina bifida with hydrocephalus

Q05.3 Sacral spina bifida with hydrocephalus

Q05.4 Unspecified spina bifida with hydrocephalus

Q05.5 Cervical spina bifida without hydrocephalus

Q05.6 Thoracic spina bifida without hydrocephalus
Spina bifida:
- dorsal NOS
- thoracolumbar NOS

Q05.7 Lumbar spina bifida without hydrocephalus
Lumbosacral spina bifida NOS

Q05.8 Sacral spina bifida without hydrocephalus

Q05.9 Spina bifida, unspecified

Q06 Other congenital malformations of spinal cord

Q06.0 Amyelia

Q06.1 Hypoplasia and dysplasia of spinal cord
Atelomyelia
Myelatelia
Myelodysplasia of spinal cord

Q06.2 Diastematomyelia

Q06.3 Other congenital cauda equina malformations

Q06.4 Hydromyelia
Hydrorachis
Isolated hydromelia
Excludes: hydromelia associated with syringomyelia and syringobulbia (G95.0)

Q06.8 Other specified congenital malformations of spinal cord

Q06.80 Diplomyelia
Q06.81 Tethered spinal cord

Q06.9 Congenital malformation of spinal cord, unspecified
Congenital:
- anomaly
- deformity
- disease or lesion

} NOS of spinal cord or meninges

Q07 Other congenital malformations of nervous system

Excludes: familial dysautonomia [Riley–Day] (G90.1)
neurofibromatosis (nonmalignant) (Q85.0)

Q07.0 Arnold–Chiari syndrome

Q07.00 Chiari malformation, type I
Q07.01 Chiari malformation, type II
Q07.02 Chiari malformation, type III

Q07.8 Other specified congenital malformations of nervous system

Q07.80 Agenesis of nerve
Q07.81 Displacement of brachial plexus
Q07.82 Jaw-winking syndrome [Marcus Gunn]

Q07.9 Congenital malformation of nervous system, unspecified

Congenital:
- anomaly
- deformity
- disease or lesion

} NOS of nervous system

Congenital malformations of eye, ear, face and neck (Q10–Q18)

Q10 Congenital malformations of eyelid, lacrimal apparatus and orbit

Q10.0 Congenital ptosis

Q10.7 Congenital malformation of orbit

Q11 Anophthalmos, microphthalmos and macrophthalmos

Q11.0 Cystic eyeball

Q11.1 Other anophthalmos

Agenesis
Aplasia
} of eye

Q11.2 Microphthalmos

Cryptophthalmos NOS
Dysplasia of eye
Hypoplasia of eye
Rudimentary eye
Excludes: cryptophthalmos syndrome (Q87.082)

Q11.3 Macrophthalmos

Excludes: macrophthalmos in congenital glaucoma (Q15.0)

Q14 Congenital malformations of posterior segment of eye

Q14.0 Congenital malformation of vitreous humour
Congenital vitreous opacity

Q14.1 Congenital malformation of retina
Congenital retinal aneurysm

Q14.2 Congenital malformation of optic disc
Coloboma of optic disc

Q14.3 Congenital malformation of choroid

Q14.8 Other congenital malformations of posterior segment of eye
Coloboma of fundus

Q14.9 Congenital malformation of posterior segment of eye, unspecified

Q15 Other congenital malformations of eye

Excludes: congenital nystagmus (H55)
ocular albinism (E70.31)
retinitis pigmentosa (H35.5)

Q15.0 Congenital glaucoma

Q16 Congenital malformations of ear causing impairment of hearing

Excludes: congenital deafness (H90.–)

Q16.0 Congenital absence of (ear) auricle

Q16.1 Congenital absence, atresia and stricture of auditory canal (external)

Q16.2 Absence of eustachian tube

Q16.3 Congenital malformation of ear ossicles
Fusion of ear ossicles

Q16.4 Other congenital malformations of middle ear
Congenital malformation of middle ear NOS

Q16.5 Congenital malformation of inner ear
Anomaly:
- membranous labyrinth
- organ of Corti

Q16.9 Congenital malformation of ear causing impairment of hearing, unspecified
Congenital absence of ear NOS

Q18 Other congenital malformations of face and neck

Excludes: conditions classified to Q67.0–Q67.4
congenital malformation of skull and face bones (Q75.–)
cyclopia (Q87.02)
dentofacial anomalies [including malocclusion] (K07.–)
malformation syndromes affecting facial appearance (Q87.0)

Q18.0 Sinus, fistula and cyst of branchial cleft
Branchial vestige

Q18.1 Preauricular sinus and cyst
Fistula (of):
- auricle, congenital
- cervicoaural

Q18.2 Other branchial cleft malformations
Branchial cleft malformation NOS
Cervical auricle
Otocephaly

Q18.3 Webbing of neck
Pterygium colli

Q18.4 Macrostomia

Q18.5 Microstomia

Q18.6 Macrocheilia
Hypertrophy of lip, congenital

Q18.7 Microcheilia

Q18.8 Other specified congenital malformations of face and neck
Medial:
- cyst } of face and neck
- fistula } of face and neck
- sinus } of face and neck

Q18.9 Congenital malformation of face and neck, unspecified
Congenital anomaly NOS of face and neck

Congenital malformations of the circulatory system (Q20–Q28)

Q27 Other congenital malformations of peripheral vascular system

Excludes: anomalies of cerebral and precerebral vessels (Q28.0–Q28.3)
congenital retinal aneurysm (Q14.1)
haemangioma and lymphangioma (D18.–)

Q27.4 Congenital phlebectasia

Q28 Other congenital malformations of circulatory system

Excludes: congenital retinal aneurysm (Q14.1)
ruptured:
- cerebral aneurysms (I60.1–I60.7, I60.9)
- cerebral arteriovenous malformation (I60.8)
- malformation of precerebral vessels (I72.–)

Q28.0 Arteriovenous malformation of precerebral vessels

Congenital arteriovenous precerebral aneurysm (nonruptured)

Q28.1 Other malformations of precerebral vessels

Congenital:
- malformation of precerebral vessels NOS
- precerebral aneurysm (nonruptured)

Q28.2 Arteriovenous malformation of cerebral vessels

Includes: arteriovenous malformation of brain NOS
congenital arteriovenous cerebral aneurysm (nonruptured)

Use additional fifth and sixth characters, if desired, for location of arteriovenous malformation:

Q28.20 Arteriovenous malformation in hemisphere, cortical
- Q28.200 Frontal
- Q28.201 Temporal
- Q28.202 Parietal
- Q28.203 Occipital
- Q28.207 Involving more than one lobe

Q28.21 Arteriovenous malformation in hemisphere, subcortical
- Q28.210 Basal ganglia
- Q28.211 Internal capsule
- Q28.212 Thalamus
- Q28.213 Hypothalamus

Q28.214 Corpus callosum

Q28.217 Involving more than one subcortical structure

Q28.22 Arteriovenous malformation in hemisphere, unspecified

Q28.23 Arteriovenous malformation in brain stem

Q28.230 Midbrain

Q28.231 Pons

Q28.232 Medulla

Q28.237 Involving more than one subdivision of brain stem

Q28.24 Arteriovenous malformation in cerebellum

Q28.25 Arteriovenous malformation in choroid plexus

Q28.250 Choroid plexus of lateral ventricle

Q28.251 Choroid plexus of third ventricle

Q28.252 Choroid plexus of fourth ventricle

Q28.257 Multiple locations in choroid plexus

Q28.26 Arteriovenous malformation in spinal cord

Q28.260 Cervical spinal cord

Q28.261 Thoracic spinal cord

Q28.262 Lumbosacral spinal cord

Q28.267 More than one subdivision of spinal cord

Q28.27 Multiple or widespread arteriovenous malformation

Q28.3 Other malformations of cerebral vessels

Includes: congenital:

- cerebral aneurysm (nonruptured)
- malformation of cerebral vessels NOS

Q28.30 Carotid siphon and internal carotid artery bifurcation

Q28.300 Aneurysm at origin of ophthalmic artery

Q28.301 Aneurysm at origin of anterior choroidal artery

Q28.302 Aneurysm at origin of posterior communicating artery

Q28.303 Aneurysm at bifurcation of internal carotid artery

Q28.31 Middle cerebral artery

Q28.310 Proximal (M1-horizontal segment) middle cerebral artery aneurysm

Q28.311 Aneurysm at major bi- or trifurcation of middle cerebral artery

Q28.312 Distal middle cerebral artery aneurysm

Q28.32 Anterior cerebral and communicating artery

Q28.320 Anterior communicating artery aneurysm

Q28.321 Proximal (A1-horizontal segment) anterior cerebral artery aneurysm

Q28.322 Distal (A2-vertical segment) anterior cerebral artery aneurysm

Q28.33 Posterior communicating artery
Distal posterior communicating artery aneurysm

Q28.34 Basilar artery

Q28.340 Proximal basilar artery (vertebral artery confluence) aneurysm
Q28.341 Midbasilar artery aneurysm
Q28.342 Top of basilar artery aneurysm
Q28.343 Bifid basilar artery aneurysm
Q28.344 Aneurysm at origin of superior cerebellar artery
Q28.345 Aneurysm at origin of anterior inferior cerebellar artery

Q28.35 Vertebral artery
Includes: intracranial vertebral artery aneurysm

Q28.350 Aneurysm at origin of posterior inferior cerebellar artery

Q28.37 Multiple intracranial aneurysms, unspecified

Q28.38 Other specified intracranial arteries

Q28.380 Distal superior cerebellar artery
Q28.381 Distal anterior inferior cerebellar artery
Q28.382 Distal posterior inferior cerebellar artery
Q28.383 Internal auditory artery
Q28.384 Proximal posterior cerebral artery
Q28.385 Distal posterior cerebral artery

Q28.8 Other specified congenital malformations of circulatory system
Congenital aneurysm, specified site NEC

Q28.9 Congenital malformation of circulatory system, unspecified

Congenital malformations of the urinary system (Q60–Q64)

Q61.– Cystic kidney disease

Congenital malformations and deformations of the musculoskeletal system (Q65–Q79)

Q66 Congenital deformities of feet

Q66.0 Talipes equinovarus

Q66.1 Talipes calcaneovarus

Q66.2 Metatarsus varus

Q66.3 Other congenital varus deformities of feet
Hallux varus, congenital

Q66.4 Talipes calcaneovalgus

Q66.5 Congenital pes planus
Flat foot:
- congenital
- rigid
- spastic (everted)

Q66.6 Other congenital valgus deformities of feet
Metatarsus valgus

Q66.7 Pes cavus

Q66.8 Other congenital deformities of feet
Clubfoot NOS
Hammer toe, congenital
Talipes:
- NOS
- asymmetric

Tarsal coalition
Vertical talus

Q66.9 Congenital deformity of feet, unspecified

Q67 Congenital musculoskeletal deformities of head, face, spine and chest

Q67.0 Facial asymmetry

Q67.1 Compression facies

Q67.2 Dolichocephaly

Q67.3 Plagiocephaly

Q67.4 Other congenital deformities of skull, face and jaw
Depressions in skull
Deviation of nasal septum, congenital
Hemifacial atrophy or hypertrophy
Squashed or bent nose, congenital
Excludes: dentofacial anomalies [including malocclusion] (K07.–)

Q67.5 Congenital deformity of spine
Congenital scoliosis:
- NOS
- postural

Excludes: infantile idiopathic scoliosis (M41.0)
scoliosis due to congenital bony malformation (Q76.3)

Q68 Other congenital musculoskeletal deformities

Q68.0 Congenital deformity of sternocleidomastoid muscle
Congenital (sternomastoid) torticollis

Q74 Other congenital malformations of limb(s)

Q74.3 Arthrogryposis multiplex congenita

Q75 Other congenital malformations of skull and face bones

Excludes: congenital malformation (of):
- face NOS (Q18.–)
- predominantly affecting facial appearance (Q87.0)

dentofacial anomalies [including malocclusion] (K07.–)
musculoskeletal deformities of head and face (Q67.0–Q67.4)
skull defects associated with congenital anomalies of brain such as:
- anencephaly (Q00.0)
- encephalocele (Q01.–)
- hydrocephalus (Q03.–)
- microcephaly (Q02)

Q75.0 Craniosynostosis

Q75.00 Acrocephaly
Q75.01 Imperfect fusion of skull
Q75.02 Oxycephaly
Q75.03 Trigonocephaly

Q75.1 Craniofacial dysostosis
Crouzon's disease
Excludes: Apert's syndrome (Q87.01)
Carpenter's syndrome (Q87.083)

Q75.2 Hypertelorism

Q75.3 Macrocephaly

Q75.4 Mandibulofacial dysostosis

Q75.5 Oculomandibular dysostosis

Q75.8 Other specified congenital malformations of skull and face bones

Q75.80 Absence of skull bone, congenital
Q75.81 Congenital deformity of forehead
Q75.82 Platybasia
Q75.83 Hypotelorism

Q75.9 Congenital malformation of skull and face bones, unspecified

Congenital anomaly of:
- face bones NOS
- skull NOS

Q76 Congenital malformations of spine and bony thorax

Excludes: congenital musculoskeletal deformities of spine (Q67.5)

Q76.0 Spina bifida occulta

Excludes: meningocele (spinal) (Q05.–)
spina bifida (aperta)(cystica) (Q05.–)

Q76.1 Klippel–Feil syndrome

Cervical fusion syndrome

Q76.2 Congenital spondylolisthesis

Congenital spondylolysis
Excludes: spondylolisthesis (acquired) (M43.1)
spondylolysis (acquired) (M43.0)

Q76.3 Congenital scoliosis due to congenital bony malformation

Q76.30 Hemivertebra fusion with scoliosis
Q76.31 Hemivertebra failure of segmentation with scoliosis
Q76.38 Other congenital scoliosis due to congenital bony malformation

Q76.4 Other congenital malformations of spine, not associated with scoliosis

Q76.40 Congenital absence of vertebra, not associated with scoliosis
Q76.41 Congenital fusion of spine, not associated with scoliosis
Q76.42 Congenital kyphosis, not associated with scoliosis
Q76.43 Congenital lordosis, not associated with scoliosis

Q76.44 Congenital malformation of lumbosacral (joint)(region), not associated with scoliosis
Q76.45 Hemivertebra, not associated with scoliosis
Q76.46 Supernumerary vertebra, not associated with scoliosis
Q76.47 Platyspondylisis

Q76.5 Cervical rib
Supernumerary rib in cervical region

Q76.6 Other congenital malformations of ribs
Accessory rib
Congenital:
- absence of rib
- fusion of ribs
- malformation of ribs NOS

Excludes: short rib syndrome (Q77.2)

Q76.7 Congenital malformation of sternum
Congenital absence of sternum
Sternum bifidum

Q76.8 Other congenital malformations of bony thorax

Q76.9 Congenital malformation of bony thorax, unspecified

Q77 Osteochondrodysplasia with defects of growth of tubular bones and spine

Excludes: mucopolysaccharidosis (E76.0–E76.3)

Q77.0 Achondrogenesis
Hypochondrogenesis

Q77.1 Thanatophoric short stature

Q77.2 Short rib syndrome
Asphyxiating thoracic dysplasia [Jeune]

Q77.3 Chondrodysplasia punctata

Q77.4 Achondroplasia
Achondroplastic short stature
Hypochondroplasia

Q77.5 Diastrophic dysplasia

Q78 Other osteochondrodysplasias

Q78.0 Osteogenesis imperfecta
Fragilitas ossium
Osteopsathyrosis

Q78.1 Polyostotic fibrous dysplasia
Albright(–McCune)(–Sternberg) syndrome

Q78.2 Osteopetrosis
Albers–Schönberg syndrome

Q78.3 Progressive diaphyseal dysplasia
Camurati–Engelmann syndrome

Q78.4 Enchondromatosis
Maffucci's syndrome
Ollier's disease

Q78.8 Other specified osteochondrodysplasias
Osteopoikilosis

Q79 Congenital malformations of musculoskeletal system, not elsewhere classified

Excludes: congenital (sternomastoid) torticollis (Q68.0)

Q79.0 Congenital diaphragmatic hernia

Q79.1 Other congenital malformations of diaphragm
Absence of diaphragm
Congenital malformation of diaphragm NOS
Eventration of diaphragm

Q79.2 Exomphalos
Omphalocele

Q79.3 Gastroschisis

Q79.4 Prune belly syndrome

Q79.5 Other congenital malformations of abdominal wall

Q79.6 Ehlers–Danlos syndrome

Q79.8 Other congenital malformations of musculoskeletal system

Q79.80 Absence of muscle or tendon
Q79.81 Accessory muscle
Q79.82 Amyotrophia congenita
Q79.83 Congenital constricting bands and shortening of tendon
Q79.84 Poland's syndrome

Q79.9 Congenital malformation of musculoskeletal system, unspecified

Congenital:
- anomaly NOS } of musculoskeletal system NOS
- deformity NOS } of musculoskeletal system NOS

Other congenital malformations (Q80–Q89)

Q82 Other congenital malformations of skin

Q82.1 Xeroderma pigmentosum

Q85 Phakomatoses, not elsewhere classified

Excludes: ataxia telangiectasia [Louis–Bar] (G11.30)
familial dysautonomia [Riley–Day] (G90.1)

Q85.0 Neurofibromatosis (nonmalignant)

Includes: von Recklinghausen's disease

Q85.00 Neurofibromatosis, type 1
Q85.01 Neurofibromatosis, type 2

Q85.1 Tuberous sclerosis

Bourneville's disease
Epiloia

Q85.8 Other phakomatoses, not elsewhere classified

Q85.80 Peutz–Jeghers syndrome
Q85.81 Sturge–Weber(–Dimitri) syndrome
Q85.82 Von Hippel–Lindau syndrome

Q85.9 Phakomatosis, unspecified

Hamartosis NOS

Q86 Congenital malformation syndromes due to known exogenous causes, not elsewhere classified

Excludes: iodine-deficiency-related hypothyroidism (E00–E02)

Q86.0 Fetal alcohol syndrome (dysmorphic)

Q86.1 Fetal hydantoin syndrome

Birth defects due to hydantoin and other antiepileptic drugs
Meadow's syndrome

Use additional code, if desired, to identify antiepileptic drug.

Q86.2 Dysmorphism due to warfarin

Q86.8 Other congenital malformation syndromes due to known exogenous causes
Use additional code, if desired, to identify exogenous cause.

Q87 Other specified congenital malformation syndromes affecting multiple systems

Q87.0 Congenital malformation syndromes predominantly affecting facial appearance
Excludes: cryptophthalmos NOS (Q11.2)

Q87.00 Acrocephalopolysyndactyly
Q87.01 Acrocephalosyndactyly [Apert]
Q87.02 Cyclopia
Q87.03 Goldenhar's syndrome
Q87.04 Moebius' syndrome
Q87.05 Congenital agenesis of brain stem nuclei
Q87.06 Oro-facial-digital syndrome
Q87.07 Robin's syndrome
Q87.08 Other specified congenital malformation syndromes predominantly affecting facial appearance
Q87.080 Treacher Collins' syndrome
Q87.081 Whistling face syndrome
Q87.082 Cryptophthalmos syndrome
Q87.083 Carpenter's syndrome

Q87.1 Congenital malformation syndromes predominantly associated with short stature

Q87.10 Aarskog's syndrome
Q87.11 Cockayne's syndrome
Q87.12 De Lange's syndrome
Q87.13 Dubowitz' syndrome
Q87.14 Noonan's syndrome
Q87.15 Prader–Willi syndrome
Q87.16 Robinow–Silverman–Smith syndrome
Q87.17 Russell-Silver syndrome
Q87.18 Other specified congenital malformation syndromes predominantly associated with short stature
Q87.180 Seckel's syndrome
Q87.181 Smith–Lemli–Opitz syndrome

Q87.2 Congenital malformation syndromes predominantly involving limbs
Excludes: arthrogryposis multiplex congenita (Q74.3)

Q87.20 Holt–Oram syndrome
Q87.21 Klippel–Trénaunay–Weber syndrome
Q87.22 Nail patella syndrome
Q87.23 Rubinstein–Taybi syndrome
Q87.24 Sirenomelia syndrome
Q87.25 Thrombocytopenia with absent radius syndrome [TAR]
Q87.26 VATER syndrome
Q87.28 Other specified congenital malformation syndromes predominantly involving limbs

Q87.3 Congenital malformation syndromes involving early overgrowth

Q87.30 Beckwith–Wiedmann syndrome
Q87.31 Sotos' syndrome
Q87.32 Weaver's syndrome

Q87.4 Marfan's syndrome

Q87.5 Other congenital malformation syndromes with other skeletal changes

Q87.8 Other specified congenital malformation syndromes, not elsewhere classified

Q87.80 Alport's syndrome
Q87.81 Laurence–Moon(–Bardet)–Biedl syndrome
Q87.82 Zellweger's syndrome

Q89 Other congenital malformations, not elsewhere classified

Q89.4 Conjoined twins
Craniopagus
Dicephaly
Double monster
Pygopagus
Thoracopagus

Q89.7 Multiple congenital malformations, not elsewhere classified
Monster NOS
Multiple congenital:
- anomalies NOS
- deformities NOS

Excludes: congenital malformation syndromes affecting multiple systems (Q87.–)

Chromosomal abnormalities, not elsewhere classified (Q90–Q99)

Q90 Down's syndrome

Q90.0 **Trisomy 21, meiotic nondisjunction**

Q90.1 **Trisomy 21, mosaicism (mitotic nondisjunction)**

Q90.2 **Trisomy 21, translocation**

Q90.9 **Down's syndrome, unspecified**
Trisomy 21 NOS

Q91 Edwards' syndrome and Patau's syndrome

Q91.0 **Trisomy 18, meiotic nondisjunction**

Q91.1 **Trisomy 18, mosaicism (mitotic nondisjunction)**

Q91.2 **Trisomy 18, translocation**

Q91.3 **Edwards' syndrome, unspecified**

Q91.4 **Trisomy 13, meiotic nondisjunction**

Q91.5 **Trisomy 13, mosaicism (mitotic nondisjunction)**

Q91.6 **Trisomy 13, translocation**

Q91.7 **Patau's syndrome, unspecified**

Q92 Other trisomies and partial trisomies of the autosomes, not elsewhere classified

Includes: unbalanced translocations and insertions
Excludes: trisomies of chromosomes 13, 18, 21 (Q90–Q91)

Q92.0 **Whole chromosome trisomy, meiotic nondisjunction**

Q92.1 **Whole chromosome trisomy, mosaicism (mitotic nondisjunction)**

Q92.2 **Major partial trisomy**
Whole arm or more duplicated.

Q92.3 **Minor partial trisomy**
Less than whole arm duplicated.

Q92.4 **Duplications seen only at prometaphase**

Q92.5 **Duplications with other complex rearrangements**

Q92.6 **Extra marker chromosomes**

Q92.7 **Triploidy and polyploidy**

Q92.8 **Other specified trisomies and partial trisomies of autosomes**

Q92.9 **Trisomy and partial trisomy of autosomes, unspecified**

Q93 Monosomies and deletions from the autosomes, not elsewhere classified

Q93.0 **Whole chromosome monosomy, meiotic nondisjunction**

Q93.1 **Whole chromosome monosomy, mosaicism (mitotic nondisjunction)**

Q93.2 **Chromosome replaced with ring or dicentric**

Q93.3 **Deletion of short arm of chromosome 4**
Wolff–Hirschorn syndrome

Q93.4 **Deletion of short arm of chromosome 5**
Cri-du-chat syndrome

Q93.5 **Other deletions of part of a chromosome**

Q93.6 **Deletions seen only at prometaphase**

Q93.7 **Deletions with other complex rearrangements**

Q93.8 **Other deletions from the autosomes**

Q93.9 **Deletion from autosomes, unspecified**

Q95 Balanced rearrangements and structural markers, not elsewhere classified

Includes: Robertsonian and balanced reciprocal translocations and insertions

Q95.0 **Balanced translocation and insertion in normal individual**

Q95.1 **Chromosome inversion in normal individual**

Q95.2 **Balanced autosomal rearrangement in abnormal individual**

Q95.3 **Balanced sex/autosomal rearrangement in abnormal individual**

Q95.4 **Individuals with marker heterochromatin**

Q95.5 **Individuals with autosomal fragile site**

Q95.8 **Other balanced rearrangements and structural markers**

Q95.9 **Balanced rearrangement and structural marker, unspecified**

Q96 Turner's syndrome

Excludes: Noonan's syndrome (Q87.14)

Q96.0 Karyotype 45,X

Q96.1 Karyotype 46,X iso (Xq)

Q96.2 Karyotype 46,X with abnormal sex chromosome, except iso (Xq)

Q96.3 Mosaicism, 45,X/46,XX or XY

Q96.4 Mosaicism, 45,X/other cell line(s) with abnormal sex chromosome

Q96.8 Other variants of Turner's syndrome

Q96.9 Turner's syndrome, unspecified

Q97 Other sex chromosome abnormalities, female phenotype, not elsewhere classified

Excludes: Turner's syndrome (Q96.–)

Q97.0 Karyotype 47,XXX

Q97.1 Female with more than three X chromosomes

Q97.2 Mosaicism, lines with various numbers of X chromosomes

Q97.3 Female with 46,XY karyotype

Q97.8 Other specified sex chromosome abnormalities, female phenotype

Q97.9 Sex chromosome abnormality, female phenotype, unspecified

Q98 Other sex chromosome abnormalities, male phenotype, not elsewhere classified

Q98.0 Klinefelter's syndrome karyotype 47,XXY

Q98.1 Klinefelter's syndrome, male with more than two X chromosomes

Q98.2 Klinefelter's syndrome, male with 46,XX karyotype

Q98.3 Other male with 46,XX karyotype

Q98.4 Klinefelter's syndrome, unspecified

Q98.5 Karyotype 47,XYY

Q98.6 Male with structurally abnormal sex chromosome

Q98.7 Male with sex chromosome mosaicism

Q98.8 Other specified sex chromosome abnormalities, male phenotype

Q98.9 Sex chromosome abnormality, male phenotype, unspecified

Q99 Other chromosome abnormalities, not elsewhere classified

Q99.0 Chimera 46,XX/46,XY
Chimera 46,XX/46,XY true hermaphrodite

Q99.1 46,XX true hermaphrodite
46,XX with streak gonads
46,XY with streak gonads
Pure gonadal dysgenesis

Q99.2 Fragile X chromosome
Fragile X syndrome

Q99.8 Other specified chromosome abnormalities

Q99.80 Specified chromosomal deletions
Q99.81 Specified DNA deletions

Q99.9 Chromosomal abnormality, unspecified

CHAPTER XVIII

Symptoms, signs and abnormal clinical and laboratory findings, not elsewhere classified (R00–R99)

This chapter includes symptoms, signs, abnormal results of clinical or other investigative procedures, and ill-defined conditions regarding which no diagnosis classifiable elsewhere is recorded.

Signs and symptoms that point rather definitively to a given diagnosis have been assigned to a category in other chapters of the classification. In general, categories in this chapter include the less well-defined conditions and symptoms that, without the necessary study of the case to establish a final diagnosis, point perhaps equally to two or more diseases or to two or more systems of the body. Practically all categories in the chapter could be designated "not otherwise specified", "unknown etiology", or "transient". The alphabetical index should be consulted to determine which symptoms and signs are to be allocated here and which to other chapters. The residual subcategories, numbered .8, are generally provided for other relevant symptoms that cannot be allocated elsewhere in the classification.

The conditions and signs or symptoms included in categories R00–R99 consist of: (a) cases for which no more specific diagnosis can be made even after all the facts bearing on the case have been investigated; (b) signs or symptoms existing at the time of initial encounter that proved to be transient and whose causes could not be determined; (c) provisional diagnoses in a patient who failed to return for further investigation or care; (d) cases referred elsewhere for investigation or treatment before the diagnosis was made; (e) cases in which a more precise diagnosis was not available for any other reason; (f) certain symptoms, for which supplementary information is provided, that represent important problems in medical care in their own right.

Excludes: certain conditions originating in the perinatal period (P00–P96)

Symptoms and signs involving the circulatory and respiratory systems (R00–R09)

R06 Abnormalities of breathing

R06.0 Dyspnoea
Orthopnoea
Shortness of breath

R06.1 Stridor

R06.2 Wheezing

R06.3 Periodic breathing

R06.30 Cheyne–Stokes breathing
R06.31 Kussmaul breathing
R06.32 Central hyperpnoea
R06.33 Apneustic breathing
R06.38 Other periodic breathing pattern

R06.4 Hyperventilation
Excludes: psychogenic hyperventilation (F45.3)

R06.5 Mouth breathing
Snoring

R06.6 Hiccough
Excludes: psychogenic hiccough (F45.3)

R06.7 Sneezing

R06.8 Other and unspecified abnormalities of breathing

R06.80 Apnoea, unspecified
R06.81 Breath-holding (spells)
R06.82 Choking sensation
R06.83 Sighing

R07 Pain in throat and chest

Excludes: dysphagia (R13)
epidemic myalgia (B33.0)
pain in neck (M54.2)

R07.0 Pain in throat

R07.1 Chest pain on breathing

R07.2 Precordial pain

R07.3 **Other chest pain**

R09 Other symptoms and signs involving the circulatory and respiratory systems

R09.0 **Asphyxia**
Excludes: asphyxia (due to):
- birth (P21.–)
- carbon monoxide (T58)
- intrauterine (P20.–)

R09.2 **Respiratory arrest**
Cardiorespiratory failure

R09.8 **Other specified symptoms and signs involving the circulatory and respiratory systems**
Bruit (arterial)
Weak pulse

Symptoms and signs involving the digestive system and abdomen (R10–R19)

R10 Abdominal and pelvic pain
Excludes: dorsalgia (M54.–)

R10.1 **Pain localized to upper abdomen**

R10.2 **Pelvic and perineal pain**

R10.3 **Pain localized to other parts of lower abdomen**

R10.4 **Other and unspecified abdominal pain**

R11 Nausea and vomiting

R13 Dysphagia
Difficulty in swallowing

R15 Faecal incontinence
Encopresis NOS
Excludes: that of nonorganic origin (F98.1)

Symptoms and signs involving the skin and subcutaneous tissue (R20–R23)

R20 Disturbances of skin sensation

Excludes: dissociative anaesthesia and sensory loss (F44.6)
psychogenic disturbances of skin sensation (F45.8)

R20.0 Anaesthesia of skin
Excludes: psychogenic anaesthesia (F44.6)

R20.1 Hypoaesthesia of skin

R20.2 Paraesthesia of skin
Formication
Pins and needles
Tingling skin
Excludes: acroparaesthesia (I73.8)

R20.3 Hyperaesthesia
Dysaesthesia

R20.8 Other and unspecified disturbances of skin sensation

Symptoms and signs involving the nervous and musculoskeletal systems (R25–R29)

R25 Abnormal involuntary movements

Excludes: specific movement disorders (G20–G26)
stereotyped movement disorders (F98.4)
tic disorders (F95.–)

R25.0 Abnormal head movements

R25.00 Titubation, familial
R25.01 Titubation, nonfamilial

R25.1 Tremor, unspecified
Excludes: chorea NOS (G25.5)
tremor:
- essential (G25.0)
- hysterical (F44.4)
- intention (G25.2)

R25.2 Cramp and spasm

Use additional code(s), if desired, to identify associated condition.

Excludes: carpopedal spasm (R29.0)
infantile spasms (G40.40)

R25.20 Nocturnal cramps
R25.21 Aches, cramps and pains syndrome associated with exertion
Exertional myalgia
R25.22 Aches, cramps and pains syndrome not associated with exertion
R25.28 Other specified cramps and spasms

R25.3 Fasciculation

Includes: twitching NOS

Use additional code(s), if desired, to identify associated condition.

Excludes: amyotrophic lateral sclerosis (G12.20)
paramyoclonus multiplex (G25.32)
spinal muscular atrophy (G12.–)

R25.30 Benign fasciculation syndrome
R25.38 Other fasciculations

R25.8 Other and unspecified abnormal involuntary movements

R26 Abnormalities of gait and mobility

Excludes: ataxia:
- NOS (R27.0)
- hereditary (G11.–)
- locomotor (syphilitic) (A52.1)

immobility syndrome (paraplegic) (M62.3)
late walker (R62.01)

R26.0 Ataxic gait

Includes: staggering gait

R26.00 Cerebellar ataxia of gait
R26.01 Sensory ataxia of gait
R26.02 Vestibular ataxia of gait
R26.03 Frontal lobe ataxia of gait
Frontal lobe gait apraxia [Bruns]

R26.1 Paralytic gait

R26.10 Spastic gait
R26.11 Cerebello-spastic gait

R26.12 Gait disorder from muscle weakness
Paretic gait

R26.2 Difficulty in walking, not elsewhere classified
Excludes: that in vertebro-basilar syndrome (G45.0)

R26.20 Gait disturbance due to loss of postural reflexes
R26.21 Senile gait disturbance
R26.22 Drop attack
R26.23 Gait apraxia
R26.24 Toe walking

R26.8 Other and unspecified abnormalities of gait and mobility
Unsteadiness on feet NOS

R27 Other lack of coordination

Excludes: ataxic gait (R26.0)
hereditary ataxia (G11.–)
vertigo NOS (R42)

R27.0 Ataxia, unspecified

R27.8 Other and unspecified lack of coordination

R29 Other symptoms and signs involving the nervous and musculoskeletal systems

R29.0 Tetany
Carpopedal spasm
Excludes: tetany:
- hysterical (F44.5)
- neonatal (P71.3)
- parathyroid (E20.9)
- post-thyroidectomy (E89.2)

R29.1 Meningismus

R29.2 Abnormal reflex
Excludes: abnormal pupillary reflex (H57.0)
vasovagal reaction or syncope (R55)

R29.3 Abnormal posture

R29.8 Other and unspecified symptoms and signs involving the nervous and musculoskeletal systems

Symptoms and signs involving the urinary system (R30–R39)

R30 **Pain associated with micturition**
Excludes: psychogenic pain (F45.3)

R30.0 **Dysuria**
Strangury

R32 **Unspecified urinary incontinence**
Enuresis NOS

R33 **Retention of urine**

R34 **Anuria and oliguria**

R35 **Polyuria**
Frequency of micturition
Nocturia
Excludes: psychogenic polyuria (F45.3)

Symptoms and signs involving cognition, perception, emotional state and behaviour (R40–R46)

R40 **Somnolence, stupor and coma**
Excludes: coma:
- diabetic (E10–E14 with common fourth character .0)
- hepatic (K72.–)
- hypoglycaemic (nondiabetic) (E15)
- neonatal (P91.5)
- uraemic (N19)

R40.0 **Somnolence**
Drowsiness

R40.1 **Stupor**
Semicoma
Excludes: dissociative stupor (F44.2)

R40.2 **Coma, unspecified**
Unconsciousness NOS

R41 Other symptoms and signs involving cognitive functions and awareness

Excludes: dissociative [conversion] disorders (F44.–)

R41.0 Disorientation, unspecified
Confusion NOS

R41.1 Anterograde amnesia

R41.2 Retrograde amnesia

R41.3 Other amnesia
Amnesia NOS
Excludes: amnesic syndrome:
- due to psychoactive substance use (F10–F19 with common fourth character .6)
- organic (F04)

transient global amnesia (G45.4)

R41.8 Other and unspecified symptoms and signs involving cognitive functions and awareness
Excludes: delirium NOS (F05.9)

R42 Dizziness and giddiness

Light headedness
Vertigo NOS
Excludes: vertiginous syndromes (H81.–)

R43 Disturbances of smell and taste

R43.0 Anosmia

R43.1 Parosmia

R43.2 Parageusia

R43.20 Ageusia
R43.21 Dysgeusia

R43.8 Other and unspecified disturbances of smell and taste
Mixed disturbance of smell and taste

R44 Other symptoms and signs involving general sensations and perceptions

Excludes: disturbances of skin sensation (R20.–)

R44.0 Auditory hallucinations

R44.1 Visual hallucinations

R44.2 Other hallucinations

R44.20 Olfactory hallucinations
R44.21 Gustatory hallucinations
R44.22 Mixed olfactory and gustatory hallucinations

R44.3 Hallucinations, unspecified

R44.8 Other and unspecified symptoms and signs involving general sensations and perceptions

R45 Symptoms and signs involving emotional state

R45.0 Nervousness
Nervous tension

R45.1 Restlessness and agitation

R45.2 Unhappiness
Worries NOS

R45.3 Demoralization and apathy
Demotivation
Excludes: that in depression (F32.–)

R45.4 Irritability and anger

R45.5 Hostility

R45.6 Physical violence

R45.7 State of emotional shock and stress, unspecified

R45.8 Other symptoms and signs involving emotional state

R46 Symptoms and signs involving appearance and behaviour

R46.0 Very low level of personal hygiene

R46.1 Bizarre personal appearance

R46.2 Strange and inexplicable behaviour

R46.3 Overactivity

R46.4 Slowness and poor responsiveness
Excludes: stupor (R40.1)

R46.5 Suspiciousness and marked evasiveness

R46.6 Undue concern and preoccupation with stressful events

R46.7 Verbosity and circumstantial detail obscuring reason for contact

R46.8 Other symptoms and signs involving appearance and behaviour

Symptoms and signs involving speech and voice (R47–R49)

R47 Speech disturbances, not elsewhere classified

Excludes: autism (F84.0–F84.1)
specific developmental disorders of speech and language (F80.–)

R47.0 Dysphasia and aphasia

Excludes: progressive isolated aphasia [Mesulam] (G31.01)

R47.00 Motor aphasia [Broca]
R47.01 Receptive aphasia [Wernicke]
R47.02 Global aphasia [Déjerine]
R47.03 Conduction aphasia
R47.04 Transcortical aphasia [Goldstein]
R47.05 Dynamic aphasia [Luria]
R47.06 Amnesic aphasia
R47.08 Other aphasia

R47.1 Dysarthria and anarthria

R47.10 Spastic dysarthria (upper motor neuron type)
R47.11 Ataxic dysarthria (cerebellar type)
R47.12 Flaccid paralytic dysarthria (lower motor neuron type)
R47.13 Hypokinetic dysarthria (basal ganglia type)
R47.14 Hyperkinetic dysarthria
R47.18 Other dysarthria

R47.8 Other and unspecified speech disturbances

R47.80 Stammering and stuttering of organic origin
Excludes: psychogenic stuttering [stammering] (F98.5)
R47.81 Cluttering of organic origin
Excludes: psychogenic cluttering (F98.6)

R48 Dyslexia and other symbolic dysfunctions, not elsewhere classified

Excludes: specific developmental disorders of scholastic skills (F81.–)

R48.0 Dyslexia and alexia

R48.00 Pure alexia
Alexia without agraphia
R48.01 Alexia with agraphia
R48.08 Other alexia

R48.1 Agnosia

R48.10 Visual agnosia
R48.100 Object agnosia
R48.101 Image agnosia
R48.102 Colour agnosia
R48.103 Prosopagnosia
R48.104 Simultanagnosia
R48.108 Other visual agnosia
R48.11 Auditory agnosia
R48.110 Amusia
R48.111 Word deafness
R48.118 Other auditory agnosia
R48.12 Somatosensory agnosia
R48.120 Autotopagnosia
R48.121 Finger agnosia
R48.122 Hemiasomatognosia
R48.123 Anosognosia
R48.124 Anosodiaphoria
R48.125 Astereognosia
R48.128 Other somatosensory agnosia

R48.2 Apraxia

R48.20 Ideomotor apraxia
R48.21 Ideatory apraxia
R48.22 Reflexive apraxia
R48.23 Dressing apraxia
R48.24 Constructional apraxia
R48.28 Other apraxia

R48.8 Other and unspecified symbolic dysfunctions

R48.80 Acalculia
R48.81 Pure agraphia
R48.82 Left–right confusion

R49 Voice disturbances

Excludes: psychogenic voice disturbance (F44.4)

R49.0 Dysphonia
Hoarseness

R49.1 Aphonia
Loss of voice

R49.2 Hypernasality and hyponasality

R49.8 Other and unspecified voice disturbances
Change in voice NOS

General symptoms and signs (R50–R69)

R51 Headache

Facial pain NOS
Excludes: atypical face pain (G50.1)
migraine and other headache syndromes (G43–G44)
trigeminal neuralgia (G50.0)

R52 Pain, not elsewhere classified

Includes: pain not referable to any one organ or body region
Excludes: headache (R51)
pain (in):
- abdomen (R10.–)
- back (M54.9)
- chest (R07.1–R07.4)
- ear [otalgia] (H92.0)
- eye (H57.1)
- lumbar region [lumbago] (M54.4–M54.5)
- pelvic and perineal (R10.2)
- psychogenic (F45.4)
- spine (M54.–)
- throat (R07.0)

R52.0 Acute pain

R52.1 Chronic intractable pain

R52.2 Other chronic pain

R52.9 Pain, unspecified
Generalized pain NOS

R53 Malaise and fatigue

Asthenia NOS
Debility:
- chronic
- nervous

General physical deterioration
Lethargy
Tiredness
Excludes: exhaustion and fatigue (due to)(in):
- neurasthenia (F48.0)
- senile asthenia (R54)

fatigue syndrome (F48.0)
- postviral (G93.3)

R54 Senility

Old age } without mention of psychosis
Senescence }
Senile:
- asthenia
- debility

Excludes: senile psychosis (F03)

R55 Syncope and collapse

Blackout
Fainting
Vasovagal attack
Excludes: neurocirculatory asthenia (F45.3)
orthostatic hypotension (I95.1)
- in Shy–Drager syndrome (G90.31)
- isolated (G90.30)
- neurogenic:

shock:
- NOS (R57.9)
- cardiogenic (R57.0)
- complicating or following:
  - abortion or ectopic or molar pregnancy (O08.3)
  - labour and delivery (O75.1)
- postoperative (T81.1)

Stokes–Adams syndrome (I45.9)
syncope:
- carotid sinus (G90.03)
- heat (T67.1)
- psychogenic (F48.84)

unconsciousness NOS (R40.2)

R56 Convulsions, not elsewhere classified

Excludes: convulsions and seizures (in):
- dissociative (F44.5)
- epilepsy (G40–G41)
- newborn (P90.–)

pseudoseizures (F44.5)

R56.0 Febrile convulsions

R56.8 Other and unspecified convulsions

Fit NOS
Isolated (first) seizure
Seizure (convulsive) NOS

R57 Shock, not elsewhere classified

Excludes: shock (due to):
- anaesthesia (T88.2)
- anaphylactic, due to:
  - NOS (T78.2)
  - adverse food reaction (T78.0)
  - serum (T80.5)
- complicating or following abortion or ectopic or molar pregnancy (O08.3)
- electric (T75.4)
- lightning (T75.0)
- obstetric (O75.1)
- postoperative (T81.1)
- septic (A41.9)
- traumatic (T79.4)

toxic shock syndrome (A48.3)

R57.0 Cardiogenic shock

R57.1 Hypovolaemic shock

R57.8 Other shock

Endotoxic shock

R57.9 Shock, unspecified

Failure of peripheral circulation NOS

R62 Lack of expected normal physiological development

Excludes: delayed puberty (E30.0)

R62.0 Delayed milestone

Includes: delayed attainment of expected physiological developmental stage

R62.00 Late talker
R62.01 Late walker

R62.8 Other lack of expected normal physiological development

Failure to:
- gain weight
- thrive

Lack of growth
Physical retardation
Excludes: HIV disease resulting in failure to thrive (B22.2)
physical retardation due to malnutrition (E45)

R63 Symptoms and signs concerning food and fluid intake

R63.0 Anorexia

Loss of appetite

R63.1 Polydipsia

Excessive thirst

R63.2 Polyphagia

Excessive eating
Hyperalimentation NOS

R63.3 Feeding difficulties and mismanagement

Feeding problem NOS

R63.4 Abnormal weight loss

R63.5 Abnormal weight gain

R63.8 Other symptoms and signs concerning food and fluid intake

R63.80 Adipsia
R63.81 Eating strike

R64 Cachexia

Excludes: HIV disease resulting in wasting syndrome (B22.2)
malignant cachexia (C80)
nutritional marasmus (E41)

R68 Other general symptoms and signs

R68.0 Hypothermia, not associated with low environmental temperature

Excludes: hypothermia due to low environmental temperature (T68)

R68.1 Nonspecific symptoms peculiar to infancy
Excessive crying of infant
Irritable infant
Excludes: neonatal cerebral irritability (P91.3)

R68.2 Dry mouth, unspecified
Excludes: when due to sicca syndrome [Sjögren] (M35.0)

Abnormal findings on examination of blood, without diagnosis (R70–R79)

R70 Elevated erythrocyte sedimentation rate and abnormality of plasma viscosity

R70.0 Elevated erythrocyte sedimentation rate

R70.1 Abnormal plasma viscosity

R73 Elevated blood glucose level

Excludes: diabetes mellitus (E10–E14)
neonatal disorders (P70.0–P70.2)
postsurgical hypoinsulinaemia (E89.1)

R73.0 Abnormal glucose tolerance test
Diabetes:
- chemical
- latent

Impaired glucose tolerance
Prediabetes

R73.9 Hyperglycaemia, unspecified

R74 Abnormal serum enzyme levels

R74.0 Elevation of levels of transaminase and lactic acid dehydrogenase [LDH]

R74.8 Abnormal levels of other serum enzymes

R74.80 Abnormal serum level of acid phosphatase
R74.81 Abnormal serum level of alkaline phosphatase
R74.82 Abnormal serum level of amylase
R74.83 Abnormal serum level of creatine kinase
R74.84 Abnormal serum level of lipase [triacylglycerol lipase]

R75 Laboratory evidence of human immunodeficiency virus [HIV]

Excludes: asymptomatic human immunodeficiency virus [HIV] infection status (Z21)
human immunodeficiency virus [HIV] disease (B20–B24)

R76 Other abnormal immunological findings in serum

R76.0 Raised antibody titre

R76.2 False-positive serological test for syphilis
False-positive Wassermann reaction

R76.8 Other specified abnormal immunological findings in serum

R76.80 Raised acetylcholine receptor antibody titre
R76.81 Raised muscle antistriational antibody titre
R76.82 Raised antineuronal antibody titre
R76.83 Raised rheumatological antibody [ANA/rheumatoid factor] titre
R76.84 Raised anti-GM1 ganglioside antibody titre
R76.87 Raised immunoglobulin level, unspecified
R76.88 Other abnormal immunological findings in serum

R76.9 Abnormal immunological finding in serum, unspecified

R78 Findings of drugs and other substances, not normally found in blood

Excludes: mental and behavioural disorders due to psychoactive substance use (F10–F19)

R78.0 Finding of alcohol in blood
Use additional external cause code (Y90.–), if desired, for detail regarding alcohol level.

R78.1 Finding of opiate drug in blood

R78.2 Finding of cocaine in blood

R78.3 Finding of hallucinogen in blood

R78.4 Finding of other drug of addictive potential in blood

R78.5 Finding of psychotropic drug in blood

R78.6 Finding of steroid agent in blood

R78.7 Finding of abnormal level of heavy metals in blood

R78.8 Finding of other specified substances, not normally found in blood

Finding of abnormal level of lithium in blood

R78.9 Finding of unspecified substance, not normally found in blood

Abnormal findings on examination of other body fluids, substances and tissues, without diagnosis (R83–R89)

R83 Abnormal findings in cerebrospinal fluid

R83.4 Abnormal immunological findings in cerebrospinal fluid

R83.40 Increased gammaglobulin in cerebrospinal fluid
R83.41 Increased oligoclonal bands in cerebrospinal fluid

R83.6 Abnormal cytological findings in cerebrospinal fluid

R83.60 Malignant cells in cerebrospinal fluid
R83.61 Increased lymphocytes in cerebrospinal fluid
R83.62 Increased polymorphs in cerebrospinal fluid

R83.8 Other abnormal findings in cerebrospinal fluid

R83.80 Increased protein in cerebrospinal fluid
R83.81 Decreased glucose in cerebrospinal fluid
R83.82 Abnormal electrolytes in cerebrospinal fluid

Abnormal findings on diagnostic imaging and in function studies, without diagnosis (R90–R94)

Includes: nonspecific abnormal findings on diagnostic imaging by:
- computerized axial tomography [CAT scan]
- magnetic resonance imaging [MRI] [NMR]
- positive electron emission tomography [PET scan]
- thermography
- ultrasound [echogram]
- X-ray examination

R90 Abnormal findings on diagnostic imaging of central nervous system

R90.0 Intracranial space-occupying lesion

R90.8 Other abnormal findings on diagnostic imaging of central nervous system

Excludes: intracranial space-occupying lesion (R90.0)

R90.80 Ventricular enlargement
R90.81 Enlarged sulci
R90.82 Abnormalities of white matter of brain on CAT scan or MRI, single, multiple or widespread (leucomalacia)
R90.83 Clinically silent cerebral infarction(s)
R90.84 Asymptomatic spinal artery aneurysm or arteriovenous malformation
R90.85 Other central nervous system artery abnormality, not elsewhere classified
R90.86 Cerebral blood flow imaging abnormality
R90.87 Cerebral metabolism imaging abnormality
R90.88 Magnetic cerebral imaging abnormality
R90.89 Other specified abnormal findings on diagnostic imaging of brain and spinal cord

R93 Abnormal findings on diagnostic imaging of other body structures

R93.0 Abnormal findings on diagnostic imaging of skull and head, not elsewhere classified

Excludes: intracranial space-occupying lesion (R90.0)

R94 Abnormal results of function studies

Includes: abnormal results of:
- radionuclide [radioisotope] uptake studies
- scintigraphy

R94.0 Abnormal results of function studies of central nervous system

R94.00 Abnormal electroencephalogram [EEG]
R94.000 Abnormal paroxysmal activity in EEG
R94.001 Abnormal spike activity in EEG
R94.002 Abnormal reactivity in EEG
R94.003 Excess beta activity in EEG
R94.004 Excess theta activity in EEG
R94.005 Excess delta activity in EEG

R94.006 Abnormal brain activity map
R94.008 Other abnormal EEG
R94.009 Abnormal EEG, unspecified

R94.01 Abnormal cerebral blood flow
Excludes: imaging (R90.86)

R94.02 Abnormal positron emission tomogram
Excludes: imaging (R90.87)

R94.03 Abnormal radionuclide brain scan

R94.08 Other abnormal results of function study of central nervous system

R94.1 Abnormal results of function studies of peripheral nervous system and special senses

R94.10 Abnormal electromyogram [EMG]
R94.100 Acute denervation changes
R94.101 Chronic denervation/reinnervation changes
R94.102 Myopathic changes
R94.103 Myotonic discharge
R94.104 Bizarre repetitive discharge
R94.105 Fasciculation
R94.106 Increased EMG single fibre density
R94.107 Increased EMG single fibre jitter
R94.108 Other abnormal EMG
R94.109 Abnormal EMG, unspecified

R94.11 Abnormal electro-oculogram (EOG)

R94.12 Abnormal electroretinogram (ERG)

R94.13 Abnormal electronystagmogram

R94.14 Abnormal evoked potential
R94.140 Abnormal visual evoked potential
R94.141 Abnormal brainstem auditory evoked response
R94.142 Abnormal somatosensory evoked potential
R94.148 Other abnormal evoked potential

R94.15 Abnormal response to nerve stimulation
R94.150 Motor nerve conduction velocity below lower limit of normal but above 50%
R94.151 Motor nerve conduction velocity below 50% of normal
R94.152 Sensory nerve conduction velocity below lower limit of normal but above 50%
R94.153 Sensory nerve conduction velocity below 50% of normal
R94.154 Multifocal conduction block
R94.155 Muscle evoked action potential amplitude below lower limit of normal

R94.156 Sensory nerve action potential amplitude below lower limit of normal

R94.157 Abnormal decrement on repetitive nerve stimulation

R94.158 Abnormal increment on repetitive nerve stimulation

R94.159 Other abnormal response to nerve stimulation

R94.16 Abnormal audiogram

R94.18 Other abnormal results of function study of peripheral nervous system or special senses

Ill-defined and unknown causes of mortality (R95–R99)

R95 Sudden infant death syndrome

R96 Other sudden death, cause unknown

Excludes: sudden infant death syndrome (R95)

R96.0 Instantaneous death

R96.1 Death occurring less than 24 hours from onset of symptoms, not otherwise explained

Death known not to be violent or instantaneous for which no cause can be discovered

Death without sign of disease

R98 Unattended death

Death in circumstances where the body of the deceased was found and no cause could be discovered

Found dead

R99 Other ill-defined and unspecified causes of mortality

Death NOS

Unknown cause of mortality

CHAPTER XIX

Injury, poisoning and certain other consequences of external causes (S00–T98)

Excludes: birth trauma (P10–P14)

Injuries to the head (S00–S09)

S00 Superficial injury of head

Excludes: cerebral contusion (diffuse) (S06.2)
• focal (S06.3)
injury of eye and orbit (S05.–)

S00.0 Superficial injury of scalp

S00.1 Contusion of eyelid and periocular area
Black eye
Excludes: contusion of eyeball and orbital tissue (S05.1)

S00.2 Other superficial injuries of eyelid and periocular area
Excludes: superficial injury of conjunctiva and cornea (S05.0)

S00.3 Superficial injury of nose

S00.4 Superficial injury of ear

S00.5 Superficial injury of lip and oral cavity

S00.7 Multiple superficial injuries of head

S00.8 Superficial injury of other parts of head

S00.9 Superficial injury of head, part unspecified

S01 Open wound of head

Excludes: decapitation (S18)
injury of eye and orbit (S05.–)

S01.0 Open wound of scalp

S01.1 **Open wound of eyelid and periocular area**
Open wound of eyelid and periocular area with or without involvement of lacrimal passages

S01.2 **Open wound of nose**

S01.3 **Open wound of ear**

S01.4 **Open wound of cheek and temporomandibular area**

S01.5 **Open wound of lip and oral cavity**
Excludes: dislocation of tooth (S03.2)

S01.7 **Multiple open wounds of head**

S01.8 **Open wound of other parts of head**

S01.9 **Open wound of head, part unspecified**

S02 Fracture of skull and facial bones

The following subdivisions are provided for optional use where it is not possible or not desired to use multiple coding to identify fracture and open wound. A fracture not indicated as closed or open should be classified as closed.

S02.*x*0 Closed
S02.*x*1 Open

S02.0 **Fracture of vault of skull**
Use additional sixth character, if desired, to indicate localization:
S02.0*x*0 Frontal bone
S02.0*x*1 Parietal bone

S02.1 **Fracture of base of skull**
Excludes: orbit NOS (S02.8)
orbital floor (S02.3)

Use additional sixth character, if desired, to indicate localization:
S02.1*x*0 Anterior fossa
S02.1*x*1 Middle fossa
S02.1*x*2 Posterior fossa
S02.1*x*3 Occiput
S02.1*x*4 Orbital roof
S02.1*x*5 Ethmoid sinus
S02.1*x*6 Frontal sinus
S02.1*x*7 Sphenoid
S02.1*x*8 Temporal bone

S02.2 **Fracture of nasal bones**

S02.3 Fracture of orbital floor
Excludes: orbit NOS (S02.8)
orbital roof (S02.1)

S02.7 Multiple fractures involving skull and facial bones

S02.8 Fractures of other skull and facial bones
Alveolus
Orbit NOS
Palate
Excludes: orbital:
- floor (S02.3)
- roof (S02.1)

S03 Dislocation, sprain and strain of joints and ligaments of head

S03.0 Dislocation of jaw
Jaw (cartilage)(meniscus)
Mandible
Temporomandibular (joint)

S03.1 Dislocation of septal cartilage of nose

S03.2 Dislocation of tooth

S03.3 Dislocation of other and unspecified parts of head

S03.4 Sprain and strain of jaw
Temporomandibular (joint)(ligament)

S03.5 Sprain and strain of joint and ligaments of other and unspecified parts of head

S04 Injury of cranial nerves

S04.0 Injury of optic nerve and pathways

S04.00 2nd cranial nerve
S04.01 Optic chiasm
S04.02 Optic tract
S04.03 Optic radiations
S04.04 Visual cortex

S04.1 Injury of oculomotor nerve
3rd cranial nerve

S04.2 Injury of trochlear nerve
4th cranial nerve

S04.3 Injury of trigeminal nerve
5th cranial nerve

S04.4 Injury of abducent nerve
6th cranial nerve

S04.5 Injury of facial nerve
7th cranial nerve

S04.6 Injury of acoustic nerve
Auditory nerve
8th cranial nerve

S04.7 Injury of accessory nerve
11th cranial nerve

S04.8 Injury of other cranial nerves

S04.80 Olfactory [1st cranial] nerve
S04.81 Glossopharyngeal [9th cranial] nerve
S04.82 Vagus [10th cranial] nerve
S04.83 Hypoglossal [12th cranial] nerve

S04.9 Injury of unspecified cranial nerve

S05 Injury of eye and orbit

Excludes: injury of:
- oculomotor [3rd] nerve (S04.1)
- optic [2nd] nerve (S04.0)

open wound of eyelid and periocular area (S01.1)
orbital bone fracture (S02.1, S02.3, S02.8)
superficial injury of eyelid (S00.1–S00.3)

S05.0 Injury of conjunctiva and corneal abrasion without mention of foreign body

S05.1 Contusion of eyeball and orbital tissues

S05.2 Ocular laceration and rupture with prolapse or loss of intraocular tissue

S05.3 Ocular laceration without prolapse or loss of intraocular tissue
Laceration of eye NOS

S05.4 Penetrating wound of orbit with or without foreign body
Excludes: retained (old) foreign body following penetrating wound of orbit (H05.5)

S05.5 Penetrating wound of eyeball with foreign body
Excludes: retained (old) intraocular foreign body, nonmagnetic (H44.7)

S05.6 Penetrating wound of eyeball without foreign body
Ocular penetration NOS

S05.7 Avulsion of eye
Traumatic enucleation

S05.8 Other injuries of eye and orbit
Lacrimal duct injury

S05.9 Injury of eye and orbit, part unspecified

S06 Intracranial injury

The following subdivisions are provided for optional use where it is not possible or not desired to use multiple coding to identify intracranial injury and open wound:

S06.*x*0 Without open intracranial wound
S06.*x*1 With open intracranial wound

S06.0 Concussion
Commotio cerebri

S06.1 Traumatic cerebral oedema

S06.2 Diffuse brain injury
Cerebral:
- contusion NOS
- laceration NOS

S06.3 Focal brain injury
Focal:
- cerebral contusion and laceration
- traumatic intracerebral haemorrhage

Use additional sixth character, if desired, to indicate localization:

S06.3*x*0 Frontal
S06.3*x*1 Temporal
S06.3*x*2 Parietal
S06.3*x*3 Occipital
S06.3*x*4 Deep cerebral hemisphere
S06.3*x*5 Corpus callosum
S06.3*x*6 Brainstem
S06.3*x*7 Cerebellar

S06.4 Epidural haemorrhage
Extradural haemorrhage (traumatic)

S06.5 Traumatic subdural haemorrhage
Use additional sixth character, if desired, to indicate onset of haemorrhage:

S06.5*x*0 Acute traumatic subdural haemorrhage (within 48 hours of trauma)
S06.5*x*1 Subacute traumatic subdural haemorrhage (48 hours to 8 days after trauma)
S06.5*x*2 Chronic traumatic subdural haemorrhage (after 8th day)

S06.6 Traumatic subarachnoid haemorrhage

S06.7 Intracranial injury with prolonged coma

S06.8 Other intracranial injuries

S06.8*x*0 Traumatic intracranial haemorrhage, unspecified
S06.8*x*1 Injury to pituitary stalk and gland

S06.9 Intracranial injury, unspecified
Brain injury NOS

S07 Crushing injury of head

S07.0 Crushing injury of face

S07.1 Crushing injury of skull

S09 Other and unspecified injuries of head

S09.0 Injury of blood vessels of head, not elsewhere classified
Excludes: injury of:
- cerebral blood vessels (S06.–)
- precerebral blood vessels (S15.–)

S09.1 Injury of muscle and tendon of head

S09.2 Traumatic rupture of ear drum

S09.7 Multiple injuries of head
Injuries classifiable to more than one of the categories S00–S09.2

S09.8 Other specified injuries of head

Injuries to the neck (S10–S19)

S11.– Open wound of neck

Excludes: decapitation (S18)

S12 Fracture of neck

Includes: cervical:
- spine
- spinous process
- transverse process
- vertebra

The following subdivisions are provided for optional use where it is not possible or not desired to use multiple coding to identify fracture and open wound. A fracture not indicated as closed or open should be classified as closed.

S12.*x*0 Closed
S12.*x*1 Open

S12.0 Fracture of first cervical vertebra
Atlas

S12.1 Fracture of second cervical vertebra
Axis

S12.2 Fracture of other specified cervical vertebra

S12.2*x*0 Fracture of C3
S12.2*x*1 Fracture of C4
S12.2*x*2 Fracture of C5
S12.2*x*3 Fracture of C6
S12.2*x*4 Fracture of C7

S12.7 Multiple fractures of cervical spine

S12.8 Fracture of other parts of neck
Hyoid bone
Larynx
Thyroid cartilage
Trachea

S12.9 Fracture of neck, part unspecified
Fracture of cervical:
- spine NOS
- vertebra NOS

S13 Dislocation, sprain and strain of joints and ligaments at neck level

Excludes: rupture or displacement (nontraumatic) of cervical intervertebral disc (M50.–)

S13.0 Traumatic rupture of cervical intervertebral disc

S13.00 Traumatic rupture of C2/3 disc
S13.01 Traumatic rupture of C3/4 disc
S13.02 Traumatic rupture of C4/5 disc
S13.03 Traumatic rupture of C5/6 disc
S13.04 Traumatic rupture of C6/7 disc
S13.05 Traumatic rupture of C7/T1 disc
S13.07 Multiple traumatic ruptures of cervical intervertebral discs

S13.1 Dislocation of cervical vertebra

Includes: dislocation of cervical spine NOS

S13.10 Dislocation of C1
S13.11 Dislocation of C2
S13.12 Dislocation of C3
S13.13 Dislocation of C4
S13.14 Dislocation of C5
S13.15 Dislocation of C6
S13.16 Dislocation of C7

S13.2 Dislocation of other and unspecified parts of neck

S13.3 Multiple dislocations of neck

S13.4 Sprain and strain of cervical spine

S13.40 Anterior longitudinal (ligament), cervical
S13.41 Atlantoaxial (joints)
S13.42 Atlanto-occipital (joints)
S13.43 Whiplash injury

S13.5 Sprain and strain of thyroid region

Cricoarytenoid (joint)(ligament)
Cricothyroid (joint)(ligament)
Thyroid cartilage

S13.6 Sprain and strain of joints and ligaments of other and unspecified parts of neck

S14 Injury of nerves and spinal cord at neck level

S14.0 Concussion and oedema of cervical spinal cord

S14.00 Concussion and oedema at C1 level
S14.01 Concussion and oedema at C2 level
S14.02 Concussion and oedema at C3 level
S14.03 Concussion and oedema at C4 level
S14.04 Concussion and oedema at C5 level
S14.05 Concussion and oedema at C6 level
S14.06 Concussion and oedema at C7 level
S14.07 Concussion and oedema at C8 level
S14.08 Multiple and overlapping concussion and oedema of cervical spinal cord

S14.1 Other and unspecified injuries of cervical spinal cord

Injury of cervical spinal cord NOS

S14.2 Injury of nerve root of cervical spine

S14.20 Injury of nerve root of C1
S14.21 Injury of nerve root of C2
S14.22 Injury of nerve root of C3
S14.23 Injury of nerve root of C4
S14.24 Injury of nerve root of C5
S14.25 Injury of nerve root of C6
S14.26 Injury of nerve root of C7
S14.27 Injury of nerve root of C8
S14.28 Multiple and bilateral injury of nerve roots of cervical spine

S14.3 Injury of brachial plexus

S14.30 Injury of brachial plexus trunk
- S14.300 Upper trunk
- S14.301 Middle trunk
- S14.302 Lower trunk
- S14.307 Multiple levels

S14.31 Injury of brachial plexus division
- S14.310 Anterior division
- S14.311 Posterior division
- S14.312 Anterior and posterior

S14.32 Injury of brachial plexus cord
- S14.320 Lateral cord
- S14.321 Posterior cord
- S14.322 Medial cord
- S14.327 Multiple levels

S14.4 Injury of peripheral nerves of neck

S14.40 Nerves supplying scalp and ear
- S14.400 Occipital nerve(s)
- S14.401 Great auricular nerve

S14.41 Nerves supplying neck and chest
- S14.410 Anterior cutaneous nerve of neck
- S14.411 Supraclavicular nerve(s)

S14.42 Phrenic nerve

S14.43 Nerves arising proximally from brachial plexus
- S14.430 Suprascapular nerve
- S14.431 Nerve to subclavius
- S14.432 Nerve to rhomboids
- S14.433 Nerve to serratus anterior
- S14.434 Nerve to latissimus dorsi
- S14.435 Subscapular nerve

S14.47 Multiple injury of peripheral nerves of neck

S14.5 Injury of cervical sympathetic nerves

S14.6 Injury of other and unspecified nerves of neck

S15 Injury of blood vessels at neck level

S15.0 Injury of carotid artery

S15.00 Innominate artery
S15.01 Common carotid artery
S15.02 Internal carotid artery in neck
S15.03 Internal carotid artery in base of skull
S15.04 External carotid artery
S15.07 Bilateral carotid artery

S15.1 Injury of vertebral artery

S15.10 Vertebral artery in root of neck
S15.11 Vertebral artery in intervertebral canal
S15.12 Vertebral artery at base of skull
S15.17 Bilateral vertebral artery

S15.2 Injury of external jugular vein

S15.3 Injury of internal jugular vein

S15.7 Injury of multiple blood vessels at neck level

S15.8 Injury of other blood vessels at neck level

S16 Injury of muscle and tendon at neck level

S17.– Crushing injury of neck

S18 Traumatic amputation at neck level

Decapitation

S19 Other and unspecified injuries of neck

S19.7 Multiple injuries of neck

Injuries classifiable to more than one of the categories S11–S18

Injuries to the thorax (S20–S29)

S22 Fracture of rib(s), sternum and thoracic spine

Includes: thoracic:

- neural arch
- spinous process
- transverse process
- vertebra
- vertebral arch

The following subdivisions are provided for optional use where it is not possible or not desired to use multiple coding to identify fracture and open wound. A fracture not indicated as closed or open should be classified as closed.

S22.*x*0 Closed
S22.*x*1 Open

S22.0 Fracture of thoracic vertebra

Includes: fracture of thoracic spine NOS

Use additional sixth character, if desired, to indicate localization:

S22.0*x*0 Fracture of T1
S22.0*x*1 Fracture of T2
S22.0*x*2 Fracture of T3 or T4
S22.0*x*3 Fracture of T5 or T6
S22.0*x*4 Fracture of T7 or T8
S22.0*x*5 Fracture of T9 or T10
S22.0*x*6 Fracture of T11
S22.0*x*7 Fracture of T12

S22.1 Multiple fractures of thoracic spine

S23 Dislocation, sprain and strain of joints and ligaments of thorax

Excludes: rupture or displacement (nontraumatic) of thoracic intervertebral disc (M51.–)

S23.0 Traumatic rupture of thoracic intervertebral disc

S23.00 Traumatic rupture of T1/T2 disc
S23.01 Traumatic rupture of T2/T3 disc
S23.02 Traumatic rupture of T3/T4 or T4/T5 disc
S23.03 Traumatic rupture of T5/T6 or T6/T7 disc
S23.04 Traumatic rupture of T7/T8 or T8/T9 disc
S23.05 Traumatic rupture of T9/T10 or T10/T11 disc
S23.06 Traumatic rupture of T11/T12 disc
S23.07 Traumatic rupture of T12/L1 disc
S23.08 Multiple traumatic ruptures of thoracic intervertebral discs

S23.1 Dislocation of thoracic vertebra

Includes: dislocation of thoracic spine NOS

S23.10 Dislocation of T1
S23.11 Dislocation of T2
S23.12 Dislocation of T3 or T4
S23.13 Dislocation of T5 or T6
S23.14 Dislocation of T7 or T8
S23.15 Dislocation of T9 or T10
S23.16 Dislocation of T11
S23.17 Dislocation of T12
S23.18 Multiple dislocations of thoracic vertebrae

S23.3 Sprain and strain of thoracic spine

S24 Injury of nerves and spinal cord at thorax level

Excludes: injury of brachial plexus (S14.3)

S24.0 Concussion and oedema of thoracic spinal cord

S24.00 Concussion and oedema at T1 level
S24.01 Concussion and oedema at T2 level
S24.02 Concussion and oedema at T3 or T4 level
S24.03 Concussion and oedema at T5 or T6 level
S24.04 Concussion and oedema at T7 or T8 level
S24.05 Concussion and oedema at T9 or T10 level
S24.06 Concussion and oedema at T11 level
S24.07 Concussion and oedema at T12 level

S24.08 Multiple and overlapping concussion and oedema of thoracic spinal cord

S24.1 Other and unspecified injuries of thoracic spinal cord

S24.2 Injury of nerve root of thoracic spine

S24.20 Injury of nerve root of T1
S24.21 Injury of nerve root of T2
S24.22 Injury of nerve root of T3 or T4
S24.23 Injury of nerve root of T5 or T6
S24.24 Injury of nerve root of T7 or T8
S24.25 Injury of nerve root of T9 or T10
S24.26 Injury of nerve root of T11
S24.27 Injury of nerve root of T12
S24.28 Multiple and bilateral injury of nerve roots of thoracic spine

S24.3 Injury of peripheral nerves of thorax

S24.4 Injury of thoracic sympathetic nerves

S24.40 Cardiac plexus
S24.41 Oesophageal plexus
S24.42 Pulmonary plexus
S24.43 Stellate ganglion
S24.44 Thoracic sympathetic ganglion
S24.47 Multiple and bilateral injury of thoracic sympathetic nerves

S24.5 Injury of other nerves of thorax

S24.6 Injury of unspecified nerve of thorax

Injuries to the abdomen, lower back, lumbar spine and pelvis (S30–S39)

S32 Fracture of lumbar spine and pelvis

Includes: lumbosacral:
- neural arch
- spinous process
- transverse process
- vertebra
- vertebral arch

The following subdivisions are provided for optional use where it is not possible or not desired to use multiple coding to identify fracture and open wound. A fracture not indicated as closed or open should be classified as closed.

S32.*x*0 Closed
S32.*x*1 Open

S32.0 Fracture of lumbar vertebra
Includes: fracture of lumbar spine

S32.0*x*0 Fracture of L1
S32.0*x*1 Fracture of L2
S32.0*x*2 Fracture of L3
S32.0*x*3 Fracture of L4
S32.0*x*4 Fracture of L5
S32.0*x*7 Fracture of multiple lumbar vertebrae

S32.1 Fracture of sacrum

S32.2 Fracture of coccyx

S32.3 Fracture of ilium

S32.4 Fracture of acetabulum

S32.5 Fracture of pubis

S32.7 Multiple fractures of lumbar spine and pelvis

S32.8 Fracture of other and unspecified parts of lumbosacral spine and pelvis
Fracture of:
- ischium
- lumbosacral spine NOS
- pelvis NOS

S33 Dislocation, sprain and strain of joints and ligaments of lumbar spine and pelvis

Excludes: rupture or displacement (nontraumatic) of lumbar intervertebral disc (M51.–)

S33.0 Traumatic rupture of lumbar intervertebral disc

S33.00 Traumatic rupture of L1/L2 disc
S33.01 Traumatic rupture of L2/L3 disc
S33.02 Traumatic rupture of L3/L4 disc
S33.03 Traumatic rupture of L4/L5 disc
S33.04 Traumatic rupture of L5/S1 disc

S33.07 Multiple traumatic ruptures of lumbar intervertebral discs

S33.1 Dislocation of lumbar vertebra
Includes: dislocation of lumbar spine NOS

S33.10 Dislocation of L1
S33.11 Dislocation of L2
S33.12 Dislocation of L3
S33.13 Dislocation of L4
S33.14 Dislocation of L5
S33.17 Dislocation of multiple lumbar vertebrae

S33.2 Dislocation of sacroiliac and sacrococcygeal joint

S33.3 Dislocation of other and unspecified parts of lumbar spine and pelvis

S33.4 Traumatic rupture of symphysis pubis

S33.5 Sprain and strain of lumbar spine

S33.6 Sprain and strain of sacroiliac joint

S33.7 Sprain and strain of other and unspecified parts of lumbar spine and pelvis

S34 Injury of nerves and lumbar spinal cord at abdomen, lower back and pelvis level

S34.0 Concussion and oedema of lumbar spinal cord
Note: This concerns the functional levels of the spinal cord, not the vertebral levels.

S34.00 Concussion and oedema at L1 level
S34.01 Concussion and oedema at L2 level
S34.02 Concussion and oedema at L3 level
S34.03 Concussion and oedema at L4 level
S34.04 Concussion and oedema at L5 level
S34.05 Concussion and oedema at S1 level
S34.06 Concussion and oedema at S2 level
S34.07 Concussion and oedema at S3 to coccygeal segment
S34.08 Multiple and overlapping concussion and oedema of lumbar spinal cord

S34.1 Other injury of lumbar spinal cord

S34.2 Injury of nerve root of lumbar and sacral spine

S34.20 Injury of nerve root of L1
S34.21 Injury of nerve root of L2

S34.22	Injury of nerve root of L3
S34.23	Injury of nerve root of L4
S34.24	Injury of nerve root of L5
S34.25	Injury of nerve root of S1
S34.26	Injury of nerve root of S2
S34.27	Injury of S3 to coccygeal nerve roots
S34.28	Multiple and bilateral injury of lumbar and sacral nerve roots

S34.3 Injury of cauda equina

S34.30	Partial injury of cauda equina
S34.31	Complete injury of cauda equina

S34.4 Injury of lumbosacral plexus

S34.40	Injury of upper part of lumbar plexus (L2–L3 roots)
S34.41	Injury of middle part of lumbar plexus (L4–L5 roots)
S34.42	Injury of sacral plexus (S1–coccyx)
S34.47	Multiple and bilateral injury of lumbosacral plexus

S34.5 Injury of lumbar, sacral and pelvic sympathetic nerves

S34.50	Coeliac ganglion or plexus
S34.51	Hypogastric plexus
S34.52	Mesenteric plexus (inferior)(superior)
S34.53	Splanchnic nerve
S34.57	Multiple and bilateral injury of lumbar, sacral and pelvic sympathetic nerves

S34.6 Injury of peripheral nerve(s) of abdomen, lower back and pelvis

S34.60	Ilio-hypogastric nerve
S34.61	Ilio-inguinal nerve
S34.62	Genito-femoral nerve
S34.63	Superior gluteal nerve
S34.64	Inferior gluteal nerve
S34.65	Obturator nerve
S34.66	Pudendal nerve
S34.67	Perineal nerve
S34.68	Multiple or bilateral injury of peripheral nerve(s) of abdomen, lower back and pelvis

S34.8 Injury of other and unspecified nerves of abdomen, lower back and pelvis level

Injuries to the shoulder and upper arm (S40–S49)

S44 Injury of nerves at shoulder and upper arm level

Excludes: injury of brachial plexus (S14.3)

S44.0 Injury of ulnar nerve at upper arm level
Excludes: ulnar nerve NOS (S54.0)

S44.1 Injury of median nerve at upper arm level
Excludes: median nerve NOS (S54.1)

S44.2 Injury of radial nerve at upper arm level
Excludes: radial nerve NOS (S54.2)

S44.3 Injury of axillary nerve

S44.4 Injury of musculocutaneous nerve

S44.6 Injury of cutaneous sensory nerve at shoulder and upper arm level

S44.7 Injury of multiple nerves at shoulder and upper arm level

S44.8 Injury of other nerves at shoulder and upper arm level

S44.80 Intercostobrachial nerve
S44.81 Lateral pectoral nerve
S44.82 Medial pectoral nerve
S44.87 Multiple nerves at shoulder and upper arm level

S44.9 Injury of unspecified nerve at shoulder and upper arm level

Injuries to the elbow and forearm (S50–S59)

S54 Injury of nerves at forearm level

Excludes: injuries of nerves at wrist and hand level (S64.–)

S54.0 Injury of ulnar nerve at forearm level
Ulnar nerve NOS

S54.1 Injury of median nerve at forearm level
Includes: median nerve NOS

S54.10 Anterior interosseous nerve

S54.2 Injury of radial nerve at forearm level

Includes: radial nerve NOS

S54.20 Posterior interosseous nerve

S54.3 Injury of cutaneous sensory nerve at forearm level

S54.7 Injury of multiple nerves at forearm level

S54.8 Injury of other nerves at forearm level

S54.9 Injury of unspecified nerve at forearm level

Injuries to the wrist and hand (S60–S69)

S64 Injury of nerves at wrist and hand level

S64.0 Injury of ulnar nerve at wrist and hand level

S64.00 Superficial branch of ulnar nerve
S64.01 Deep palmar branch of ulnar nerve

S64.1 Injury of median nerve at wrist and hand level

S64.2 Injury of radial nerve at wrist and hand level

S64.20 Superficial branch of radial nerve

S64.3 Injury of digital nerve of thumb

S64.4 Injury of digital nerve of other finger

S64.7 Injury of multiple nerves at wrist and hand level

S64.8 Injury of other nerves at wrist and hand level

S64.9 Injury of unspecified nerve at wrist and hand level

Injuries to the hip and thigh (S70–S79)

S74 Injury of nerves at hip and thigh level

S74.0 Injury of sciatic nerve at hip and thigh level

S74.1 Injury of femoral nerve at hip and thigh level

S74.2 Injury of cutaneous sensory nerve at hip and thigh level

S74.20 Lateral cutaneous nerve of thigh
S74.21 Posterior cutaneous nerve of thigh
S74.22 Intermediate and medial cutaneous nerve of thigh

S74.7 Injury of multiple nerves at hip and thigh level

S74.8 Injury of other nerves at hip and thigh level

S74.9 Injury of unspecified nerve at hip and thigh level

Injuries to the knee and lower leg (S80–S89)

S84 Injury of nerves at lower leg level

Excludes: injury of nerves at ankle and foot level (S94.–)

S84.0 Injury of tibial nerve at lower leg level

S84.1 Injury of peroneal nerve at lower leg level

S84.10 Superficial peroneal nerve
S84.11 Deep peroneal nerve
S84.12 Deep and superficial peroneal nerves

S84.2 Injury of cutaneous sensory nerve at lower leg level

S84.20 Lateral cutaneous nerve of calf
S84.21 Saphenous nerve
S84.22 Musculocutaneous nerve
S84.23 Sural nerve

S84.7 Injury of multiple nerves at lower leg level

S84.8 Injury of other nerves at lower leg level

S84.9 Injury of unspecified nerve at lower leg level

Injuries to the ankle and foot (S90–S99)

S94 Injury of nerves at ankle and foot level

S94.0 Injury of lateral plantar nerve

S94.1 Injury of medial plantar nerve

S94.2 Injury of deep peroneal nerve at ankle and foot level
Terminal, lateral branch of deep peroneal nerve

S94.3 Injury of cutaneous sensory nerve at ankle and foot level

S94.7 Injury of multiple nerves at ankle and foot level

S94.8 Injury of other nerves at ankle and foot level

S94.9 Injury of unspecified nerve at ankle and foot level

Injuries involving multiple body regions (T00–T07)

T02 Fractures involving multiple body regions

The following subdivisions are provided for optional use where it is not possible or not desired to use multiple coding to identify fracture and open wound. A fracture not indicated as closed or open should be classified as closed.

T02.*x*0 Closed
T02.*x*1 Open

T02.0 Fractures involving head with neck
Includes: fractures of sites classifiable to S02.– and S12.–

T02.1 Fractures involving thorax with lower back and pelvis
Includes: fractures of sites classifiable to S22.–, S32.– and T08
Excludes: when combined with fractures of limb(s) (T02.7)

T02.7 Fractures involving thorax with lower back and pelvis with limb(s)

T03 Dislocations, sprains and strains involving multiple body regions

T03.0 Dislocations, sprains and strains involving head with neck
Dislocations, sprains and strains of sites classifiable to S03.– and S13.–

T03.1 Dislocations, sprains and strains involving thorax with lower back and pelvis
Dislocations, sprains and strains of sites classifiable to S23.–, S33.– and T09.2

T03.8 Dislocations, sprains and strains involving other combinations of body regions

T04 Crushing injuries involving multiple body regions

T04.0 Crushing injuries involving head with neck
Crushing injuries of sites classifiable to S07.– and S17.–

T04.1 Crushing injuries involving thorax with abdomen, lower back and pelvis

T06 Other injuries involving multiple body regions, not elsewhere classified

T06.0 Injuries of brain and cranial nerves with injuries of nerves and spinal cord at neck level
Injuries classifiable to S04.– and S06.– with injuries classifiable to S14.–

T06.1 Injuries of nerves and spinal cord involving other multiple body regions

T06.2 Injuries of nerves involving multiple body regions
Multiple injuries of nerves NOS
Excludes: with spinal cord involvement (T06.0–T06.1)

Injuries to unspecified part of trunk, limb or body region (T08–T14)

T08 Fracture of spine, level unspecified

Excludes: multiple fractures of spine, level unspecified (T02.1)

The following subdivisions are provided for optional use where it is not possible or not desired to use multiple coding to identify fracture and open wound. A fracture not indicated as closed or open should be classified as closed.

T08.0 Closed

T08.1 Open

T09 Other injuries of spine and trunk, level unspecified

T09.2 Dislocation, sprain and strain of unspecified joint and ligament of trunk

T09.3 Injury of spinal cord, level unspecified

T09.4 Injury of unspecified nerve, spinal nerve root and plexus of trunk

T11 Other injuries of upper limb, level unspecified

T11.3 Injury of unspecified nerve of upper limb, level unspecified

T13 Other injuries of lower limb, level unspecified

T13.3 Injury of unspecified nerve of lower limb, level unspecified

T14 Injury of unspecified body region

Excludes: injuries involving multiple body regions (T03–T04, T06)

T14.0 Superficial injury of unspecified body region

Abrasion } NOS
Blister (nonthermal) } NOS
Bruise } NOS
Contusion } NOS
Haematoma } NOS
Injury from superficial foreign body (splinter) without major open wound } NOS
Insect bite (nonvenomous) } NOS
Superficial injury } NOS

T14.1 Open wound of unspecified body region

Animal bite } NOS
Cut } NOS
Laceration } NOS
Open wound } NOS
Puncture wound with (penetrating) foreign body } NOS

Excludes: traumatic amputation NOS (T14.7)

T14.2 Fracture of unspecified body region

Fracture:
- NOS
- closed
- dislocated
- displaced
- open

The following subdivisions are provided for optional use where it is not possible or not desired to use multiple coding to identify fracture and open wound. A fracture not indicated as closed or open should be classified as closed.

T14.20 Closed
T14.21 Open

T14.3 Dislocation, sprain and strain of unspecified body region

Avulsion, Laceration, Sprain, Strain, Traumatic:
- haemarthrosis
- rupture
- subluxation
- tear

of joint (capsule) / ligament NOS

T14.4 Injury of nerve(s) of unspecified body region

Injury of nerve, Traumatic:
- division of nerve
- haematomyelia
- paralysis (transient)

NOS

Excludes: multiple injuries of nerves NOS (T06.2)

T14.5 Injury of blood vessel(s) of unspecified body region

Avulsion, Cut, Injury, Laceration, Traumatic:
- aneurysm or fistula (arteriovenous)
- arterial haematoma
- rupture

of blood vessel(s) NOS

T14.6 Injury of tendons and muscles of unspecified body region

Avulsion, Cut, Injury, Laceration, Traumatic rupture of muscle(s) NOS and tendon(s) NOS

T14.7 Crushing injury and traumatic amputation of unspecified body region

Crushing injury NOS
Traumatic amputation NOS

T14.8 Other injuries of unspecified body region

T14.9 Injury, unspecified

Effects of foreign body entering through natural orifice (T15–T19)

T17.– **Foreign body in respiratory tract**
Includes: asphyxia due to foreign body
inhalation of liquid or vomitus NOS

Poisoning by drugs, medicaments and biological substances (T36–T50)

Includes: overdose of these substances
wrong substance given or taken in error
Excludes: adverse effects ["hypersensitivity", "reaction", etc.] of correct substance properly administered; such cases are to be classified according to the nature of the adverse effect, such as:
- aspirin gastritis (K29.–)
- blood disorders (D50–D76)
- unspecified adverse effect of drug (T88.7)

drug dependence and related mental and behavioural disorders due to psychoactive substance use (F10–F19)
drug reaction and poisoning affecting the fetus and newborn (P00–P96)
pathological drug intoxication (F10–F19)

T36 **Poisoning by systemic antibiotics**
Excludes: antineoplastic antibiotics (T45.1)

T36.0 **Penicillins**

T36.1 **Cefalosporins and other β-lactam antibiotics**

T36.2 **Chloramphenicol group**

T36.4 **Tetracyclines**

T36.5 **Aminoglycosides**
Streptomycin

T36.6 **Rifamycins**

T36.7 **Antifungal antibiotics, systemically used**

T36.8 **Other systemic antibiotics**

T36.9 **Systemic antibiotic, unspecified**

T37 Poisoning by other systemic anti-infectives and antiparasitics

T37.0 **Sulfonamides**

T37.1 **Antimycobacterial drugs**
Excludes: rifamycins (T36.6)
streptomycin (T36.5)

T37.10 Dapsone

T37.2 **Antimalarials and drugs acting on other blood protozoa**
Excludes: hydroxyquinoline derivatives (T37.8)

T37.3 **Other antiprotozoal drugs**

T37.4 **Anthelminthics**

T37.8 **Other specified systemic anti-infectives and antiparasitics**

T37.80 Hydroxyquinoline derivatives
T37.81 Clioquinol

T37.9 **Systemic anti-infective and antiparasitic, unspecified**

T38 Poisoning by hormones and their synthetic substitutes and antagonists, not elsewhere classified

Excludes: mineralocorticoids and their antagonists (T50.0)
oxytocic hormones (T48.0)
parathyroid hormones and derivatives (T50.9)

T38.0 **Glucocorticoids and synthetic analogues**

T38.1 **Thyroid hormones and substitutes**

T38.2 **Antithyroid drugs**

T38.3 **Insulin and oral hypoglycaemic [antidiabetic] drugs**

T38.4 **Oral contraceptives**
Multiple- and single-ingredient preparations

T38.5 **Other estrogens and progestogens**
Mixtures and substitutes

T38.6 Antigonadotrophins, antiestrogens, antiandrogens, not elsewhere classified
Tamoxifen

T38.7 Androgens and anabolic congeners

T38.8 Other and unspecified hormones and their synthetic substitutes
Anterior pituitary [adenohypophyseal] hormones

T39 Poisoning by nonopioid analgesics, antipyretics and antirheumatics

T39.0 Salicylates

T39.1 4-Aminophenol derivatives

T39.2 Pyrazolone derivatives

T39.3 Other nonsteroidal anti-inflammatory drugs [NSAID]

T39.4 Antirheumatics, not elsewhere classified
Excludes: glucocorticoids (T38.0)
salicylates (T39.0)

T39.8 Other nonopioid analgesics and antipyretics, not elsewhere classified

T40 Poisoning by narcotics and psychodysleptics [hallucinogens]

Excludes: drug dependence and related mental and behavioural disorders due to psychoactive substance use (F10–F19)

T40.0 Opium

T40.1 Heroin

T40.2 Other opioids
Codeine
Morphine

T40.3 Methadone

T40.4 Other synthetic narcotics
Pethidine

T40.5 Cocaine

T40.6 Other and unspecified narcotics

T40.7 Cannabis (derivatives)

T40.8 Lysergide [LSD]

T40.9 Other and unspecified psychodysleptics [hallucinogens]

T40.90 Mescaline
T40.91 Psilocin
T40.92 Psilocybine
T40.93 Phencyclidine
T40.94 1-Methyl-4-phenyl-1,2,3,6-tetrahydropyridine [MPTP]

T41 Poisoning by anaesthetics and therapeutic gases

Excludes: benzodiazepines (T42.4)
cocaine (T40.5)
opioids (T40.0–T40.2)

T41.0 Inhaled anaesthetics

T41.00 Nitrous oxide

T41.1 Intravenous anaesthetics
Thiobarbiturates

T41.2 Other and unspecified general anaesthetics

T41.3 Local anaesthetics

T41.5 Therapeutic gases
Carbon dioxide
Oxygen

T42 Poisoning by antiepileptic, sedative–hypnotic and antiparkinsonism drugs

Excludes: drug dependence and related mental and behavioural disorders due to psychoactive substance use (F10–F19)

T42.0 Hydantoin derivatives
Excludes: fetal hydantoin syndrome (Q86.1)

T42.1 Iminostilbenes
Carbamazepine

T42.2 Succinimides and oxazolidinediones

T42.3 Barbiturates
Excludes: thiobarbiturates (T41.1)

T42.4 Benzodiazepines

T42.5 Mixed antiepileptics, not elsewhere classified

T42.6 Other antiepileptic and sedative–hypnotic drugs
Methaqualone
Paraldehyde
Valproic acid
Excludes: carbamazepine (T42.1)

T42.7 Antiepileptic and sedative–hypnotic drugs, unspecified
Sleeping:
- draught } NOS
- drug } NOS
- tablet } NOS

T42.8 Antiparkinsonism drugs and other central muscle-tone depressants
Amantadine

T43 Poisoning by psychotropic drugs, not elsewhere classified

Excludes: barbiturates (T42.3)
benzodiazepines (T42.4)
methaqualone (T42.6)
psychodysleptics [hallucinogens] (T40.7–T40.9)

T43.0 Tricyclic and tetracyclic antidepressants

T43.1 Monoamine-oxidase-inhibitor antidepressants

T43.2 Other and unspecified antidepressants

T43.3 Phenothiazine antipsychotics and neuroleptics

T43.4 Butyrophenone and thioxanthene neuroleptics

T43.5 Other and unspecified antipsychotics and neuroleptics
Lithium
Excludes: rauwolfia (T46.5)

T43.6 Psychostimulants with abuse potential
Excludes: cocaine (T40.5)

T43.8 Other psychotropic drugs, not elsewhere classified

T43.9 Psychotropic drug, unspecified

T44 Poisoning by drugs primarily affecting the autonomic nervous system

T44.0 Anticholinesterase agents

T44.1 Other parasympathomimetics [cholinergics]

T44.2 Ganglionic blocking drugs, not elsewhere classified

T44.3 Other parasympatholytics [anticholinergics and antimuscarinics] and spasmolytics, not elsewhere classified
Papaverine

T44.4 Predominantly α-adrenoreceptor agonists, not elsewhere classified
Metaraminol

T44.5 Predominantly β-adrenoreceptor agonists, not elsewhere classified
Excludes: salbutamol (T48.6)

T44.6 α-Adrenoreceptor antagonists, not elsewhere classified
Excludes: ergot alkaloids (T48.0)

T44.7 β-Adrenoreceptor antagonists, not elsewhere classified

T44.8 Centrally acting and adrenergic-neuron-blocking agents, not elsewhere classified
Excludes: clonidine (T46.5)
guanethidine (T46.5)

T44.9 Other and unspecified drugs primarily affecting the autonomic nervous system
Drug stimulating both α- and β-adrenoreceptors

T45 Poisoning by primarily systemic and haematological agents, not elsewhere classified

T45.0 Antiallergic and antiemetic drugs
Cinnarizine
Excludes: phenothiazine-based neuroleptics (T43.3)

T45.1 Antineoplastic and immunosuppressive drugs
Cytarabine

T45.2 Vitamins, not elsewhere classified
Excludes: nicotinic acid (derivatives) (T46.7)
vitamin K (T45.7)

T45.3 Enzymes, not elsewhere classified

T45.4 Iron and its compounds

T45.5 Anticoagulants

T45.7 Anticoagulant antagonists, vitamin K and other coagulants

T45.8 Other primarily systemic and haematological agents
Liver preparations and other antianaemic agents
Natural blood and blood products
Plasma substitute
Excludes: immunoglobulin (T50.9)
iron (T45.4)

T46 Poisoning by agents primarily affecting the cardiovascular system

Excludes: metaraminol (T44.4)

T46.0 Cardiac-stimulant glycosides and drugs of similar action

T46.1 Calcium-channel blockers
Diltiazem

T46.2 Other antidysrhythmic drugs, not elsewhere classified

T46.3 Coronary vasodilators, not elsewhere classified
Excludes: β-adrenoreceptor antagonists (T44.7)

T46.30 Aminodarone
T46.31 Dipyridamole

T46.4 Angiotensin-converting-enzyme inhibitors

T46.5 Other antihypertensive drugs, not elsewhere classified
Clonidine
Guanethidine
Rauwolfia
Reserpine tetrabenazine

T46.50 Perhexiline

T46.6 Antihyperlipidaemic and antiarteriosclerotic drugs

T46.7 Peripheral vasodilators
Nicotinic acid (derivatives)
Flunarizine

T46.8 Antivaricose drugs, including sclerosing agents

T47 Poisoning by agents primarily affecting the gastrointestinal system

T47.0 Histamine H_2-receptor antagonists

T47.1 Other antacids and anti-gastric-secretion drugs

T47.5 Digestants

T47.6 Antidiarrhoeal drugs

Excludes: systemic antibiotics and other anti-infectives (T36–T37)

T47.7 Emetics

T48 Poisoning by agents primarily acting on smooth and skeletal muscles and the respiratory system

T48.0 Oxytocic drugs

Excludes: estrogens, progestogens and antagonists (T38.4–T38.6)

T48.1 Skeletal muscle relaxants [neuromuscular blocking agents]

Aminophylline

T48.3 Antitussives

T48.4 Expectorants

T48.5 Anti-common-cold drugs

T48.6 Antiasthmatics, not elsewhere classified

Salbutamol

Excludes: β-adrenoreceptor agonists (T44.5)
Anterior pituitary [adenohypophyseal] hormones (T38.8)

T49 Poisoning by topical agents primarily affecting skin and mucous membrane and by ophthalmological, otorhinolaryngological and dental drugs

Includes: glucocorticoids, topically used

T49.0 Local antifungal, anti-infective and anti-inflammatory drugs, not elsewhere classified

T49.1 Antipruritics

T49.2 Local astringents and local detergents

T49.3 Emollients, demulcents and protectants

T49.4 Keratolytics, keratoplastics and other hair treatment drugs and preparations

T49.5 Ophthalmological drugs and preparations

Eye anti-infectives

T49.6 Otorhinolaryngological drugs and preparations

Ear, nose and throat preparations

T49.7 Dental drugs, topically applied

T49.8 **Other topical agents**
Spermicides

T49.9 **Topical agent, unspecified**

T50 Poisoning by diuretics and other and unspecified drugs, medicaments and biological substances

T50.0 **Mineralocorticoids and their antagonists**

T50.2 **Carbonic-anhydrase inhibitors, benzothiazides and other diuretics**
Acetazolamide

T50.3 **Electrolytic, caloric and water-balance agents**
Oral rehydration salts

T50.4 **Drugs affecting uric acid metabolism**

T50.5 **Appetite depressants**

T50.6 **Antidotes and chelating agents, not elsewhere classified**
Alcohol deterrents

T50.7 **Analeptics and opioid receptor antagonists**

T50.8 **Diagnostic agents**

T50.9 **Other and unspecified drugs, medicaments and biological substances**
Acidifying agents
Alkalizing agents
Immunoglobulin
Immunologicals
Lipotropic drugs
Parathyroid hormones and derivatives

Toxic effects of substances chiefly nonmedicinal as to source (T51–T65)

T51 Toxic effect of alcohol

T51.0 **Ethanol**
Ethyl alcohol
Excludes: acute alcohol intoxication or "hangover" effects (F10.0)
drunkenness (F10.0)
pathological alcohol intoxication (F10.0)

T51.1 Methanol
Methyl alcohol

T51.2 2-Propanol
Isopropyl alcohol

T51.3 Fusel oil
Alcohol:
- amyl
- butyl [1-butanol]
- propyl [1-propanol]

T51.8 Other alcohols

T52 Toxic effect of organic solvents

T52.0 Petroleum products
Gasoline [petrol]
Kerosine [paraffin oil]
Paraffin wax
Petroleum:
- ether
- naphtha
- spirits

T52.1 Benzene
Excludes: homologues of benzene (T52.2)
nitroderivatives and aminoderivatives of benzene and its homologues (T65.3)

T52.2 Homologues of benzene
Toluene [methylbenzene]
Xylene [dimethylbenzene]

T52.3 Glycols

T52.4 Ketones

T52.40 Methyl isobutyl ketone

T52.8 Other organic solvents
Includes: adhesives

T52.80 *n*-Hexane
T52.88 Other specified hexacarbons

T53 Toxic effect of halogen derivatives of aliphatic and aromatic hydrocarbons

T53.0 **Carbon tetrachloride**
Tetrachloromethane

T53.5 **Chlorofluorocarbons**

T53.9 **Halogen derivative of aliphatic and aromatic hydrocarbons, unspecified**

T54 Toxic effect of corrosive substances

T54.0 **Phenol and phenol homologues**

T54.2 **Corrosive acids and acid-like substances**
Acid:
- hydrochloric
- sulfuric

T54.3 **Corrosive alkalis and alkali-like substances**
Potassium hydroxide
Sodium hydroxide

T54.9 **Corrosive substance, unspecified**

T55 Toxic effect of soaps and detergents

T56 Toxic effect of metals

Includes: fumes and vapours of metals
metals from all sources, except medicinal substances

Excludes: arsenic and its compounds (T57.0)
manganese and its compounds (T57.2)
thallium (T60.4)

T56.0 **Lead and its compounds**

T56.1 **Mercury and its compounds**

T56.2 **Chromium and its compounds**

T56.3 **Cadmium and its compounds**

T56.4 **Copper and its compounds**

T56.5 **Zinc and its compounds**

T56.6 **Tin and its compounds**

T56.7 **Beryllium and its compounds**

T56.8 **Other metals**

T56.9 **Metal, unspecified**

T57 Toxic effect of other inorganic substances

T57.0 **Arsenic and its compounds**

T57.1 **Phosphorus and its compounds**

T57.2 **Manganese and its compounds**

T57.3 **Hydrogen cyanide**

T57.8 **Other specified inorganic substances**

T57.9 **Inorganic substance, unspecified**

T58 Toxic effect of carbon monoxide

T59 Toxic effect of other gases, fumes and vapours

Includes: aerosol propellants

T59.0 **Nitrogen oxides**

T59.3 **Lacrimogenic gas**
Tear gas

T59.7 **Carbon dioxide**

T59.8 **Other specified gases, fumes or vapours**

T59.80 Polyester fumes
T59.81 Thylene oxide

T59.9 **Gases, fumes and vapours, unspecified**

T60 Toxic effect of pesticides

Includes: wood preservatives

T60.2 **Other insecticides**

T60.20 Pyrethroids

T60.3 **Herbicides and fungicides**

T60.4 **Rodenticides**
Pyriminil
Thallium
Excludes: strychnine and its salts (T65.1)

T60.8 **Other pesticides**

T60.9 **Pesticide, unspecified**

T61 Toxic effect of noxious substances eaten as seafood

T61.0 Ciguatera fish poisoning

T61.2 Other fish and shellfish poisoning

T61.9 Toxic effect of unspecified seafood

T62 Toxic effect of other noxious substances eaten as food

T62.2 Other ingested (parts of) plant(s)

T62.20 Toxic effect of nuts

T62.200 Garsava

T62.201 Cyead

T62.21 Toxic effect of seeds

T62.210 Lathyrus sativus

T62.8 Other specified noxious substances eaten as food

T62.9 Noxious substance eaten as food, unspecified

T63.– Toxic effect of contact with venomous animals

T64 Toxic effect of aflatoxin and other mycotoxin food contaminants

T65 Toxic effect of other and unspecified substances

T65.0 Cyanides

Excludes: hydrogen cyanide (T57.3)

T65.00 Cyanates

Toluene di-isocyanate

T65.1 Strychnine and its salts

T65.2 Tobacco and nicotine

T65.3 Nitroderivatives and aminoderivatives of benzene and its homologues

Aniline [benzenamine]

Nitrobenzene

Trinitrotoluene

T65.6 Paints and dyes, not elsewhere classified

T65.8 Toxic effect of other specified substances

T65.80 Organophosphorus compounds
T65.81 Acrylamide
T65.82 Propionitrile
T65.820 β,β′-Iminodipropionitrile
T65.821 Dimethylaminopropionitrile

Other and unspecified effects of external causes (T66–T78)

T67 Effects of heat and light

Excludes: malignant hyperthermia due to anaesthesia (T88.3)

T67.0 Heatstroke and sunstroke

Heat:
- apoplexy
- pyrexia

Siriasis
Thermoplegia

T67.1 Heat syncope

Heat collapse

T67.2 Heat cramp

T67.3 Heat exhaustion, anhydrotic

Heat prostration due to water depletion
Excludes: heat exhaustion due to salt depletion (T67.4)

T67.4 Heat exhaustion due to salt depletion

Heat prostration due to salt (and water) depletion

T67.5 Heat exhaustion, unspecified

Heat prostration NOS

T67.6 Heat fatigue, transient

T68 Hypothermia

Accidental hypothermia
Excludes: hypothermia not associated with low environmental temperature (R68.0)

T70 Effects of air pressure and water pressure

T70.0 Otitic barotrauma

Aero-otitis media

Effects of change in ambient atmospheric pressure or water pressure on ears

T70.1 Sinus barotrauma
Aerosinusitis
Effects of change in ambient atmospheric pressure on sinuses

T70.2 Other and unspecified effects of high altitude
Alpine sickness
Altitudinal insomnia
Anoxia due to high altitude
Barotrauma NOS
Hypobaropathy
Mountain sickness
Excludes: polycythaemia due to high altitude (D75.1)

T70.3 Caisson disease [decompression sickness]
Compressed-air disease
Diver's palsy or paralysis

T70.4 Effects of high-pressure fluids
Traumatic jet injection (industrial)

T70.8 Other effects of air pressure and water pressure
Blast injury syndrome

T70.9 Effects of air pressure and water pressure, unspecified

T71 Asphyxiation

Suffocation (by strangulation)
Systemic oxygen deficiency due to:
- low oxygen content in ambient air
- mechanical threat to breathing

Excludes: anoxia due to high altitude (T70.2)
asphyxia from:
- carbon monoxide (T58)
- inhalation of food or foreign body (T17)
- other gases, fumes and vapours (T59.–)

T73 Effects of other deprivation

T73.0 Effects of hunger
Deprivation of food
Starvation

T73.1 Effects of thirst
Deprivation of water

T73.2 Exhaustion due to exposure

T73.3 Exhaustion due to excessive exertion
Overexertion

T73.8 Other effects of deprivation

T73.9 Effect of deprivation, unspecified

T74 Maltreatment syndromes
Use additional code, if desired, to identify current injury.

T74.0 Neglect or abandonment

T74.1 Physical abuse
Battered:
- baby or child syndrome NOS
- spouse syndrome NOS

T74.2 Sexual abuse

T74.3 Psychological abuse

T74.8 Other maltreatment syndromes
Mixed forms

T74.9 Maltreatment syndrome, unspecified
Effects of:
- abuse of adult NOS
- child abuse NOS

T75 Effects of other external causes
Excludes: adverse effects NEC (T78.–)

T75.0 Effects of lightning
Shock from lightning
Struck by lightning NOS

T75.1 Drowning and nonfatal submersion
Immersion
Swimmer's cramp

T75.2 Effects of vibration
Pneumatic hammer syndrome
Traumatic vasospastic syndrome
Vertigo from infrasound

T75.3 Motion sickness
Airsickness
Seasickness
Travel sickness

T75.4 Effects of electric current
Electrocution
Shock from electric current

T75.8 Other specified effects of external causes
Effects of:
- abnormal gravitational [G] forces
- weightlessness

T78 Adverse effects, not elsewhere classified

Note: This category is to be used as the primary code to identify the effects, not elsewhere classifiable, of unknown, undetermined or ill-defined causes. For multiple coding purposes this category may be used as an additional code to identify the effect of conditions classified elsewhere.

Excludes: complications of surgical and medical care NEC (T80–T88)

T78.0 Anaphylactic shock due to adverse food reaction

T78.2 Anaphylactic shock, unspecified
Allergic shock NOS
Anaphylactic reaction NOS
Anaphylaxis NOS
Excludes: anaphylactic shock due to:
- adverse effect of correct medicinal substance properly administered (T88.6)
- adverse food reaction (T78.0)
- serum (T80.5)

T78.3 Angioneurotic oedema
Giant urticaria
Quincke's oedema

T78.4 Allergy, unspecified
Allergic reaction NOS
Hypersensitivity NOS
Idiosyncrasy NOS
Excludes: allergic reaction NOS to correct medicinal substance properly administered (T88.7)

T78.8 Other adverse effects, not elsewhere classified

Certain early complications of trauma (T79)

T79 Certain early complications of trauma, not elsewhere classified

Excludes: complications of surgical and medical care NEC (T80–T88)

T79.0 Air embolism (traumatic)

T79.1 Fat embolism (traumatic)

T79.2 Traumatic secondary and recurrent haemorrhage

T79.3 Post-traumatic wound infection, not elsewhere classified

T79.4 Traumatic shock

Shock (immediate)(delayed) following injury

Excludes: shock:

- anaesthetic (T88.2)
- anaphylactic:
  - NOS (T78.2)
  - due to:
    - adverse food reaction (T78.0)
    - correct medicinal substance properly administered (T88.6)
    - serum (T80.5)
- complicating abortion or ectopic or molar pregnancy (O08.3)
- electric (T75.4)
- lightning (T75.0)
- nontraumatic NEC (R57.–)
- obstetric (O75.1)
- postoperative (T81.1)

T79.6 Traumatic ischaemia of muscle

Compartment syndrome

Volkmann's ischaemic contracture

Complications of surgical and medical care, not elsewhere classified (T80–T88)

T80 Complications following infusion, transfusion and therapeutic injection

Includes: perfusion

T80.2 Infections following infusion, transfusion and therapeutic injection

Infection, Sepsis, Septicaemia, Septic shock } following infusion, transfusion and therapeutic injection

T80.5 Anaphylactic shock due to serum

T81 Complications of procedures, not elsewhere classified

Excludes: adverse effect of drug NOS (T88.7)
complication following infusion, transfusion and therapeutic injection (T80.–)
specified complications classified elsewhere, such as:
- complications of prosthetic devices, implants and grafts (T82–T85)
- poisoning and toxic effects of drugs and chemicals (T36–T65)

T81.0 Haemorrhage and haematoma complicating a procedure, not elsewhere classified

Haemorrhage at any site resulting from a procedure

T81.1 Shock during or resulting from a procedure, not elsewhere classified

Collapse NOS, Shock (endotoxic)(hypovolaemic)(septic) } during or following a procedure

Postoperative shock NOS

Excludes: shock:
- anaesthetic (T88.2)
- anaphylactic:
  - NOS (T78.2)
  - due to:
    - correct medicinal substance properly administered (T88.6)
    - serum (T80.5)

- electric (T75.4)
- following abortion or ectopic or molar pregnancy (O08.3)
- obstetric (O75.1)
- traumatic (T79.4)

T81.2 Accidental puncture and laceration during a procedure, not elsewhere classified

Accidental perforation of:

• blood vessel • nerve • organ	by	catheter endoscope instrument probe	during a procedure

T81.4 Infection following a procedure, not elsewhere classified

Abscess: • intra-abdominal • stitch • subphrenic • wound Septicaemia	postprocedural

T81.5 Foreign body accidentally left in body cavity or operation wound following a procedure

Adhesions Obstruction Perforation	due to foreign body accidentally left in operation wound or body cavity

T81.7 Vascular complications following a procedure, not elsewhere classified

Air embolism following procedure NEC

T81.8 Other complications of procedures, not elsewhere classified

Complication of inhalation therapy
Emphysema (subcutaneous) resulting from a procedure
Persistent postoperative fistula
Excludes: malignant hyperpyrexia due to anaesthesia (T88.3)

T85 Complications of other internal prosthetic devices, implants and grafts

T85.1 Mechanical complication of implanted electronic stimulator of nervous system

Breakdown (mechanical)
Displacement
Leakage
Malposition
Obstruction (mechanical)
Perforation
Protrusion
} due to electronic neurostimulator (electrode) of:
- brain
- peripheral nerve
- spinal cord

T85.6 Mechanical complication of other specified internal prosthetic devices, implants and grafts

Conditions listed in T85.1 due to:
- epidural and subdural infusion catheter
- nonabsorbable surgical material NOS
- permanent sutures

T85.7 Infection and inflammatory reaction due to other internal prosthetic devices, implants and grafts

T85.8 Other complications of internal prosthetic devices, implants and grafts, not elsewhere classified

Complication
Embolism
Fibrosis
Haemorrhage
Pain
Stenosis
Thrombosis
} due to internal prosthetic devices, implants and grafts NEC

T88 Other complications of surgical and medical care, not elsewhere classified

T88.2 Shock due to anaesthesia

Shock due to anaesthesia in which the correct substance was properly administered

Excludes: complications of anaesthesia (in):
- from overdose or wrong substance given (T36–T50)
- labour and delivery (O74.–)
- pregnancy (O29.–)
- puerperium (O89.–)

postoperative shock NOS (T81.1)

T88.3 Malignant hyperthermia due to anaesthesia

T88.6 Anaphylactic shock due to adverse effect of correct drug or medicament properly administered
Excludes: anaphylactic shock due to serum (T80.5)

T88.7 Unspecified adverse effect of drug

Adverse effect of Allergic reaction to Hypersensitivity to Idiosyncrasy to	correct drug or medicament properly administered

Drug:
- hypersensitivity NOS
- reaction NOS

Sequelae of injuries, of poisoning and of other consequences of external causes (T90–T98)

Note: These categories are to be used to indicate conditions in S00–S99 and T00–T88 as the cause of late effects, which are themselves classified elsewhere. The "sequelae" include those specified as such, or as late effects, or those present one year or more after the acute injury. (See also Section II, note 1.5: coding of late effects.)

T90 Sequelae of injuries of head

T90.2 Sequelae of fracture of skull and facial bones
Sequelae of injury classifiable to S02.–

T90.3 Sequelae of injury of cranial nerves
Sequelae of injury classifiable to S04.–

T90.5 Sequelae of intracranial injury
Sequelae of injury classifiable to S06.–

T90.8 Sequelae of other specified injuries of head
Sequelae of injury classifiable to S03.–, S07–S08 and S09.0–S09.8

T90.9 Sequelae of unspecified injury of head
Sequelae of injury classifiable to S09.9

T91 Sequelae of injuries of neck and trunk

T91.0 Sequelae of superficial injury and open wound of neck and trunk
Sequelae of injury classifiable to S11.–

T91.1 Sequelae of fracture of spine
Sequelae of injury classifiable to S12.–, S22.0–S22.1, S32.0, S32.7 and T08

T91.2 Sequelae of other fracture of thorax and pelvis
Sequelae of injury classifiable to S32.1–S32.5 and S32.8

T91.3 Sequelae of injury of spinal cord
Sequelae of injury classifiable to S14.0–S14.1, S24.0–S24.1, S34.0–S34.1 and T09.3

T91.8 Sequelae of other specified injuries of neck and trunk
Sequelae of injury classifiable to S13.–, S14.2–S14.6, S15–S18, S19.7, S23.–, S24.2–S24.6, S33.–, S34.2–S34.8, T09.2 and T09.4

T91.9 Sequelae of unspecified injury of neck and trunk

T92 Sequelae of injuries of upper limb

T92.4 Sequelae of injury of nerve of upper limb
Sequelae of injury classifiable to S44.–, S54.–, S64.– and T11.3

T93 Sequelae of injuries of lower limb

T93.4 Sequelae of injury of nerve of lower limb
Sequelae of injury classifiable to S74.–, S84.–, and S94.–

T94 Sequelae of injuries involving multiple and unspecified body regions

Sequelae of injury classifiable to T00–T01, T03–T04, T06 and T14.–

T95.– Sequelae of burns, corrosions and frostbite

T96 Sequelae of poisoning by drugs, medicaments and biological substances

Sequelae of poisoning classifiable to T36–T50

T97 Sequelae of toxic effects of substances chiefly nonmedicinal as to source

Sequelae of toxic effects classifiable to T51–T65

T98 Sequelae of other and unspecified effects of external causes

T98.1 Sequelae of other and unspecified effects of external causes
Sequelae of effects classifiable to T66–T78

T98.2 Sequelae of certain early complications of trauma
Sequelae of effects classifiable to T79.–

T98.3 Sequelae of complications of surgical and medical care, not elsewhere classified
Sequelae of complications classifiable to T80–T88

CHAPTER XX

External causes of morbidity and mortality (V01–Y98)

This chapter, which in previous revisions of ICD constituted a supplementary classification, permits the classification of environmental events and circumstances as the cause of injury, poisoning and other adverse effects. Where a code from this section is applicable, it is intended that it shall be used in addition to a code from another chapter of the Classification indicating the nature of the condition. Most often, the condition will be classifiable to Chapter XIX, Injury, poisoning and certain other consequences of external causes (S00–T98). Causes of death should preferably be tabulated according to both Chapter XIX and Chapter XX, but if only one code is tabulated then the code from Chapter XX should be used in preference. Other conditions that may be stated to be due to external causes are classified in Chapters I to XVIII. For these conditions, codes from Chapter XX should be used to provide additional information for multiple-condition analysis only.

Place of occurrence code

The following fourth-character subdivisions are for use with categories W85–X49 to identify the place of occurrence of the external cause where relevant:

.0 **Home**
.1 **Residential institution**
.2 **School, other institution and public administrative area**
.3 **Sports and athletics areas**
.4 **Street and highway**
.5 **Trade and service area**
.6 **Industrial and construction area**
.7 **Farm**
.8 **Other specified places**
.9 **Unspecified place**

Exposure to electric current, radiation and extreme ambient air temperature and pressure (W85–W99)

W85 Exposure to electric transmission lines

W86 Exposure to other specified electric current

W87 Exposure to unspecified electric current

Burns or other injury from electric current NOS
Electric shock NOS
Electrocution NOS

W88 Exposure to ionizing radiation

Radioactive isotopes
X-rays

W89 Exposure to man-made visible and ultraviolet light

Welding light (arc)

W90 Exposure to other nonionizing radiation

Infrared, Laser, Radiofrequency } radiation

W91 Exposure to unspecified type of radiation

W92 Exposure to excessive heat of man-made origin

W93 Exposure to excessive cold of man-made origin

Contact with or inhalation of:
- dry ice
- liquid:
  - air
  - hydrogen
  - nitrogen

Prolonged exposure in deep-freeze unit

W94 Exposure to high and low air pressure and changes in air pressure

High air pressure from rapid descent in water
Reduction in atmospheric pressure while surfacing from:
- deep-water diving
- underground

Residence or prolonged visit at high altitude as the cause of:
- anoxia
- barodontalgia
- barotitis

- hypoxia
- mountain sickness

Sudden change in air pressure in aircraft during ascent or descent

W99 Exposure to other and unspecified man-made environmental factors

Accidental poisoning by and exposure to noxious substances (X40–X49)

Note: Evidence of alcohol involvement in combination with substances specified below may be identified by using the supplementary codes Y90–Y91.

Includes: accidental overdose of drug, wrong drug given or taken in error, and drug taken inadvertently
accidents in the use of drugs, medicaments and biological substances in medical and surgical procedure

Excludes: correct drug properly administered in therapeutic or prophylactic dosage as the cause of any adverse effect (Y40–Y59)

X40 Accidental poisoning by and exposure to nonopioid analgesics, antipyretics and antirheumatics

4-Aminophenol derivatives
Nonsteroidal anti-inflammatory drugs [NSAID]
Pyrazolone derivatives
Salicylates

X41 Accidental poisoning by and exposure to antiepileptic, sedative–hypnotic, antiparkinsonism and psychotropic drugs, not elsewhere classified

Antidepressants
Barbiturates
Hydantoin derivatives
Iminostilbenes
Methaqualone compounds
Neuroleptics
Psychostimulants
Succinimides and oxazolidinediones
Tranquillizers

X42 Accidental poisoning by and exposure to narcotics and psychodysleptics [hallucinogens], not elsewhere classified

Cannabis (derivatives)
Cocaine
Codeine
Heroin
Lysergide [LSD]
Mescaline
Methadone
Morphine
Opium (alkaloids)

X43 Accidental poisoning by and exposure to other drugs acting on the autonomic nervous system

Parasympatholytics [anticholinergics and antimuscarinics] and spasmolytics
Parasympathomimetics [cholinergics]
Sympatholytics [antiadrenergics]
Sympathomimetics [adrenergics]

X44 Accidental poisoning by and exposure to other and unspecified drugs, medicaments and biological substances

Agents primarily acting on smooth and skeletal muscles and the respiratory system
Anaesthetics (general)(local)
Drugs affecting the:
- cardiovascular system
- gastrointestinal system

Hormones and synthetic substitutes
Systemic and haematological agents
Systemic antibiotics and other anti-infectives
Therapeutic gases
Topical preparations
Vaccines
Water-balance agents, and drugs affecting mineral and uric acid metabolism

X45 Accidental poisoning by and exposure to alcohol

Alcohol:
- NOS
- butyl [1-butanol]
- ethyl [ethanol]

- isopropyl [2-propanol]
- methyl [methanol]
- propyl [1-propanol]

Fusel oil

X46 Accidental poisoning by and exposure to organic solvents and halogenated hydrocarbons and their vapours

Benzene and homologues
Carbon tetrachloride [tetrachloromethane]
Chlorofluorocarbons
Petroleum (derivatives)

X47 Accidental poisoning by and exposure to other gases and vapours

Carbon monoxide
Lacrimogenic gas [tear gas]
Motor (vehicle) exhaust gas
Nitrogen oxides
Sulfur dioxide
Utility gas
Excludes: metal fumes and vapours (X49)

X48 Accidental poisoning by and exposure to pesticides

Fumigants
Fungicides
Herbicides
Insecticides
Rodenticides
Wood preservatives
Excludes: plant foods and fertilizers (X49)

X49 Accidental poisoning by and exposure to other and unspecified chemicals and noxious substances

Corrosive aromatics, acids and caustic alkalis
Glues and adhesives
Metals including fumes and vapours
Paints and dyes
Plant foods and fertilizers
Poisoning NOS
Poisonous foodstuffs and poisonous plants
Soaps and detergents

Drugs, medicaments and biological substances causing adverse effects in therapeutic use (Y40–Y59)

Y40 Systemic antibiotics

Excludes: antibiotics, topically used (Y56.–)
antineoplastic antibiotics (Y43.3)

Y40.0 Penicillins

Y40.1 Cefalosporins and other β-lactam antibiotics

Y40.2 Chloramphenicol group

Y40.3 Macrolides

Y40.4 Tetracyclines

Y40.5 Aminoglycosides
Streptomycin

Y40.6 Rifamycins

Y40.7 Antifungal antibiotics, systemically used

Y40.8 Other systemic antibiotics

Y40.9 Systemic antibiotic, unspecified

Y41 Other systemic anti-infectives and antiparasitics

Excludes: anti-infectives, topically used (Y56.–)

Y41.0 Sulfonamides

Y41.1 Antimycobacterial drugs
Excludes: rifamycins (Y40.6)
streptomycin (Y40.5)

Y41.2 Antimalarials and drugs acting on other blood protozoa
Chloroquine
Excludes: hydroxyquinoline derivatives (Y41.8)

Y41.3 Other antiprotozoal drugs

Y41.4 Anthelminthics

Y41.5 Antiviral drugs
Excludes: amantadine (Y46.7)
cytarabine (Y43.1)

Y41.8 Other specified anti-infectives and antiparasitics
Hydroxyquinoline derivatives
Excludes: antimalarial drugs (Y41.2)

Y41.9 Systemic anti-infective and antiparasitic, unspecified

Y42 Hormones and their synthetic substitutes and antagonists, not elsewhere classified

Excludes: mineralocorticoids and their antagonists (Y54.0–Y54.1)
oxytocic hormones (Y55.0)
parathyroid hormones and derivatives (Y54.7)

Y42.0 Glucocorticoids and synthetic analogues
Excludes: glucocorticoids, topically used (Y56.–)

Y42.1 Thyroid hormones and substitutes

Y42.2 Antithyroid drugs

Y42.3 Insulin and oral hypoglycaemic [antidiabetic] drugs

Y42.4 Oral contraceptives
Multiple- and single-ingredient preparations

Y42.5 Other estrogens and progestogens
Mixtures and substitutes

Y42.6 Antigonadotrophins, antiestrogens, antiandrogens, not elsewhere classified
Tamoxifen

Y42.7 Androgens and anabolic congeners

Y42.8 Other and unspecified hormones and their synthetic substitutes
Anterior pituitary [adenohypophyseal] hormones

Y42.9 Other and unspecified hormone antagonists

Y43 Primarily systemic agents

Excludes: vitamins NEC (Y57.7)

Y43.0 Antiallergic and antiemetic drugs
Excludes: phenothiazine-based neuroleptics (Y49.3)

Y43.1 Antineoplastic antimetabolites
Cytarabine

Y43.2 Antineoplastic natural products

Y43.3 Other antineoplastic drugs
Antineoplastic antibiotics
Excludes: tamoxifen (Y42.6)

Y43.4 Immunosuppressive agents

Y43.5 Acidifying and alkalizing agents

Y43.6 Enzymes, not elsewhere classified

Y43.8 Other primarily systemic agents, not elsewhere classified
Heavy metal antagonists

Y43.9 Primarily systemic agent, unspecified

Y44 Agents primarily affecting blood constituents

Y44.0 Iron preparations and other anti-hypochromic-anaemia preparations

Y44.1 Vitamin B_{12}, folic acid and other anti-megaloblastic-anaemia preparations

Y44.2 Anticoagulants

Y44.3 Anticoagulant antagonists, vitamin K and other coagulants

Y44.4 Antithrombotic drugs [platelet-aggregation inhibitors]
Excludes: acetylsalicylic acid (Y45.1)
dipyridamole (Y52.3)

Y44.5 Thrombolytic drugs

Y44.6 Natural blood and blood products
Excludes: immunoglobulin (Y59.3)

Y44.7 Plasma substitutes

Y44.9 Other and unspecified agents affecting blood constituents

Y45 Analgesics, antipyretics and anti-inflammatory drugs

Y45.0 Opioids and related analgesics

Y45.1 Salicylates

Y45.2 Propionic acid derivatives
Propanoic acid derivatives

Y45.3 Other nonsteroidal anti-inflammatory drugs [NSAID]

Y45.4 Antirheumatics
Excludes: chloroquine (Y41.2)
glucocorticoids (Y42.0)
salicylates (Y45.1)

Y45.4 4-Aminophenol derivatives

Y45.8 Other analgesics and antipyretics

Y45.9 Analgesic, antipyretic and anti-inflammatory drug, unspecified

Y46 Antiepileptics and antiparkinsonism drugs

Excludes: acetazolamide (Y54.2)
barbiturates NEC (Y47.0)
benzodiazepines (Y47.1)
paraldehyde (Y47.3)

Y46.0 Succinimides

Y46.1 Oxazolidinediones

Y46.2 Hydantoin derivatives

Y46.3 Deoxybarbiturates

Y46.4 Iminostilbenes
Carbamazepine

Y46.5 Valproic acid

Y46.6 Other and unspecified antiepileptics

Y46.7 Antiparkinsonism drugs
Amantadine

Y46.8 Antispasticity drugs
Excludes: benzodiazepines (Y47.1)

Y47 Sedatives, hypnotics and antianxiety drugs

Y47.0 Barbiturates, not elsewhere classified
Excludes: deoxybarbiturates (Y46.3)
thiobarbiturates (Y48.1)

Y47.1 Benzodiazepines

Y47.2 Cloral derivatives

Y47.3 Paraldehyde

Y47.4 Bromine compounds

Y47.5 **Mixed sedatives and hypnotics, not elsewhere classified**

Y47.8 **Other sedatives, hypnotics and antianxiety drugs**
Methaqualone

Y47.9 **Sedative, hypnotic and antianxiety drug, unspecified**
Sleeping:
- draught } NOS
- drug } NOS
- tablet } NOS

Y48 Anaesthetics and therapeutic gases

Y48.0 **Inhaled anaesthetics**

Y48.1 **Parenteral anaesthetics**
Thiobarbiturates

Y48.2 **Other and unspecified general anaesthetics**

Y48.3 **Local anaesthetics**

Y48.4 **Anaesthetic, unspecified**

Y48.5 **Therapeutic gases**

Y49 Psychotropic drugs, not elsewhere classified

Excludes: appetite depressants [anorectics] (Y57.0)
barbiturates NEC (Y47.0)
benzodiazepines (Y47.1)
caffeine (Y50.2)
cocaine (Y48.3)
methaqualone (Y47.8)

Y49.0 **Tricyclic and tetracyclic antidepressants**

Y49.1 **Monoamine-oxidase-inhibitor antidepressants**

Y49.2 **Other and unspecified antidepressants**

Y49.3 **Phenothiazine antipsychotics and neuroleptics**

Y49.4 **Butyrophenone and thioxanthene neuroleptics**

Y49.5 **Other antipsychotics and neuroleptics**
Excludes: rauwolfia (Y52.5)

Y49.6 **Psychodysleptics [hallucinogens]**

Y49.7 **Psychostimulants with abuse potential**

Y49.8 **Other psychotropic drugs, not elsewhere classified**

Y49.9 Psychotropic drug, unspecified

Y50 Central nervous system stimulants, not elsewhere classified

Y50.0 Analeptics

Y50.1 Opioid receptor antagonists

Y50.2 Methylxanthines, not elsewhere classified
Caffeine
Excludes: aminophylline (Y55.6)
theobromine (Y55.6)
theophylline (Y55.6)

Y50.8 Other central nervous system stimulants

Y50.9 Central nervous system stimulant, unspecified

Y51 Drugs primarily affecting the autonomic nervous system

Y51.0 Anticholinesterase agents

Y51.1 Other parasympathomimetics [cholinergics]

Y51.2 Ganglionic blocking drugs, not elsewhere classified

Y51.3 Other parasympatholytics [anticholinergics and antimuscarinics] and spasmolytics, not elsewhere classified
Papaverine

Y51.4 Predominantly α-adrenoreceptor agonists, not elsewhere classified
Metaraminol

Y51.5 Predominantly β-adrenoreceptor agonists, not elsewhere classified
Excludes: salbutamol (Y55.6)

Y51.6 α-Adrenoreceptor antagonists, not elsewhere classified
Excludes: ergot alkaloids (Y55.0)

Y51.7 β-Adrenoreceptor antagonists, not elsewhere classified

Y51.8 Centrally acting and adrenergic-neuron-blocking agents, not elsewhere classified
Excludes: clonidine (Y52.5)
guanethidine (Y52.5)

Y51.9 Other and unspecified drugs primarily affecting the autonomic nervous system
Drugs stimulating both α- and β-adrenoreceptors

Y52 Agents primarily affecting the cardiovascular system

Excludes: metaraminol (Y51.4)

Y52.0 Cardiac-stimulant glycosides and drugs of similar action

Y52.1 Calcium-channel blockers

Y52.2 Other antidysrhythmic drugs, not elsewhere classified
Excludes: β-adrenoreceptor antagonists (Y51.7)

Y52.3 Coronary vasodilators, not elsewhere classified
Aminodarone
Dipyridamole
Excludes: β-adrenoreceptor antagonists (Y51.7)
calcium-channel blockers (Y52.1)

Y52.4 Angiotensin-converting-enzyme inhibitors

Y52.5 Other antihypertensive drugs, not elsewhere classified
Clonidine
Guanethidine
Rauwolfia
Excludes: β-adrenoreceptor antagonists (Y51.7)
calcium-channel blockers (Y52.1)
diuretics (Y54.0–Y54.5)

Y52.6 Antihyperlipidaemic and antiarteriosclerotic drugs

Y52.7 Peripheral vasodilators
Nicotinic acid (derivatives)
Excludes: papaverine (Y51.3)

Y52.8 Antivaricose drugs, including sclerosing agents

Y52.9 Other and unspecified agents primarily affecting the cardiovascular system

Y53 Agents primarily affecting the gastrointestinal system

Y53.0 Histamine H_2-receptor antagonists

Y53.1 Other antacids and anti-gastric-secretion drugs

Y53.2 Stimulant laxatives

Y53.3 **Saline and osmotic laxatives**

Y53.4 **Other laxatives**
Intestinal atonia drugs

Y53.5 **Digestants**

Y53.6 **Antidiarrhoeal drugs**
Excludes: systemic antibiotics and other anti-infectives (Y40–Y41)

Y53.7 **Emetics**

Y53.8 **Other agents primarily affecting the gastrointestinal system**

Y53.9 **Agent primarily affecting the gastrointestinal system, unspecified**

Y54 Agents primarily affecting water-balance and mineral and uric acid metabolism

Y54.0 **Mineralocorticoids**

Y54.1 **Mineralocorticoid antagonists [aldosterone antagonists]**

Y54.2 **Carbonic-anhydrase inhibitors**
Acetazolamide

Y54.3 **Benzothiadiazine derivatives**

Y54.4 **Loop [high-ceiling] diuretics**

Y54.5 **Other diuretics**

Y54.6 **Electrolytic, caloric and water-balance agents**
Oral rehydration salts

Y54.7 **Agents affecting calcification**
Parathyroid hormones and derivatives
Vitamin D group

Y54.8 **Agents affecting uric acid metabolism**

Y54.9 **Mineral salts, not elsewhere classified**

Y55 Agents primarily acting on smooth and skeletal muscles and the respiratory system

Y55.0 **Oxytocic drugs**
Ergot alkaloids
Excludes: estrogens, progestogens and antagonists (Y42.5–Y42.6)

Y55.1 **Skeletal muscle relaxants [neuromuscular blocking agents]**
Excludes: antispasticity drugs (Y46.8)

Y55.2 Other and unspecified agents primarily acting on muscles

Y55.3 Antitussives

Y55.4 Expectorants

Y55.5 Anti-common-cold drugs

Y55.6 Antiasthmatics, not elsewhere classified

Aminophylline
Salbutamol
Theobromine
Theophylline

Excludes: β-adrenoreceptor agonists (Y51.5)
anterior pituitary [adenohypophyseal] hormones (Y42.8)

Y55.7 Other and unspecified agents primarily acting on the respiratory system

Y56 Topical agents primarily affecting skin and mucous membrane and ophthalmological, otorhinolaryngological and dental drugs

Includes: glucocorticoids, topically used

Y56.0 Local antifungal, anti-infective and anti-inflammatory drugs, not elsewhere classified

Y56.1 Antipruritics

Y56.2 Local astringents and local detergents

Y56.3 Emollients, demulcents and protectants

Y56.4 Keratolytics, keratoplastics and other hair treatment drugs and preparations

Y56.5 Ophthalmological drugs and preparations

Y56.6 Otorhinolaryngological drugs and preparations

Y56.7 Dental drugs, topically applied

Y56.8 Other topical agents

Spermicides

Y56.9 Topical agent, unspecified

Y57 Other and unspecified drugs and medicaments

Y57.0 Appetite depressants [anorectics]

Y57.1 Lipotropic drugs

Y57.2 **Antidotes and chelating agents, not elsewhere classified**

Y57.3 **Alcohol deterrents**

Y57.4 **Pharmaceutical excipients**

Y57.5 **X-ray contrast media**

Y57.6 **Other diagnostic agents**

Y57.7 **Vitamins, not elsewhere classified**
Excludes: nicotinic acid (Y52.7)
vitamin B_{12} (Y44.1)
vitamin D (Y54.7)
vitamin K (Y44.3)

Y57.8 **Other drugs and medicaments**

Y57.9 **Drug or medicament, unspecified**

Y58 Bacterial vaccines

Y58.0 **BCG vaccine**

Y58.1 **Typhoid and paratyphoid vaccine**

Y58.2 **Cholera vaccine**

Y58.3 **Plague vaccine**

Y58.4 **Tetanus vaccine**

Y58.5 **Diphtheria vaccine**

Y58.6 **Pertussis vaccine, including combinations with a pertussis component**

Y58.8 **Mixed bacterial vaccines, except combinations with a pertussis component**

Y58.9 **Other and unspecified bacterial vaccines**

Y59 Other and unspecified vaccines and biological substances

Y59.0 **Viral vaccines**

Y59.1 **Rickettsial vaccines**

Y59.2 **Protozoal vaccines**

Y59.3 **Immunoglobulin**

Y59.8 Other specified vaccines and biological substances

Y59.9 Vaccine or biological substance, unspecified

Misadventures to patients during surgical and medical care (Y60–Y69)

Excludes: accidental overdose of drug and wrong drug given in error (X40–X44)
neurological devices associated with adverse incidents in diagnostic and therapeutic use (Y75.–)
surgical and medical procedures as the cause of abnormal reaction by the patient, without mention of misadventure at the time of procedure (Y83–Y84)

Y60.– Unintentional cut, puncture, perforation or haemorrhage during surgical and medical care

Y61.– Foreign object accidentally left in body during surgical and medical care

Y62.– Failure of sterile precautions during surgical and medical care

Y63.– Failure in dosage during surgical and medical care

Y64.– Contaminated medical or biological substances

Y65.– Other misadventures during surgical and medical care

Y69 Unspecified misadventure during surgical and medical care

Medical devices associated with adverse incidents in diagnostic and therapeutic use (Y70–Y82)

Y75 Neurological devices associated with adverse incidents

Y75.0 **Diagnostic and monitoring devices**

Y75.1 **Therapeutic (nonsurgical) and rehabilitative devices**

Y75.2 **Prosthetic and other implants, materials and accessory devices**

Y75.3 **Surgical instruments, materials and accessory devices (including sutures)**

Y75.8 **Miscellaneous devices, not elsewhere classified**

Surgical and other medical procedures as the cause of abnormal reaction of the patient, or of later complication, without mention of misadventure at the time of the procedure (Y83–Y84)

Y83 Surgical operation and other surgical procedures as the cause of abnormal reaction of the patient, or of later complication, without mention of misadventure at the time of the procedure

Y83.0 **Surgical operation with transplant of whole organ**

Y83.1 **Surgical operation with implant of artificial internal device**

Y83.2 **Surgical operation with anastomosis, bypass or graft**

Y83.3 **Surgical operation with formation of external stoma**

Y83.4 **Other reconstructive surgery**

Y83.5 **Amputation of limb(s)**

Y83.6 **Removal of other organ (partial)(total)**

Y83.8 **Other surgical procedures**

Y83.9 **Surgical procedure, unspecified**

Y84 Other medical procedures as the cause of abnormal reaction of the patient, or of later complication, without mention of misadventure at the time of the procedure

Excludes: post-lumbar punction headache (G97.0)
spinal fluid leak (G97.0)

Y84.0 **Cardiac catheterization**

Y84.1 Kidney dialysis

Y84.2 Radiological procedure and radiotherapy

Y84.3 Shock therapy

Y84.4 Aspiration of fluid

Y84.5 Insertion of gastric or duodenal sound

Y84.6 Urinary catheterization

Y84.7 Blood-sampling

Y84.8 Other medical procedures

Y84.9 Medical procedure, unspecified

Supplementary factors related to causes of morbidity and mortality classified elsewhere (Y90–Y98)

Note: These categories may be used, if desired, to provide supplementary information concerning causes of morbidity and mortality. They are not to be used for single-condition coding in morbidity or mortality.

Y90 Evidence of alcohol involvement determined by blood alcohol level

Y90.0 Blood alcohol level of less than 20 mg/100 ml

Y90.1 Blood alcohol level of 20–39 mg/100 ml

Y90.2 Blood alcohol level of 40–59 mg/100 ml

Y90.3 Blood alcohol level of 60–79 mg/100 ml

Y90.4 Blood alcohol level of 80–99 mg/100 ml

Y90.5 Blood alcohol level of 100–119 mg/100 ml

Y90.6 Blood alcohol level of 120–199 mg/100 ml

Y90.7 Blood alcohol level of 200–239 mg/100 ml

Y90.8 Blood alcohol level of 240 mg/100 ml or more

Y90.9 Presence of alcohol in blood, level not specified

Y91 Evidence of alcohol involvement determined by level of intoxication

Excludes: evidence of alcohol involvement determined by blood alcohol content (Y90.–)

Y91.0 Mild alcohol intoxication

Smell of alcohol on breath, slight behavioural disturbance in functions and responses, or slight difficulty in coordination.

Y91.1 Moderate alcohol intoxication

Smell of alcohol on breath, moderate behavioural disturbance in functions and responses, or moderate difficulty in coordination.

Y91.2 Severe alcohol intoxication

Severe disturbance in functions and responses, severe difficulty in coordination, or impaired ability to cooperate.

Y91.3 Very severe alcohol intoxication

Very severe disturbance in functions and responses, very severe difficulty in coordination, or loss of ability to cooperate.

Y91.9 Alcohol involvement, not otherwise specified

Suspected alcohol involvement NOS

CHAPTER XXI

Factors influencing health status and contact with health services (Z00–Z99)

Note: This chapter should not be used for international comparison or for primary mortality coding.

Categories Z00–Z99 are provided for occasions when circumstances other than a disease, injury or external cause classifiable to categories A00–Y89 are recorded as "diagnoses" or "problems". This can arise in two main ways:

(a) When a person who may or may not be sick encounters the health services for some specific purpose, such as to receive limited care or service for a current condition, to donate an organ or tissue, to receive prophylactic vaccination or to discuss a problem which is in itself not a disease or injury.

(b) When some circumstance or problem is present which influences the person's health status but is not in itself a current illness or injury. Such factors may be elicited during population surveys, when the person may or may not be currently sick, or be recorded as an additional factor to be borne in mind when the person is receiving care for some illness or injury.

Persons encountering health services for examination and investigation (Z00–Z13)

Note: Nonspecific abnormal findings disclosed at the time of these examinations are classified to categories R70–R94.

Z00 General examination and investigation of persons without complaint or reported diagnosis

Excludes: examination for administrative purposes (Z02.–)
special screening examinations (Z13)

Z00.1 Routine child health examination
Development testing of infant or child

Z00.2 Examination for period of rapid growth in childhood

Z00.3 Examination for adolescent development state
Puberty development state

Z01 Other special examinations and investigations of persons without complaint or reported diagnosis

Includes: routine examination of specific system

Z01.0 Examination of eyes and vision
Excludes: examination for driving licence (Z02.4)

Z01.1 Examination of ears and hearing

Z02 Examination and encounter for administrative purposes

Z02.0 Examination for admission to educational institution
Examination for admission to preschool (education)

Z02.1 Pre-employment examination

Z02.2 Examination for admission to residential institution
Excludes: examination for admission to prison (Z02.8)

Z02.3 Examination for recruitment to armed forces

Z02.4 Examination for driving licence

Z02.5 Examination for participation in sport

Z02.6 Examination for insurance purposes

Z02.7 Issue of medical certificate
Issue of medical certificate of:
- cause of death
- fitness
- incapacity
- invalidity

Excludes: encounter for general medical examination (Z00–Z01, Z02.0–Z02.6, Z02.8–Z02.9)

Z02.8 Other examinations for administrative purposes
Examination (for):
- admission to:
  - prison
  - summer camp
- adoption
- immigration
- naturalization
- premarital

Z02.9 Examination for administrative purposes, unspecified

Z03 Medical observation and evaluation for suspected diseases and conditions

Z03.1 Observation for suspected malignant neoplasm

Z03.3 Observation for suspected nervous system disorder

Z04.– Examination and observation for other reasons

Includes: examination for medicolegal reasons

Z08 Follow-up examination after treatment for malignant neoplasm

Includes: medical surveillance following treatment

Z08.0 Follow-up examination after surgery for malignant neoplasm

Z08.1 Follow-up examination after radiotherapy for malignant neoplasm

Excludes: radiotherapy session (Z51.0)

Z08.2 Follow-up examination after chemotherapy for malignant neoplasm

Excludes: chemotherapy session (Z51.1)

Z08.7 Follow-up examination after combined treatment for malignant neoplasm

Z08.8 Follow-up examination after other treatment for malignant neoplasm

Z08.9 Follow-up examination after unspecified treatment for malignant neoplasm

Z09 Follow-up examination after treatment for conditions other than malignant neoplasms

Includes: medical surveillance following treatment

Excludes: follow-up medical care and convalescence (Z42–Z51)
medical surveillance following treatment for malignant neoplasm (Z08.–)

Z09.0 Follow-up examination after surgery for other conditions

Z09.1 Follow-up examination after radiotherapy for other conditions

Excludes: radiotherapy session (Z51.0)

Z09.2 Follow-up examination after chemotherapy for other conditions
Excludes: maintenance chemotherapy (Z51.1–Z51.2)

Z09.3 Follow-up examination after psychotherapy

Z09.4 Follow-up examination after treatment of fracture

Z09.7 Follow-up examination after combined treatment for other conditions

Z09.8 Follow-up examination after other treatment for other conditions

Z09.9 Follow-up examination after unspecified treatment for other conditions

Z13 Special screening examination for other diseases and disorders

Z13.4 Special screening examination for certain developmental disorders in childhood
Excludes: routine development testing of infant or child (Z00.1)

Z13.7 Special screening examination for congenital malformations, deformations and chromosomal abnormalities

Persons with potential health hazards related to communicable diseases (Z20–Z29)

Z21 Asymptomatic human immunodeficiency virus [HIV] infection status

Excludes: human immunodeficiency virus [HIV] disease (B20–B24)
laboratory evidence of human immunodeficiency virus [HIV] (R75)

Persons encountering health services in circumstances related to reproduction (Z30–Z39)

Z31 Procreative management

Z31.5 **Genetic counselling**

Z31.6 **Genetic counselling and advice on procreation**

Z36 Antenatal screening

Z36.0 **Antenatal screening for chromosomal anomalies**
Amniocentesis
Placental sample (taken vaginally)

Z36.1 **Antenatal screening for raised alphafetoprotein level**

Z36.2 **Other antenatal screening based on amniocentesis**

Z36.3 **Antenatal screening for malformations using ultrasound and other physical methods**

Z36.4 **Antenatal screening for fetal growth retardation using ultrasound and other physical methods**

Z36.5 **Antenatal screening for isoimmunization**

Z36.8 **Other antenatal screening**
Screening for haemoglobinopathy

Z36.9 **Antenatal screening, unspecified**

Persons encountering health services for specific procedures and health care (Z40–Z54)

Z42 Follow-up care involving plastic surgery

Z42.0 **Follow-up care involving plastic surgery of head and neck**

Z46 Fitting and adjustment of other devices

Z46.2 **Fitting and adjustment of other devices related to nervous system and special senses**

Z50 Care involving use of rehabilitation procedures

Z50.4 **Psychotherapy, not elsewhere classified**

Z50.5 **Speech therapy**

Z50.6 **Orthoptic training**

Z50.7 **Occupational therapy and vocational rehabilitation, not elsewhere classified**

Z50.8 Care involving use of other rehabilitation procedures
Tobacco rehabilitation
Training in activities of daily living [ADL] NEC

Z50.9 Care involving use of rehabilitation procedure, unspecified
Rehabilitation NOS

Z51 Other medical care

Z51.0 Radiotherapy session

Z51.1 Chemotherapy session for neoplasm

Z51.2 Other chemotherapy
Maintenance chemotherapy NOS

Persons encountering health services in other circumstances (Z70–Z76)

Z71 Persons encountering health services for other counselling and medical advice, not elsewhere classified

Excludes: procreation counselling (Z31.–)

Z71.8 Other specified counselling
Consanguinity counselling

Z73 Problems related to life-management difficulty

Z73.0 Burn-out
State of vital exhaustion

Z73.1 Accentuation of personality traits
Type A behaviour pattern (characterized by unbridled ambition, a need for high achievement, impatience, competitiveness and a sense of urgency)

Z73.2 Lack of relaxation and leisure

Z73.3 Stress, not elsewhere classified
Physical and mental strain NOS

Z73.4 Inadequate social skills, not elsewhere classified

Z73.5 Social role conflict, not elsewhere classified

Z73.6 Limitation of activities due to disability
Excludes: care-provider dependency (Z74.–)

Z73.8 Other problems related to life-management difficulty

Z73.9 Problems related to life-management difficulty, unspecified

Z74 Problems related to care-provider dependency

Excludes: dependence on enabling machines or devices NEC (Z99.–)

Z74.0 Reduced mobility
Bedfast
Chairfast

Z74.1 Need for assistance with personal care

Z74.2 Need for assistance at home and no other household member able to render care

Z74.8 Other problems related to care-provider dependency

Z74.9 Problems related to care-provider dependency, unspecified

Z76 Persons encountering health services in other circumstances

Z76.0 Issue of repeat prescription

Z76.5 Malingerer [conscious simulation]
Person feigning illness (with obvious motivation)
Excludes: factitious disorder (F68.1)
peregrinating patient (F68.1)

Persons with potential health hazards related to family and personal history and certain conditions influencing health status (Z80–Z99)

Z80.– Family history of malignant neoplasm

Z81.– Family history of mental and behavioural disorders

Z82 Family history of certain disabilities and chronic diseases leading to disablement

Z82.0 Family history of epilepsy and other diseases of the nervous system
Conditions classifiable to G00–G99, e.g. Huntington's chorea

Z82.1 Family history of blindness and visual loss
Conditions classifiable to H54.–

Z82.2 Family history of deafness and hearing loss
Conditions classifiable to H90–H91

Z82.3 Family history of stroke
Conditions classifiable to I60–I64

Z82.7 Family history of congenital malformations, deformations and chromosomal abnormalities
Conditions classifiable to Q00–Q99

Z83 Family history of other specific disorders

Z83.0 Family history of human immunodeficiency virus [HIV] disease
Conditions classifiable to B20–B24

Z83.5 Family history of eye and ear disorders
Conditions classifiable to H00–H53, H55–H83, H92–H95
Excludes: family history of:
- blindness and visual loss (Z82.1)
- deafness and hearing loss (Z82.2)

Z84 Family history of other conditions

Z84.3 Family history of consanguinity

Z85.– Personal history of malignant neoplasm

Z86 Personal history of certain other diseases

Z86.0 Personal history of other neoplasms
Conditions classifiable to D00–D48

Z86.6 Personal history of diseases of the nervous system and sense organs
Conditions classifiable to G00–G99, H00–H95

Z87 Personal history of other diseases and conditions

Z87.3 Personal history of diseases of the musculoskeletal system and connective tissue
Conditions classifiable to M00–M99

Z87.7 Personal history of congenital malformations, deformations and chromosomal abnormalities
Conditions classifiable to Q00–Q99

Z88.– Personal history of allergy to drugs, medicaments and biological substances

Z98 Other postsurgical states

Z98.2 Presence of cerebrospinal fluid drainage device
CSF shunt

Z99 Dependence on enabling machines and devices, not elsewhere classified

Z99.0 Dependence on aspirator

Z99.1 Dependence on respirator

Z99.2 Dependence on renal dialysis
Presence of arteriovenous shunt for dialysis
Renal dialysis status

Z99.3 Dependence on wheelchair

Z99.8 Dependence on other enabling machines and devices

Z99.9 Dependence on unspecified enabling machine and device

SECTION V

Morphology of neoplasms

Morphology of neoplasms

The second edition of the International Classification of Diseases for Oncology (ICD-O) was published in 1990. It contains a coded nomenclature for the morphology of neoplasms, which is reproduced here for those who wish to use it in conjunction with Chapter II.

The morphology code numbers consist of five digits; the first four identify the histological type of the neoplasm and the fifth, following a slash or solidus, indicates its behaviour. The one-digit behaviour code is as follows:

/0 Benign

/1 Uncertain whether benign or malignant
Borderline malignancy
Low malignant potential

/2 Carcinoma in situ
Intraepithelial
Noninfiltrating
Noninvasive

/3 Malignant, primary site

/6 Malignant, metastatic site
Malignant, secondary site

/9 Malignant, uncertain whether primary or metastatic site

In the nomenclature given here, the morphology code numbers include the behaviour code appropriate to the histological type of neoplasm; this behaviour code should be changed if the other reported information makes this appropriate. For example, chordoma is assumed to be malignant and is therefore assigned the code number M9370/3; the term "benign chordoma" should, however, be coded M9370/0.

The following table shows the correspondence between the behaviour code and the different sections of Chapter II:

Behaviour code		Chapter II categories
/0	Benign neoplasms	D10–D36
/1	Neoplasms of uncertain or unknown behaviour	D37–D48
/2	In situ neoplasms	D00–D09
/3	Malignant neoplasms, stated or presumed to be primary	C00–C76 C80–C97
/6	Malignant neoplasms, stated or presumed to be secondary	C77–C79

The ICD-O behaviour digit /9 is not applicable in the ICD context, since all malignant neoplasms are presumed to be primary (/3) or secondary (/6), according to other information on the medical record.

Some types of neoplasm are specific to certain sites or types of tissue; in such cases, the appropriate code from Chapter II has been added in parentheses in the nomenclature, and the appropriate fourth character for the reported site should be used. The Chapter II codes assigned to the morphological terms should be used when the site of the neoplasm is not given in the diagnosis. Chapter II codes have not been assigned to many of the morphology terms because the histological types can arise in more than one organ or type of tissue.

Occasionally a problem arises when a site given in a diagnosis is different from the site indicated by the site-specific code. In such instances, the given Chapter II code should be ignored and the appropriate code for the site included in the diagnosis should be used.

For neoplasms of lymphoid, haematopoietic and related tissue (M959–M998) the relevant codes from C81–C96 and D45–D47 are given. These Chapter II codes should be used irrespective of the stated site of the neoplasm.

Further information about the coding of morphology is provided in Volume 2 of ICD-10.

Coded nomenclature for morphology of neoplasms

M801–M804 Epithelial neoplasms NOS

M8010/6 Carcinoma, metastatic NOS
  Secondary carcinoma

M8010/9 Carcinomatosis

M814–M838 Adenomas and adenocarcinomas

M8140/0 Adenoma NOS
M8140/6 Adenocarcinoma, metastatic NOS
M8248/1 Apudoma
M8270/0 Chromophobe adenoma (D35.2)
M8270/3 Chromophobe carcinoma (C75.1)
  Chromophobe adenocarcinoma
M8271/0 Prolactinoma (D35.2)
M8280/0 Acidophil adenoma (D35.2)
  Eosinophil adenoma
M8280/3 Acidophil carcinoma (C75.1)
  Acidophil adenocarcinoma
  Eosinophil adenocarcinoma
  Eosinophil carcinoma

M868–M871 Paragangliomas and glomus tumours

M8680/1 Paraganglioma NOS
M8680/3 Paraganglioma, malignant
M8681/1 Sympathetic paraganglioma
M8682/1 Parasympathetic paraganglioma
M8683/0 Gangliocytic paraganglioma (D13.2)
M8690/1 Glomus jugulare tumour (D44.7)
  Jugular paraganglioma
M8691/1 Aortic body tumour (D44.7)
  Aortic body paraganglioma
M8692/1 Carotid body tumour (D44.6)
  Carotid body paraganglioma
M8693/1 Extra-adrenal paraganglioma NOS
  Chemodectoma
  Nonchromaffin paraganglioma NOS
M8693/3 Extra-adrenal paraganglioma, malignant
  Nonchromaffin paraganglioma, malignant
M8700/0 Phaeochromocytoma NOS (D35.0)
  Chromaffinoma
  Chromaffin phaeochromocytoma
  Chromaffin tumour
M8700/3 Phaeochromocytoma, malignant (C74.1)
  Phaeochromoblastoma
M8710/3 Glomangiosarcoma
  Glomoid sarcoma
M8711/0 Glomus tumour
M8712/0 Glomangioma

M889–M892 Myomatous neoplasms

M8900/0 Rhabdomyoma NOS
M8900/3 Rhabdomyosarcoma NOS
Rhabdosarcoma
M8901/3 Pleomorphic rhabdomyosarcoma
M8902/3 Mixed type rhabdomyosarcoma
M8903/0 Fetal rhabdomyoma
M8904/0 Adult rhabdomyoma
Glycogenic rhabdomyoma
M8910/3 Embryonal rhabdomyosarcoma
Botryoid sarcoma
Sarcoma botryoides
M8920/3 Alveolar rhabdomyosarcoma

M906–M909 Germ cell neoplasms

M9060/3 Dysgerminoma
M9064/3 Germinoma
Germ cell tumour NOS
M9070/3 Embryonal carcinoma NOS
Embryonal adenocarcinoma
M9080/0 Teratoma, benign
Adult cystic teratoma
Adult teratoma NOS
Cystic teratoma NOS
Teratoma, differentiated
M9080/1 Teratoma NOS
Mature teratoma
Solid teratoma
M9080/3 Teratoma, malignant NOS
Embryonal teratoma
Immature teratoma
Teratoblastoma, malignant
M9081/3 Teratocarcinoma
Mixed embryonal carcinoma and teratoma
M9082/3 Malignant teratoma, undifferentiated
Malignant teratoma, anaplastic
M9083/3 Malignant teratoma, intermediate
M9084/0 Dermoid cyst NOS
Dermoid NOS
M9084/3 Teratoma with malignant transformation
Dermoid cyst with malignant transformation

M912–M916 Blood vessel tumours

M9120/0 Haemangioma NOS (D18.0)
  Angioma NOS
  Chorioangioma
M9120/3 Haemangiosarcoma
  Angiosarcoma
M9121/0 Cavernous haemangioma (D18.0)
M9122/0 Venous haemangioma (D18.0)
M9123/0 Racemose haemangioma (D18.0)
  Arteriovenous haemangioma
M9124/3 Kupffer cell sarcoma (C22.3)
M9125/0 Epithelioid haemangioma (D18.0)
M9126/0 Histiocytoid haemangioma (D18.0)
M9130/0 Haemangioendothelioma, benign (D18.0)
M9130/1 Haemangioendothelioma NOS
  Angioendothelioma
M9130/3 Haemangioendothelioma, malignant
  Haemangioendothelial sarcoma
M9131/0 Capillary haemangioma (D18.0)
  Haemangioma simplex
  Infantile haemangioma
  Juvenile haemangioma
  Plexiform haemangioma
M9132/0 Intramuscular haemangioma (D18.0)
M9133/1 Epithelioid haemangioendothelioma NOS
M9133/3 Epithelioid haemangioendothelioma, malignant
M9134/1 Intravascular bronchial alveolar tumour (D38.1)
M9140/3 Kaposi's sarcoma (C46.–)
  Multiple haemorrhagic sarcoma
M9141/0 Angiokeratoma
M9142/0 Verrucous keratotic haemangioma (D18.0)
M9150/0 Haemangiopericytoma, benign
M9150/1 Haemangiopericytoma NOS
M9150/3 Haemangiopericytoma, malignant
M9161/1 Haemangioblastoma
  Angioblastoma

M918–M924 Osseous and chondromatous neoplasms

M9220/0 Chondroma NOS (D16.–)
  Endochondroma

M935–M937 Miscellaneous tumours

M9350/1 Craniopharyngioma (D44.3, D44.4)
  Rathke's pouch tumour
M9360/1 Pinealoma (D44.5)
M9361/1 Pineocytoma (D44.5)
M9362/3 Pineoblastoma (C75.3)
M9363/0 Melanotic neuroectodermal tumour
  Melanomeloblastoma
  Melanotic progonoma
  Retinal anlage tumour
M9364/3 Peripheral neuroectodermal tumour
  Neuroectodermal tumour NOS
M9370/3 Chordoma

M938–M948 Gliomas

M9380/3 Glioma, malignant (C71.–)
  Glioma NOS
M9381/3 Gliomatosis cerebri (C71.–)
M9382/3 Mixed glioma (C71.–)
  Mixed oligoastrocytoma
M9383/1 Subependymal glioma (D43.–)
  Subependymal astrocytoma NOS
  Subependymoma
M9384/1 Subependymal giant cell astrocytoma (D43.–)
M9390/0 Choroid plexus papilloma NOS (D33.0)
M9390/3 Choroid plexus papilloma, malignant (C71.5)
  Choroid plexus papilloma, anaplastic
M9391/3 Ependymoma NOS (C71.–)
  Epithelial ependymoma
M9392/3 Ependymoma, anaplastic (C71.–)
  Ependymoblastoma
M9393/1 Papillary ependymoma (D43.–)
M9394/1 Myxopapillary ependymoma (D43.–)
M9400/3 Astrocytoma NOS (C71.–)
  Astrocytic glioma
  Astroglioma
  Cystic astrocytoma
M9401/3 Astrocytoma, anaplastic (C71.–)
M9410/3 Protoplasmic astrocytoma (C71.–)
M9411/3 Gemistocytic astrocytoma (C71.–)
  Gemistocytoma
M9420/3 Fibrillary astrocytoma (C71.–)
  Fibrous astrocytoma

M9421/3 Pilocytic astrocytoma (C71.–)
Juvenile astrocytoma
Piloid astrocytoma
M9422/3 Spongioblastoma NOS (C71.–)
M9423/3 Spongioblastoma polare (C71.–)
M9424/3 Pleomorphic xanthoastrocytoma (C71.–)
M9430/3 Astroblastoma (C71.–)
M9440/3 Glioblastoma NOS (C71.–)
Glioblastoma multiforme
Spongioblastoma multiforme
M9441/3 Giant cell glioblastoma (C71.–)
M9442/3 Gliosarcoma (C71.–)
M9443/3 Primitive polar spongioblastoma (C71.–)
M9450/3 Oligodendroglioma NOS (C71.–)
M9451/3 Oligodendroglioma, anaplastic (C71.–)
M9460/3 Oligodendroblastoma (C71.–)
M9470/3 Medulloblastoma NOS (C71.6)
M9471/3 Desmoplastic medulloblastoma (C71.6)
Circumscribed arachnoidal cerebellar sarcoma
M9472/3 Medullomyoblastoma (C71.6)
M9473/3 Primitive neuroectodermal tumour (C71.–)
M9480/3 Cerebellar sarcoma NOS (C71.6)
M9481/3 Monstrocellular sarcoma (C71.–)

M949–M952 Neuroepitheliomatous neoplasms

M9490/0 Ganglioneuroma
Gangliocytoma
M9490/3 Ganglioneuroblastoma
M9491/0 Ganglioneuromatosis
M9500/3 Neuroblastoma NOS
Sympathicoblastoma
M9501/3 Medulloepithelioma NOS
Diktyoma
M9502/3 Teratoid medulloepithelioma
M9503/3 Neuroepithelioma NOS
M9504/3 Spongioneuroblastoma
M9505/1 Ganglioglioma
Glioneuroma
Neuroastrocytoma
M9506/0 Neurocytoma
M9507/0 Pacinian tumour
M9510/3 Retinoblastoma NOS (C69.2)
M9511/3 Retinoblastoma, differentiated (C69.2)
M9512/3 Retinoblastoma, undifferentiated (C69.2)

M9520/3 Olfactory neurogenic tumour
M9521/3 Esthesioneurocytoma (C30.0)
M9522/3 Esthesioneuroblastoma (C30.0)
  Olfactory neuroblastoma
M9523/3 Esthesioneuroepithelioma (C30.0)
  Olfactory neuroepithelioma

M953 Meningiomas

M9530/0 Meningioma NOS (D32.–)
M9530/1 Meningiomatosis NOS (D42.–)
  Diffuse meningiomatosis
  Multiple meningiomatosis
M9530/3 Meningioma, malignant (C70.–)
  Leptomeningeal sarcoma
  Meningeal sarcoma
  Meningiothelial sarcoma
M9531/0 Meningotheliomatous meningioma (D32.–)
  Endotheliomatous meningioma
  Syncytial meningioma
M9532/0 Fibrous meningioma (D32.–)
  Fibroblastic meningioma
M9533/0 Psammomatous meningioma (D32.–)
M9534/0 Angiomatous meningioma (D32.–)
M9535/0 Haemangioblastic meningioma (D32.–)
  Angioblastic meningioma
M9536/0 Haemangiopericytic meningioma (D32.–)
M9537/0 Transitional meningioma (D32.–)
  Mixed meningioma
M9538/1 Papillary meningioma (D42.–)
M9539/3 Meningeal sarcomatosis (C70.–)

M954–M957 Nerve sheath tumours

M9540/0 Neurofibroma NOS
M9540/1 Neurofibromatosis NOS (Q85.0)
  Multiple neurofibromatosis
  Von Recklinghausen's disease (*except of bone*)
M9540/3 Neurofibrosarcoma
  Neurogenic sarcoma
  Neurosarcoma
M9541/0 Melanotic neurofibroma
M9550/0 Plexiform neurofibroma
  Plexiform neuroma

M9560/0 Neurilemmoma NOS
Acoustic neuroma
Melanocytic schwannoma
Neurinoma
Pigmented neuroma
Schwannoma
M9560/1 Neurinomatosis
M9560/3 Neurilemmoma, malignant
Malignant schwannoma NOS
Neurilemmosarcoma
M9561/3 Triton tumour, malignant
Malignant schwannoma with rhabdomyoblastic differentiation
M9562/0 Neurothekeoma
Nerve sheath myxoma
M9570/0 Neuroma NOS

M958 Granular cell tumours and alveolar soft part sarcoma
M9580/0 Granular cell tumour NOS
Granular cell myoblastoma NOS
M9580/3 Granular cell tumour, malignant
Granular cell myoblastoma, malignant
M9581/3 Alveolar soft part sarcoma

M959–M971 Hodgkin's and non-Hodgkin's lymphoma

M959 Malignant lymphomas NOS or diffuse
M9590/3 Malignant lymphoma NOS (C84.5, C85.9)
Lymphoma NOS
M9591/3 Malignant lymphoma, non-Hodgkin's NOS (C84.5, C85.9)
Non-Hodgkin's lymphoma NOS
M9592/3 Lymphosarcoma NOS (C85.0)
Lymphosarcoma, diffuse
M9593/3 Reticulosarcoma NOS (C83.3, C83.9)
Reticulosarcoma, diffuse
Reticulum cell sarcoma, diffuse
Reticulum cell sarcoma NOS
M9594/3 Microglioma (C85.7)
M9595/3 Malignant lymphoma, diffuse NOS (C83.9)

M965–M966 Hodgkin's disease
M9650/3 Hodgkin's disease NOS (C81.9)
Malignant lymphoma, Hodgkin's

M9652/3 Hodgkin's disease, mixed cellularity NOS (C81.2)
M9653/3 Hodgkin's disease, lymphocytic depletion NOS (C81.3)
M9654/3 Hodgkin's disease, lymphocytic depletion, diffuse fibrosis (C81.3)
M9655/3 Hodgkin's disease, lymphocytic depletion, reticular (C81.3)
M9657/3 Hodgkin's disease, lymphocytic predominance NOS (C81.0)
  Hodgkin's disease, lymphocytic–histiocytic predominance
M9658/3 Hodgkin's disease, lymphocytic predominance, diffuse (C81.0)
M9659/3 Hodgkin's disease, lymphocytic predominance, nodular (C81.0)
M9660/3 Hodgkin's paragranuloma NOS (C81.7)
  Hodgkin's paragranuloma, nodular
M9661/3 Hodgkin's granuloma (C81.7)
M9662/3 Hodgkin's sarcoma (C81.7)
M9663/3 Hodgkin's disease, nodular sclerosis NOS (C81.1)
M9664/3 Hodgkin's disease, nodular sclerosis, cellular phase (C81.1)
M9665/3 Hodgkin's disease, nodular sclerosis, lymphocytic predominance (C81.1)
M9666/3 Hodgkin's disease, nodular sclerosis, mixed cellularity (C81.1)
M9667/3 Hodgkin's disease, nodular sclerosis, lymphocytic depletion (C81.1)
  Hodgkin's disease, nodular sclerosis, syncytial variant

M967–M968 Malignant lymphoma, diffuse or NOS, specified type

M9670/3 Malignant lymphoma, small lymphocytic NOS (C83.0)
  Malignant lymphoma, lymphocytic NOS
  Malignant lymphoma, lymphocytic, diffuse NOS
  Malignant lymphoma, lymphocytic, well differentiated, diffuse
  Malignant lymphoma, small cell NOS
  Malignant lymphoma, small cell, diffuse NOS
  Malignant lymphoma, small cell, lymphocytic, diffuse NOS
M9671/3 Malignant lymphoma, lymphoplasmacytic (C83.8)
  Immunocytoma
  Malignant lymphoma, lymphoplasmacytoid
  Malignant lymphoma, plasmacytoid
  Plasmacytic lymphoma
M9672/3 Malignant lymphoma, small cleaved cell, diffuse (C83.1)
  Malignant lymphoma, cleaved cell NOS
  Malignant lymphoma, lymphocytic, poorly differentiated, diffuse
  Malignant lymphoma, small cleaved cell NOS
M9673/3 Malignant lymphoma, lymphocytic, intermediate differentiation, diffuse (C83.8)
  Mantle zone lymphoma
M9674/3 Malignant lymphoma, centrocytic (C83.8)

M9675/3 Malignant lymphoma, mixed small and large cell, diffuse (C83.2)
Malignant lymphoma, mixed cell type, diffuse
Malignant lymphoma, mixed lymphocytic–histiocytic, diffuse
M9676/3 Malignant lymphoma, centroblastic–centrocytic, diffuse (C83.8)
Malignant lymphoma, centroblastic–centrocytic NOS
M9680/3 Malignant lymphoma, large cell, diffuse NOS (C83.3)
Malignant lymphoma, histiocytic NOS
Malignant lymphoma, histiocytic, diffuse
Malignant lymphoma, large cell NOS
Malignant lymphoma, large cell, cleaved and noncleaved
M9681/3 Malignant lymphoma, large cell, cleaved, diffuse (C83.3)
Malignant lymphoma, large cleaved cell NOS
M9682/3 Malignant lymphoma, large cell, noncleaved, diffuse (C83.3)
Malignant lymphoma, large cell, noncleaved NOS
Malignant lymphoma, noncleaved NOS
Malignant lymphoma, noncleaved, diffuse NOS
M9683/3 Malignant lymphoma, centroblastic, diffuse (C83.8)
Malignant lymphoma, centroblastic NOS
M9684/3 Malignant lymphoma, immunoblastic NOS (C83.4)
Immunoblastic sarcoma
Malignant lymphoma, large cell, immunoblastic
M9685/3 Malignant lymphoma, lymphoblastic (C83.5)
Lymphoblastoma
Malignant lymphoma, convoluted cell
M9686/3 Malignant lymphoma, small cell, noncleaved, diffuse (C83.0, C83.6)
Malignant lymphoma, undifferentiated cell, non-Burkitt's
Malignant lymphoma, undifferentiated cell type NOS
M9687/3 Burkitt's lymphoma NOS (C83.7)
Burkitt's tumour
Malignant lymphoma, small noncleaved, Burkitt's, diffuse
Malignant lymphoma, undifferentiated, Burkitt's type

M969 Malignant lymphoma, follicular or nodular, with or without diffuse areas

M9690/3 Malignant lymphoma, follicular NOS (C82.9)
Malignant lymphoma, lymphocytic, nodular NOS
Malignant lymphoma, nodular NOS
M9691/3 Malignant lymphoma, mixed small cleaved and large cell, follicular (C82.1)
Malignant lymphoma, mixed cell type, follicular
Malignant lymphoma, mixed cell type, nodular
Malignant lymphoma, mixed lymphocytic–histiocytic, nodular

M9692/3 Malignant lymphoma, centroblastic–centrocytic, follicular (C82.8)
M9693/3 Malignant lymphoma, lymphocytic, well differentiated, nodular (C82.8)
M9694/3 Malignant lymphoma, lymphocytic, intermediate differentiation, nodular (C82.8)
M9695/3 Malignant lymphoma, small cleaved cell, follicular (C82.0)
M9696/3 Malignant lymphoma, lymphocytic, poorly differentiated, nodular (C82.8)
M9697/3 Malignant lymphoma, centroblastic, follicular (C82.8)
M9698/3 Malignant lymphoma, large cell, follicular NOS (C82.2)
    Malignant lymphoma, histiocytic, nodular
    Malignant lymphoma, large cell, noncleaved, follicular
    Malignant lymphoma, large cleaved cell, follicular
    Malignant lymphoma, noncleaved, follicular NOS

M970 Specified cutaneous and peripheral T-cell lymphomas
M9703/3 T-zone lymphoma (C84.2)
M9704/3 Lymphoepithelioid lymphoma (C84.3)
    Lennert's lymphoma

M971 Other specified non-Hodgkin's lymphomas
M9711/3 Monocytoid B-cell lymphoma (C85.7)
M9712/3 Angioendotheliomatosis (C85.7)
M9713/3 Angiocentric T-cell lymphoma (C84.7)
    Malignant midline reticulosis
    Malignant reticulosis NOS
    Polymorphic reticulosis
M9714/3 Large cell (Ki-1+) lymphoma (C85.7)

M972 Other lymphoreticular neoplasms
M9720/3 Malignant histiocytosis (C96.1)
    Histiocytic medullary reticulosis
M9722/3 Letterer–Siwe disease (C96.0)
    Acute differentiated progressive histiocytosis
    Acute progressive histiocytosis X
    Nonlipid reticuloendotheliosis
M9723/3 True histiocytic lymphoma (C96.3)

M973 Plasma cell tumours
M9731/3 Plasmacytoma NOS (C90.2)
    Extramedullary plasmacytoma
    Plasma cell tumour
    Solitary myeloma
    Solitary plasmacytoma

M9732/3 Multiple myeloma (C90.0)
  Myeloma NOS
  Myelomatosis
  Plasma cell myeloma

M974 Mast cell tumours

M9740/1 Mastocytoma NOS (D47.0)
  Mast cell tumour NOS
M9740/3 Mast cell sarcoma (C96.2)
  Malignant mast cell tumour
  Malignant mastocytoma
M9741/3 Malignant mastocytosis (C96.2)
  Systemic tissue mast cell disease

M976 Immunoproliferative diseases

M9760/3 Immunoproliferative disease NOS (C88.9)
M9761/3 Waldenström's macroglobulinaemia (C88.0)
M9762/3 Alpha heavy chain disease (C88.1)
M9763/3 Gamma heavy chain disease (C88.2)
  Franklin's disease
M9764/3 Immunoproliferative small intestinal disease (C88.3)
  Mediterranean lymphoma
M9765/1 Monoclonal gammopathy (D47.2)
M9766/1 Angiocentric immunoproliferative lesion (D47.7)
  Lymphoid granulomatosis
M9767/1 Angioimmunoblastic lymphadenopathy (D47.7)
  Lymphoid granulomatosis
M9768/1 T-gamma lymphoproliferative disease (D47.7)

M980–M994 Leukaemias

M980 Leukaemias NOS

M9800/3 Leukaemia NOS (C95.9)
M9801/3 Acute leukaemia NOS (C95.0)
  Blast cell leukaemia
  Undifferentiated leukaemia
M9802/3 Subacute leukaemia NOS (C95.2)
M9803/3 Chronic leukaemia NOS (C95.1)
M9804/3 Aleukaemic leukaemia NOS (C95.7)

M982 Lymphoid leukaemias

M9820/3 Lymphoid leukaemia NOS (C91.9)
  Lymphatic leukaemia NOS
  Lymphocytic leukaemia NOS

M9821/3 Acute lymphoblastic leukaemia NOS (C91.0)
Acute lymphatic leukaemia
Acute lymphocytic leukaemia
Acute lymphoid leukaemia
Lymphoblastic leukaemia NOS
M9822/3 Subacute lymphoid leukaemia (C91.2)
Subacute lymphatic leukaemia
Subacute lymphocytic leukaemia
M9823/3 Chronic lymphocytic leukaemia (C91.1)
Chronic lymphatic leukaemia
Chronic lymphoid leukaemia
M9824/3 Aleukaemic lymphoid leukaemia (C91.7)
Aleukaemic lymphatic leukaemia
Aleukaemic lymphocytic leukaemia
M9825/3 Prolymphocytic leukaemia (C91.3)
M9826/3 Burkitt's cell leukaemia (C91.7)
Acute lymphoblastic leukaemia, Burkitt's type
M9827/3 Adult T-cell leukaemia/lymphoma (C91.5)
Adult T-cell leukaemia
Adult T-cell lymphoma

M983 Plasma cell leukaemia
M9830/3 Plasma cell leukaemia (C90.1)
Plasmacytic leukaemia

M984 Erythroleukaemias
M9840/3 Erythroleukaemia (C94.0)
Erythraemic myelosis NOS
M9841/3 Acute erythraemia (C94.0)
Acute erythraemic myelosis
Di Guglielmo's disease
M9842/3 Chronic erythraemia (C94.0)

M985 Lymphosarcoma cell leukaemia
M9850/3 Lymphosarcoma cell leukaemia (C94.7)

M986 Myeloid (granulocytic) leukaemias
M9860/3 Myeloid leukaemia NOS (C92.9)
Granulocytic leukaemia NOS
Myelocytic leukaemia NOS
Myelogenous leukaemia NOS
Myelomonocytic leukaemia NOS

M9861/3 Acute myeloid leukaemia (C92.0)
    Acute granulocytic leukaemia
    Acute myeloblastic leukaemia
    Acute myelocytic leukaemia
    Acute myelogenous leukaemia
M9862/3 Subacute myeloid leukaemia (C92.2)
    Subacute granulocytic leukaemia
    Subacute myelogenous leukaemia
M9863/3 Chronic myeloid leukaemia (C92.1)
    Chronic granulocytic leukaemia
    Chronic myelocytic leukaemia
    Chronic myelogenous leukaemia
M9864/3 Aleukaemic myeloid leukaemia (C92.7)
    Aleukaemic granulocytic leukaemia
    Aleukaemic myelocytic leukaemia
M9866/3 Acute promyelocytic leukaemia (C92.4)
M9867/3 Acute myelomonocytic leukaemia (C92.5)
M9868/3 Chronic myelomonocytic leukaemia (C92.7)

M987 Basophilic leukaemia
M9870/3 Basophilic leukaemia (C92.–)

M988 Eosinophilic leukaemia
M9880/3 Eosinophilic leukaemia (C92.–)

M989 Monocytic leukaemias
M9890/3 Monocytic leukaemia NOS (C93.9)
M9891/3 Acute monocytic leukaemia (C93.0)
    Acute monoblastic leukaemia
    Monoblastic leukaemia NOS
M9892/3 Subacute monocytic leukaemia (C93.2)
M9893/3 Chronic monocytic leukaemia (C93.1)
M9894/3 Aleukaemic monocytic leukaemia (C93.7)

M990–M994 Other leukaemias
M9900/3 Mast cell leukaemia (C94.3)
M9910/3 Acute megakaryoblastic leukaemia (C94.2)
    Megakaryocytic leukaemia
M9930/3 Myeloid sarcoma (C92.3)
    Chloroma
    Granulocytic sarcoma
M9931/3 Acute panmyelosis (C94.4)
M9932/3 Acute myelofibrosis (C94.5)
M9940/3 Hairy cell leukaemia (C91.4)

M995–M997 Miscellaneous myeloproliferative and lymphoproliferative disorders

M9950/1 Polycythaemia vera (D45)
  Polycythaemia rubra vera
M9960/1 Chronic myeloproliferative disease (D47.1)
  Myeloproliferative disease NOS
M9961/1 Myelosclerosis with myeloid metaplasia (D47.1)
  Megakaryocytic myelosclerosis
  Myelofibrosis with myeloid metaplasia
M9962/1 Idiopathic thrombocythaemia (D47.3)
  Essential haemorrhagic thrombocythaemia
  Essential thrombocythaemia
  Idiopathic haemorrhagic thrombocythaemia
M9970/1 Lymphoproliferative disease NOS (D47.9)

Index

A

Absence — *continued*
- skull bone, congenital Q75.80
- sternum, congenital Q76.7
- vertebra, congenital, not associated with scoliosis Q76.40

Abuse
- adult or child, effects of T74.9
- drugs — *see* Use, harmful
- physical T74.1
- psychological T74.3
- sexual T74.2

Acalculia R48.80
- developmental F81.2

Acatalasaemia, acatalasia E80.310
Accessory
- muscle Q79.81
- rib Q76.6

Accident, cerebrovascular I64
Acephaly Q00.01
Achondrogenesis Q77.0
Achondroplasia Q77.4
Achromatopsia H53.5
Acidaemia
- glutaric E88.820
- γ-hydroxybutyric E72.815
- hyperpipecolic E80.301
- isovaleric E71.11
- methylmalonic E71.12
- orotic E79.8
- phytanic, hereditary G60.1
- propionic E71.13
- pyroglutamic E72.811

Acidosis E87.2
- diabetic — *see* E10–E14 with fourth character .1
- fetal P20.–
- intrauterine P20.–
- lactic E87.22
- metabolic E87.20
- - late, of newborn P74.0
- renal tubular N25.8

Aciduria
- argininosuccinic E72.20
- glutaric E72.30

Acquired immunodeficiency syndrome B24
Acrania Q00.00
Acrocephalopolysyndactyly Q87.00
Acrocephalosyndactyly Q87.01
Acrocephaly Q75.00
Acrocyanosis I73.8
Acrodermatitis enteropathica E83.20
Acromegaly E22.0
Acroparaesthesia I73.8
Actinomycosis A42
Addiction — *see* Syndrome, dependence
Addisonian crisis E27.2
Addison's disease E27.1
Addison–Schilder complex E71.320
Adenolipomatosis, Launois–Bensaude E88.80
Adenomatosis, multiple endocrine D44.8
Adhesions (due to)
- foreign body accidentally left in operation wound or body cavity T81.5
- meningeal G96.1

Adie's (myotonic) pupil H57.00
Adipsia R63.80
Adjustment of devices NEC Z46
Adrenal gland disorder — *see* Disorder, adrenal gland
Adrenalitis, autoimmune E27.1
Adrenocortical
- crisis E27.2
- insufficiency E27.4
- - drug-induced E27.3
- - primary E27.1
- overactivity NEC E27.0

Adrenogenital disorder E25.9
- congenital, associated with enzyme deficiency E25.0
- idiopathic E25.8
- specified NEC E25.8

Adrenoleukodystrophy E71.32
Adrenomyeloleukodystrophy E71.32
Adrenomyeloneuropathy E71.32
Adverse
- effects — *see* Table of drugs and chemicals, page 565
- incident associated with neurological device Y75.–

Aero-otitis media T70.0
Aerosinusitis T70.1
Afibrinogenaemia D65
- congenital D68.2

Agenesis (of)
- brain stem nuclei, congenital Q87.05
- corpus callosum
- partial Q04.01
- total Q04.00
- eye Q11.1
- nerve Q07.80
- septum pellucidum Q04.82

Ageusia R43.20
Agitation R45.1
Agnosia
- auditory R48.11
- developmental F88
- somatosensory R48.12
- visual R48.10

Agranulocytosis D70
Agraphia R48.8
- with alexia R48.01

Agyria Q04.30
AIDS–dementia complex F02.4
AIDS-related complex B24
Air pressure, effects T70.–

Aneurysm — *continued*
- artery — *continued*
- - - specified NEC — *continued*
- - - - ruptured I60.6
- - renal I72.2
- - specified NEC I72.8
- - vertebral I67.15
- - - congenital Q28.35
- - - ruptured I60.5
- berry, ruptured (congenital) I60.7
- cerebral I67.1
- - congenital Q28.–
- - ruptured I60.9
- congenital, specified site NEC Q28.8
- heart I25.3
- mural I25.3
- precerebral, congenital Q28.1
- - arteriovenous Q28.2
- retina H35.0
- - congenital Q14.1
- ventricular I25.3
Anger R45.4
Angiitis
- cerebral
- - primary I67.70
- - specified NEC I67.78
- granulomatous
- - allergic M30.1
- - of nervous system I67.70
- hypersensitivity M31.0
Angina pectoris I20
Angiohaemophilia D68.0
Angioid streaks of macula H35.3
Angiopathy
- amyloid, cerebral E85.–† I68.0*
- congophilic E85.–† I68.0*
Angiostrongyliasis B83.2
Anhidrosis, chronic idiopathic G90.82
Aniseikonia H52.3
Anisocoria H57.03
Anisometropia H52.3
Ankylosis of spinal joint M43.2
Anomaly — *see also* Abnormal, abnormality
- dental arch relationship K07.2
- dentofacial K07.–
- jaw–cranial base relationship K07.1
- jaw size K07.0
- pupillary function H57.0
- tooth position K07.3
Anophthalmos Q11.–
Anopsia, quadrant H53.4
Anosmia R43.0
Anosodiaphoria R48.124
Anosognosia R48.123
Anorexia R63.0
Anoxia
- altitudinal T70.2

Anoxia — *continued*
- birth P21.9
- cerebral
- - due to anaesthesia, during
- - - labour and delivery O74.3
- - - the puerperium O89.2
- - following caesarean or other obstetric surgery or procedures O75.4
- fetal or intrauterine P20.–
Anoxic brain damage G93.1
Anterocollis, spasmodic G24.32
Anthrax A22.–
- meningitis A22.8† G01*
- septicaemia A22.7
Antritis
- acute J01.0
- chronic J32.0
Anuria R34
Anxiety disorder, dream F51.5
Aortitis I77.6
- syphilitic A52.0† I79.1*
Apathy R45.3
Apert's syndrome Q87.01
Aphasia R47.0
- acquired, with epilepsy F80.3
- developmental
- - expressive type F80.1
- - receptive type F80.2
- dynamic, Luria's R47.05
- global, Déjerine's R47.02
- Goldstein's R47.0
- progressive isolated G31.01
- Wernicke's
- - developmental F80.2
- - receptive R47.01
Aphonia R49.1
- psychogenic F44.4
Aphthae
- Bednar's K12.0
- oral, recurrent K12.0
Aplasia
- cerebellar G11.00
- eye Q11.1
- thyroid (with myxoedema) E03.1
Apnoea R06.8
- sleep G47.3
Apoplexy I64
- heat T67.0
- pituitary E23.63
Appearance, bizarre R46.1
Apraxia R48.2
- gait R26.23
- oculomotor H51.80
Arachnoiditis G03.9
- bacterial G00.–
- opto-chiasmatic G96.10
Argininaemia E72.25

Argyll Robertson phenomenon or pupil, syphilitic A52.1† H58.0*
Arhinencephaly Q04.1
Ariboflavinosis E53.0
Arnold–Chiari syndrome Q07.0
Arnold's occipital neuralgia G52.80
Arousal, confusional G47.82
Arrest
- cardiac
- - sinus, REM-sleep-related G47.803
- - with successful resuscitation I46.1
- - due to anaesthesia during labour and delivery O74.2
- - following caesarean or other obstetric surgery or procedures O75.4
- respiratory R09.2
Arrhythmia
- cardiac I49.9
- extrasystolic I49.4
- ventricular, re-entry I47.0
Arteriosclerosis — *see also* Atherosclerosis
- kidney I12
Arteritis I77.6
- cerebral I67.7
- - listerial A32.8† I68.1*
- - syphilitic A52.0† I68.1*
- - tuberculous A18.8† I68.1*
- giant cell, with polymyalgia rheumatica M31.5
Arthritis
- postmeningococcal A39.8† M03.0*
- rheumatic (*see also* Fever, rheumatic) I00
- rheumatoid, seropositive M05
Arthropathy
- Charcot's A52.1†, M14.6*
- crystal
- - in hyperparathyroidism E21.–† M14.2*
- - specified NEC M11
- diabetic (*see also* E10–E14 with fourth character .6) E14.6† M14.2*
- - neuropathic E14.6† M14.6*
- gouty
- - in
- - - Lesch–Nyhan syndrome E79.1† M14.0*
- - - sickle-cell disorders D57.–† M14.0*
- in
- - erythema
- - - multiforme L51.–† M14.8*
- - - nodosum L52† M14.8*
- - leukaemia C95† M36.1*
- - malignant histiocytosis C96.1† M36.1*
- - multiple myeloma C90.0† M36.1*
- - sarcoidosis D86.8† M14.8*
- - Whipple's disease K90.8† M14.8*
- postinfective in syphilis A50.5† M03.1*
- tabetic A52.1† M14.6*
Arthrosis of spine M47.–
Ascariasis B77.–
Ascaridiasis B77.–
Aspartylglucosaminuria E77.13
Asperger's syndrome F84.5
Aspergillosis B44.–
Asphyxia R09.0
- birth P21.9
- - blue P21.1
- - mild and moderate P21.1
- - severe P21.0
- - white P21.0
- carbon monoxide T58
- due to foreign body T17
- fetal P20.–
- gases, fumes and vapours NEC T59.8
- inhalation of food or foreign body T17
- intrauterine P20.–
Asphyxiation T71
Astereognosia R48.125
Asthenia R53
- neurocirculatory F45.3
- senile R54
Asthenopia H53.1
Asthma J45
- - acute severe J46
Astigmatism H52.2
Asymmetry
- facial Q67.0
- jaw K07.1
Ataxia, ataxic R27.0
- cerebellar G11
- - alcoholic G31.20
- - congenital G11.01
- - early-onset G11.1
- - late-onset G11.2
- - with defective DNA repair G11.3
- congenital nonprogressive G11.0
- gait R26.0
- Gillespie's G11.05
- hereditary G11.9
- Holmes' G11.12
- Ramsay–Hunt G11.13
- Sanger–Brown G11.23
- telangiectasia G11.30
Atelencephaly
- aperta Q00.03
- clausa Q00.02
Atelomyelia Q06.1
Atheroma
- cerebral arteries I67.2
- coronary I25.1
Atherosclerosis, atherosclerotic (*see also* Arteriosclerosis) I70.9
- aorta I70.0
- cardiovascular disease I25.0
- cerebral I67.2

Atherosclerosis, atherosclerotic — *continued*
- coronary (artery) I25.1
- gangrene I70.2
- heart disease I25.1
- ophthalmic artery I70.81
- renal artery I70.1
- retinopathy I70.81† H36.8*

Atmospheric pressure change, effects T70.–

Atresia
- auditory canal, congenital Q16.1
- foramina of Magendie and Luschka Q03.1

Atrophy
- brain, circumscribed G31.0
- choroid H31.1
- disuse M62.5
- hemifacial Q67.4
- muscle fibre
- – type I G71.807
- – type II G71.805
- muscular
- – peroneal G60.0
- – – axonal G60.01
- – – hypertrophic G60.00
- – progressive G12.24
- – – post-polio B91.–0
- – spinal G12.9
- – – inherited G12.1
- – – specified NEC G12.8
- olivopontocerebellar G11.2

Atrophy — *continued*
- optic H47.2
- – late syphilitic A52.1† H48.0*
- orbit H05.3
- Sudeck's M89.0
- thyroid E03.4
- – congenital E03.1
- yellow liver K72

Attack
- drop R26.22
- ischaemic, transient cerebral G45.9
- salaam G40.40
- shuddering, of childhood G25.04
- vasovagal R55

Attention deficit syndrome F90.0

Auricle, cervical Q18.2

Autism
- atypical F84.1
- childhood F84.0

Autotopagnosia R48.120

Avulsion
- blood vessel T14.5
- eye S05.7
- joint (capsule) T14.3
- ligament T14.3
- muscle T14.6
- nerve root G54.81
- tendon T14.6

B

Blindness — *continued*
- night — *continued*
- - due to vitamin A deficiency E50.5
- one eye H54.4
- - low vision, other eye H54.1
- psychogenic F44.6
- river B73
Blind spot, enlarged H53.4
Blister (nonthermal) T14.0
Block
- atrioventricular I44.3
- complete I44.2
- first-degree I44.0
- second-degree I44.1
- bifascicular I45.2
- bundle-branch I45.4
- - left I44.7
- - - hemiblock I44.6
- - right I45.1
- fascicular
- - left
- - - anterior I44.4
- - - posterior I44.5
- - right I45.0
- heart I45.9
- - complete I44.2
- intraventricular, nonspecific I45.4
- sinoatrial I45.5
- sinoauricular I45.5
- - third-degree I44.2
- trifascicular I45.3
- Wenckebach's I44.1
Bornholm disease B33.0
Boston exanthem A88.0
Botulism A05.1
Bourneville's disease Q85.1
Bouveret(–Hoffmann) syndrome I47.9
Bowel, neurogenic NEC K59.2
Brain damage
- anoxic G93.1
- birth injury P11.2
Branchial vestige Q18.0
Breath
- holding (spells) R06.81
- shortness R06.0
Breathing
- abnormality R06.8
- apneustic R06.33
- Cheyne–Stokes R06.30
- Kussmaul R06.31
- mouth R06.5
- periodic NEC R06.38
Briquet's disorder F48.80
Broca's aphasia R47.00
Brodie's myopathy G71.85
Bronchiectasis J47
Bronchitis J40
- chronic J42
Brown's sheath syndrome H50.6
Brucellosis A23.–
Bruise T14.0
Bruit (arterial) R09.8
Bruns' apraxia R26.03
Bruxism F45.8
- sleep-related G47.810
Buerger's disease I73.1
Bundle-branch block I45.4
Burn
- electric current W87
- sequelae T95
Burn-out Z73.0

C

Chiari malformation Q07.0
Chickenpox B01.–
– congenital P35.8
Child abuse
– effects T74.9
– physical T74.1
– psychological T74.3
– sexual T74.2
Chimera 46,XX/46,XY Q99.0
Choking sensation R06.82
Cholera A00
Cholestasis K71.0
Cholesteatoma
– middle ear H71
– recurrent postprocedural H95.0
Cholesterosis, cerebrotendinous E75.50
Chondrodysplasia punctata Q77.3
Chorea G25.5
– associated with hormone therapy G25.51
– benign hereditary G25.54
– drug-induced G25.4
– gravidarum G25.50
– Huntington's G10
– in
– – hyperthyroidism E05.–† G26.–1*
– – neurocanthocytosis G25.53† G26.–1*
– – systemic lupus erythematosus M32.–† G26.–1*
– rheumatic I02.9
– – with heart involvement I02.0
– senile G25.55
– Sydenham's I02.–
– with heart involvement I02.0
Choreathetosis, kinesiogenic G25.56
Choreoacanthocytosis G25.53
Choriocarcinoma C58
Chorioiditis H30.9
– disseminated H30.1
– focal H30.0
Choriomeningitis, lymphocytic A87.2
Chorionepithelioma C58
Chorioretinitis H30.9
– disseminated H30.1
– focal H30.0
– in toxoplasma B58.0† H32.0*
– syphilitic A52.7† H32.0*
– tuberculous A18.5† H32.0*
Chorioretinopathy, central serous H35.7
Choroideremia H31.2
Christmas disease D67
Chromosome abnormality — *see* Abnormality, chromosome
Chromomycosis B43.–
Churg–Strauss syndrome M30.1
Circadian rhythm inversion
– organic G47.2
– psychogenic F51.2
Cirrhosis of liver, alcoholic K70.3
Citrullinaemia E72.21
Claude's disease or syndrome I67.9† G46.30*
Claudication, intermittent I73.9
Clubfoot Q66.8
Clumsy child syndrome F82
Cluttering
– organic origin R47.81
– psychogenic origin F98.6
Clutton's joints A50.5† M03.1*
Coagulation
– defect D68.9
– – specified NEC D68.8
– intravascular disseminated D65
Coagulopathy, consumption D65
Coats' retinopathy H35.0
Coccidioidomycosis meningitis B38.4† G02.1*
Coccygodynia M53.3
Cockayne's syndrome Q87.11
Colitis, ulcerative K51
Collapse, collapsed R55
– during or following a procedure T81.1
– heat T67.1
– vertebra NEC M48.5
Coloboma
– fundus Q14.8
– optic disc Q14.2
Colour blindness H53.5
Coma R40
– diabetic — *code to* E10–E14 with fourth character .0
– hepatic K72
– hypoglycaemic, nondiabetic E15
– in hepatitis
– – A B15.0
– – viral B19.0
– insulin, in nondiabetic E15
– myxoedema E03.5
– neonatal P91.5
Commotio cerebri S06.0
Complex
– Addison–Schilder E71.320
– Costen's K07.6
Complications (due to) (following) (of)
– abortion and ectopic and molar pregnancy O08.8
– anaesthesia (during) (from) (in)
– – labour and delivery O74.–
– – pregnancy O29.–
– – puerperium O89.–
– graft NEC T85.8
– implant NEC T85.8
– infusion T80.–
– inhalation therapy T81.8
– injection, therapeutic T80.–
– internal prosthetic device NEC T85.8
– labour and delivery NEC O75.–

Cryptophthalmos — *continued*
– syndrome Q87.082
Curvature, spine M43.9
– congenital Q67.5
Cushing's disease or syndrome E24.9
– alcohol-induced E24.4
– drug-induced E24.2
– pituitary-dependent E24.0
– specified NEC E24.8
Cut T14.1
– blood vessel T14.5
– tendon and muscle T14.6
– unintentional, during surgical or medical care Y60
Cyclitis H20.0
– posterior H30.2
Cyclopia Q87.02
Cyclothymia F34.0
Cyclotropia H50.4
Cyst
– arachnoid G93.00
– cerebral G93.0
– – congenital Q04.6
– branchial cleft Q18.0
– leptomeningeal, congenital Q04.63

Cyst — *continued*
– macula H35.3
– medial, face and neck Q18.8
– nerve root G54.80
– orbit H05.8
– perineural G54.80
– periventricular, acquired, of newborn P91.1
– porencephalic, acquired G93.01
– preauricular Q18.1
– Rathke's pouch E23.62
Cystathioninuria E72.12
Cystic
– eyeball (congenital) Q11.0
– fibrosis E84.9
Cysticercosis B69.–
Cystinosis E72.02
Cystinuria E72.06
Cytomegalovirus, cytomegaloviral
– disease B25.8
– infection
– – congenital P35.1
– – maternal care for O35.3
– mononucleosis B27.1

D

Damage, brain
- anoxic G93.1
- birth injury P11.2

Dandy–Walker syndrome Q03.1

Davidenkow's spinal muscular atrophy G12.114

Dawson's inclusion body encephalitis A81.1

Deafness H91.9
- conductive H90.2
- congenital H90.–
- high frequency H91.9
- ischaemic, transient H93.0
- low frequency H91.9
- psychogenic F44.6
- sensorineural H90.5
- word R48.111

Death
- instantaneous R96.0
- sudden (cause unknown) R96.0
- – infant R95
- – without sign of disease R96.1
- unattended R98

Debility
- chronic R53
- nervous R53
- senile R54

Decapitation S18

Decompression sickness T70.3

Decreased glucose in cerebrospinal fluid R83.81

Defect
- catalase E80.3
- coagulation D68.9
- – specified NEC D68.8
- glycoprotein degradation E77.1
- lysosomal enzyme, post-translational modification E77.0
- mitochondrial respiratory chain E88.83
- peroxidase E80.3
- platelet, qualitative D69.1
- visual field H53.4

Deficiency (of)
- acetyl CoA *C*-acyltransferase E88.820
- acetyl CoA-α-glucosaminide *N*-acetyltransferase E76.202
- *N*-acetyl-galactosamine-4-sulfatase E76.22
- *N*-acetyl glucosaminephosphotransferase E77.00
- α-*N*-acetyl glucosaminidase E76.201
- *N*-acetyl-α-D-glucosaminide-6-sulfatase E76.203
- *N*-acetylglutamate synthetase E72.24

Deficiency (of) — *continued*
- *N*-acetyltransferase E72.24
- acid β-gangliosidase E75.10
- acid phosphatase E83.30
- ACTH
- – drug-induced E23.10
- – isolated E23.06
- adrenocorticotropic hormone
- – drug-induced E23.10
- – isolated E23.06
- alanine–glyoxylate transaminase E80.311
- β-alanine transaminase E70.803
- aminomethyltransferase E72.55
- amylo-1,6-glucosidase (debrancher) E74.02
- 1,4-α-glucan branching enzyme E74.03
- α-1-antitrypsin E88.0
- arginase E72.23
- argininosuccinate
- – lysase E72.20
- – synthetase E72.21
- aryl-sulphatase A E75.23
- ascorbic acid E54
- β-aspartyl-*N*-acetyl glucosaminidase E77.13
- biotin E53.82
- biotinidase E88.822
- calcium, dietary E58
- carbamoylphosphate synthetase I E72.22
- carboxylase (multiple) E88.821
- carnitine E71.314
- – muscle E71.312
- – systemic E71.313
- carnitine *O*-acetyltransferase E71.310
- carnitine *O*-palmitoyltransferase E71.311
- carnosinase E70.801
- cholesterol ester hydrolase E75.51
- clotting factors NEC, hereditary D68.2
- coagulation factor, acquired D68.4
- coenzyme A (CoA)
- – lyase E71.30
- – mutase E71.12
- colour vision, acquired H53.5
- copper E61.0
- coproporphyrinogen oxidase E80.21
- cystathionine β-synthase E72.100
- dihydrobiopterin synthetase E70.03
- dihydrolipoamide dehydrogenase E74.402
- dihydropteridine reductase E70.02
- endplate acetylcholinesterase G70.20
- – receptor G70.21
- exo-α-sialidase E77.12

Deficiency (of) — *continued*
- factor
- - VIII D66
- - - with vascular defect D68.0
- - IX D67
- - XI D68
- ferrochetalase E80.01
- folate (folic acid) E53.81
- follicle-stimulating hormone E23.05
- fructokinase E74.10
- fructose-bisphosphatase E74.12
- fructose-bisphosphate aldolase E74.11
- FSH E23.05
- α-L-fucosidase E77.11
- fumarylacetoacetase E70.20
- galactocerebroside β-galactosidase E75.21
- galactokinase E74.21
- galactosamine-6-sulfate sulfatase E76.210
- galactose-1-phosphate uridylyl transferase E74.20
- α-galactosidase E75.22
- β-galactosidase E76.211
- glucocerebrosidase E75.20
- glucose-6-phosphatase E74.00
- β-glucuronidase E76.24
- glutamate–cysteine ligase E72.810
- glutamate decarboxylase E72.814
- glutamate formiminotransferase E70.804
- γ-glutamyltransferase E72.813
- glutaryl-CoA dehydrogenase E72.30
- glutathione synthetase E72.812
- glycerate dehydrogenase E74.81
- glycine dehydrogenase (decarboxylating) E72.53
- gonadotropin E23.02
- growth hormone E23.02
- guanosine triphosphate cyclohydrolase I E70.04
- heparan-*N*-sulfatase E76.200
- β-hexosaminidase E75.0
- histidase E70.800
- histidinase E70.800
- histidine ammonia-lyase E70.800
- hydroxymethylbilane synthase E80.20
- hydroxymethylglutaryl-CoA lysase E88.820
- 4-hydroxyphenylpyruvate dioxygenase E70.10
- hypoxanthine phosphoribosyltransferase E79.1
- L-iduronidase E76.0
- imidazole E70.802
- iron E61.1
- isoleucine transaminase E71.15
- isovaleryl-CoA dehydrogenase E71.11
- kalium E87.6
- ketoacid, branched-chain
- - dehydrogenase

Deficiency (of) — *continued*
- ketoacid, branched-chain — *continued*
- - dehydrogenase — *continued*
- - - partial E71.01
- - - severe E71.00
- - dihydrolipoyltransacetylase E71.02
- kynureninase E70.812
- lactase
- - congenital E73.0
- - secondary E73.1
- lecithin cholesterol acyltransferase E78.65
- leucine transaminase E71.15
- LH E23.05
- lipoprotein E78.6
- liver phosphorylase E74.05
- luteinizing hormone E23.05
- lysosomal α-glucosidase E74.01
- mannose-6-phosphate isomerase E74.83
- α-mannosidase E77.10
- 3-methyl crotonyl-CoA carboxylase E88.820
- methylmalonyl-CoA mutase E71.12
- muscle
- - carnitine E71.312
- - lactate dehydrogenase E74.86
- - phosphorylase E74.040
- - - kinase E74.041
- myoadenylate deaminase E79.83
- natrium E87.10
- NADH-coenzyme Q reductase E88.830
- niacin(-tryptophan) E52
- - sequelae E64.–
- nicotinamide E52
- nutrient element specified NEC E61.–
- nutritional, sequelae E64.–
- ornithine carbamoyltransferase E72.40
- ornithine–ketoacid aminotransferase E72.41
- ornithine transcarbamylase E72.40
- orotate phosphoribosyl transferase E79.81
- orotidine-5′-phosphate decarboxylase E79.82
- 5-oxoprolinase E72.811
- oxygen, systemic T71
- oxytocin E23.31
- pantothenic acid E53.83
- phenylalanine 4-monooxygenase
- - partial E70.01
- - severe E70.00
- phosphoenolpyruvate carboxykinase E74.411
- 6-phosphofructokinase E74.06
- phosphoglycerate
- - kinase E74.85
- - mutase E74.84
- pituitary hormones
- - anterior, multiple E23.07
- - multiple E23.00

Déjerine–Sottas disease or neuropathy G60.02
Déjerine's global aphasia R47.02
De Lange's syndrome Q87.12
Delay, delayed
- development, physiological R62.0
- milestone R62.0
- muscle maturation G72.82
- puberty E30.0
Deletion
- autosome Q93.9
- - specified NEC Q93.8
- chromosome
- - at prometaphase Q93.6
- - part Q93.5
- - short arm
- - - 4 Q93.3
- - - 5 Q93.4
- mitochondrial DNA E88.833
Delirium
- alcohol-induced F10.4
- mixed origin F05.8
- not superimposed on dementia F05.0
- superimposed on dementia F05.1
- tremens (alcohol-induced) F10.4
- withdrawal state F1*x*.4
Delivery, complications affecting fetus and newborn P03.–
Dementia F03
- alcoholic F10.73
- Alzheimer's type G30.9† F00.9*
- - - atypical G30.8† F00.8*
- - - presenile G30.0† F00.0*
- - - senile G30.1† F00.1*
- arteriosclerotic F01.9
- frontal lobe G31.02
- in (due to)
- - Alzheimer's disease G30.9† F00.9*
- - - atypical G30.8† F00.2*
- - - early onset G30.0† F00.0*
- - - late onset G30.1† F00.1*
- - brain atrophy, circumscribed G31.0† F02.8*
- - carbon monoxide poisoning T58† F02.8*
- - ceroid lipofuscinosis, adult E75.43† F02.8*
- - Creutzfeldt–Jakob disease A81.0† F02.1*
- - epilepsy G40.–† F02.8*
- - human immunodeficiency virus disease B22.0† F02.4*
- - Huntington's disease G10.–† F02.2*
- - hypercalcaemia E83.5† F02.8*
- - hyperthyroidism, acquired E03.–† F02.8*
- - Lewy body disease G31.85† F02.8
- - multiple sclerosis G35.–† F02.8*
Dementia — *continued*
- in (due to) — *continued*
- - neurosyphilis A52.1† F02.8*
- - niacin deficiency E52† F02.8*
- - paralysis agitans G20.–† F02.3*
- - parkinsonism G20.–† F02.3*
- - Pick's disease G31.00† F02.0*
- - polyarteritis nodosa M30.0† F02.8*
- - systemic lupus erythematosus M32.–† F02.8*
- - trypanosomiasis
- - - African B56.9† F02.8*
- - - American B57.–† F02.8*
- - vitamin B_{12} deficiency E53.80† F02.8*
- infantilis F84.3
- paralytica juvenilis A50.40
- presenile F03
- senile F03
- - with delirium F05.1
- vascular F01.9
- - acute onset F01.0
- - mixed cortical and subcortical F01.3
- - multi-infarct F01.1
- - predominantly cortical F01.1
- - specified NEC F01.8
- - subcortical F01.2
Demoralization R45.3
Demotivation R45.3
Demyelination
- central nervous system G37.9
- - specified NEC G37.8
- corpus callosum G37.1
- disseminated, acute G36.9
- - specified NEC G36.8
- spinal cord, in optic neuritis G36.0
Dengue fever
- classical A90
- haemorrhagic A91
Denny–Brown syndrome D48.9† G13.01*
Dependence
- due to
- - alcohol F10.2
- - caffeine F15.2
- - cannabinoids F12.2
- - cocaine F14.2
- - hallucinogens F16.2
- - hypnotics F13.2
- - opioids F11.2
- - psychoactive substances NEC F19.2
- - sedatives F13.2
- - stimulants NEC F15.2
- - tobacco F17.2
- - volatile solvents F18.2
- on
- - aspirator Z99.0
- - care-provider, problems related to Z74.–
- - enabling machine or device NEC Z99.8

Dependence — *continued*
– on — *continued*
– – renal dialysis Z99.2
– – respirator Z99.1
– – wheelchair Z99.3
Depletion, volume E86
Depolarization, premature I49.–
Depression F32.9
– agitated, single episode F32.2
– anxiety, persistent F34.1
– atypical F32.8
– cerebral, neonatal P91.4
– endogenous F33.2
– – with psychotic symptoms F33.3
– major
– – recurrent F33.2
– – – with psychotic symptoms F33.3
– – single episode F32.2
– – – with psychotic symptoms F32.3
– masked F32.8
– monopolar F33.9
– neurotic F34.1
– psychogenic
– – recurrent F33.9
– – single episode F32.9
– psychotic
– – recurrent F33.3
– – single episode F32.3
– reactive
– – recurrent F33.9
– – single episode F32.9
– recurrent F33.9
– – specified NEC F33.8
– single episode F32.9
– – specified NEC F32.8
– skull, congenital Q67.4
– vital
– – recurrent F33.2
– – single episode F32.9
Deprivation effect T73.–
Dermatomyositis M33.–
– paraneoplastic M36.00
Dermatopolymyositis M33.9
– specified NEC M33.28
Detachment
– choroid H31.4
– retina H33.–
– – pigment epithelium H35.7
– – rhegmatogenous H33.0
– – traction H33.4
– – with
– – – proliferative vitreo-retinopathy H33.4
– – – retinal break H33.0
Deterioration, general physical R53
Deuteranomaly H53.5
Deuteranopia H53.5
Development
– physiological, delayed R62.0
Development — *continued*
– retarded, following protein-energy malnutrition E45
– sexual, delayed E30.0
Deviation
– midline, of dental arch K07.2
– nasal septum, congenital Q67.4
Devic's syndrome G36.0
Dhat syndrome F48.81
Diabetes
– chemical R73.0
– insipidus E23.2
– – nephrogenic N25.1
– latent R73.0
– mellitus E14.–
– – insulin-dependent E10.–
– – malnutrition-related E12.–
– – maternal (pre-existing), affecting fetus and newborn P70.1
– – neonatal P70.2
– – non-insulin-dependent E11.–
– – specified NEC E13.–
Diaphragmatitis J98.6
Diarrhoea, functional K59.1
Diastasis of muscle M62.0
Diastematomyelia Q06.2
Dicephaly Q89.4
Diencephalic syndrome E23.30
Difficulty (in)
– feeding R63.3
– life-management Z73.–
– swallowing R13
– walking R26.2
Dilatation, aorta I71.9
Diphtheria A36.–
Diphyllobothriasis B70.0
Diplacusis H93.2
Diplegia
– ataxic, congenital G11.02
– spastic G80.1
– upper limbs G83.0
Diplomyelia Q06.80
Diplopia H53.2
Dipsomania F10.2
Disability
– knowledge acquisition F81.9
– learning F81.9
– limiting activities Z73.6
Discitis M46.4
Disease — *see also* Syndrome
– Addison's E27.1
– Alpers' G31.80
– alpha heavy chain C88.1
– Alzheimer's G30.9
– – dementia in G30.9† F00.9*
– – Guamanian-type G30.80
– Andersen's E74.03
– autoimmune (systemic) M35.9

Disease — *continued*
- atherosclerotic
- - cardiovascular I25.0
- - coronary (heart) I25.1
- atticoantral, chronic H66.2
- bacterial, specified NEC A48.–
- Baló's G37.5
- Bassen–Kornzweig E78.62
- Batten's E75.4
- Behçet's M35.2
- Bielschowsky–Jansky E75.41
- Binswanger's I67.3
- Bornholm B33.0
- Bourneville's Q85.1
- brain, congenital Q04.9
- Buerger's I73.1
- caisson T70.3
- Calvé's M42.0
- capillaries I78.–
- central nervous system, demyelinating G37.–
- cerebellar, hereditary G11.9
- cerebrovascular, specified NEC I67.–
- - sequelae I69.–
- Chagas' B57.–
- Chanarin's E75.52
- Charcot–Marie–Tooth
- - hypertrophic demyelinative G60.00
- - neuronal G60.01
- Charcot's G12.20
- Christmas D67
- Claude's I67.9† G46.30*
- collagen (vascular) M35.9
- compressed-air T70.3
- connective tissue, mixed M35.1
- Cori's E74.02
- coronary (artery) I25.1
- Creutzfeldt–Jakob A81.0
- - dementia in A81.0† F02.1*
- Crohn's K50
- Crouzon's Q75.1
- Cushing's, pituitary-dependent E24.0
- cytomegaloviral B25.–
- - congenital P35.1
- degenerative (of) (*see also* Degeneration)
- - basal ganglia G23.–
- - nervous system, specified NEC G31.–
- Déjerine–Sottas G60.02
- demyelinating, central nervous system G37.–
- digestive system K92.–
- ear, inner H83.–
- Ebola virus A98.4
- Erb's G71.03
- Fabry(–Anderson) E75.22
- Fahr's G23.850
- Fazio–Londe G12.110
- Forbes' E74.02

Disease — *continued*
- Forestier's M48.1
- Franklin's C88.2
- gamma heavy chain C88.2
- Gaucher's E75.20
- Gerstmann–Straussler–Scheinker's A81.81
- glomerular N05
- glycogen storage E74.0
- Graves' E05.0
- - ophthalmic H05.22
- haemoglobin-M D74.0
- haemorrhagic, fetus and newborn P53
- Hageman's D68.2
- Hallervorden–Spatz G23.0
- Hand–Schüller–Christian D76.0
- Hansen's A30.–
- Harada's H30.8
- Hartnup's E70.810
- Hb-M D74.0
- Hb-SS, with crisis D57.0
- heart
- - atherosclerotic I25.1
- - hypertensive I11
- - ischaemic
- - - acute I24
- - - chronic I25.–
- - meningococcal A39.5
- - rheumatic NEC I09.–
- - - acute or active I01.9
- - thyrotoxic E05.9† I43.*
- herpesviral, disseminated B00.7
- Hers' E74.05
- Heubner's I66.1† G46.11*
- HIV — *see* Human immunodeficiency virus (HIV) disease
- Hodgkin's C81
- Huntington's G10.–
- - dementia in G10.–† F02.2*
- Hurler's E76.00
- Hurst's G36.1
- hyaline membrane P22.0
- I-cell E77.00
- immunoproliferative, malignant C88.–
- infectious, congenital NEC P37.–
- ischaemic heart
- - acute I24
- - chronic I25.–
- Jeune's Q77.2
- Jordan's E75.53
- Kahler's C90.0
- Krabbe's E75.21
- Kuf's E75.43
- Kugelberg–Welander G12.101
- Kunjin virus A83.4
- Kyasanur Forest A98.2
- larynx J38.–
- Leigh's G31.81
- Letterer–Siwe C96.0

Disease — *continued*
- Lewy body, diffuse G31.85
- Libman–Sacks M32.1† I39*
- Little's G80.–
- liver
- – alcoholic K70.–
- – toxic K71.–
- Luft's G71.33
- Lutz' B41.–
- Lyme A69.2
- lymphoproliferative D47.9
- lymphoreticular tissue D76.–
- Machado–Joseph G11.24
- maple-syrup-urine E71.00
- Marburg virus A98.3
- Marchiafava–Bignami G37.1
- McArdle's E74.04
- Ménière's H81.0
- Menkes' E83.00
- motor neuron G12.2
- – paraneoplastic G13.12
- moyamoya I67.5
- nervous system
- – congenital Q07.9
- – maternal, complicating pregnancy, childbirth and the puerperium O99.3
- Niemann–Pick E75.26
- oasthouse E72.03
- Ollier's Q78.4
- Owren's D68.2
- Paget's, of bone M88.–
- pancreas NEC K86.–
- parasitic, congenital NEC P37.–
- Parkinson's G20.–
- – dementia in G20.–† F02.3*
- Pick's G31.00
- – dementia in G31.00† F02.0*
- Pompe's E74.010
- Pott's A18.0† M49.0*
- Powassan virus A84.8
- prion, of central nervous system A81.–
- protozoal NEC B60.–
- pulp, dental, and periapical tissues K04
- Raynaud's I73.0
- Refsum's G60.1
- – infantile E80.300
- renal, hypertensive I12
- Rendu–Osler–Weber I78.0
- reticulohistiocytic system D76.–
- rheumatic (of)
- – aortic valve I06
- – endocardium I09.1
- – heart I09.–
- – mitral valve I05.–
- – pulmonary valve I09.8
- – tricuspid valve I07
- Rocio virus A83.6
- Ross River B33.1

Disease — *continued*
- Sandhoff's E75.03
- Scheuermann's M42.0
- Schilder's G37.0
- Segawa's G24.13
- simian B B00.4† G05.1*
- Simmonds' E23.00
- slim B22.2
- Spielmeyer–Vogt E75.42
- spinal cord
- – congenital Q06.9
- – specified NEC G95.–
- spleen D73.–
- Stargardt's H35.5
- Steele–Richardson–Olszewski G23.10
- Steinert's G71.12
- stomach NEC K31.–
- Stuart–Prower D68.2
- Takahara's E80.310
- Tangier E78.60
- Tauri's E74.06
- Tay–Sachs E75.00
- Thomsen's G71.130
- thymus E32.–
- thyrotoxic heart E05.9† I43.–*
- tubotympanic, chronic H66.1
- Unverricht–Lundborg G40.37
- valve (*see also* Disorder, valve) I08.–
- rheumatic
- – aortic I06
- – mitral I05
- – tricuspid I07
- van Bogaert–Scherer–Epstein E75.50
- vascular, peripheral NEC I73.–
- Venezuelan equine encephalitis virus A92.2
- viral, virus — *see also* Disease, by type of virus
- – congenital P35.–
- vocal cords J38.–
- Von Economo–Cruchet A85.8
- Von Gierke's E74.00
- Von Recklinghausen's Q85.0
- – of bone E21.0
- von Willebrand's D68.0
- Weber–Christian M35.6
- Werdnig–Hoffmann G12.0
- Whipple's K90.8† M14.8*
- Wilson's E83.01
- Wolman's E75.51

Dislocation (articular) T14.3
- head, part NEC S03.3
- jaw S03.0
- mandible S03.0
- multiple
- – body regions NEC T03.8
- – head with neck T03.0
- – thorax with lower back and pelvis T03.1

Dislocation (articular) — *continued*
- neck S13.2
- – multiple S13.3
- nose, septal cartilage S03.1
- pelvis, part NEC S33.3
- spine
- – cervical S13.1
- – lumbar S33.1
- – – part NEC S33.3
- – thoracic S23.1
- temporomandibular (joint) S03.0
- tooth S03.2
- vertebra
- – cervical S13.1
- – lumbar S33.1
- – thoracic S23.1

Disorder (of) — *see also* Disease
- absorption, intestinal carbohydrate NEC E74
- accommodation H52.5
- acid–base balance, mixed E87.4
- adrenal gland E27.9
- – specified NEC E27.8
- adrenogenital E25.9
- – idiopathic E25.8
- – specified NEC E25.8
- – with enzyme deficiency E25.0
- affective (*see also* Disorder, mood) F39
- – bipolar F31.9
- – – specified NEC F31.8
- – organic F06.3
- – – right hemispheric F07.8
- – persistent F34.9
- – – specified NEC F34.8
- – personality F34.0
- – recurrent NEC F38.1
- – single NEC F38.0
- – specified NEC F38.8
- amnesic, amnestic
- – alcohol-induced F10.6
- – organic F04
- – psychoactive substance-induced — code to F11–F19 with fourth character .6
- anxiety, organic F06.4
- arithmetical skills, specific F81.2
- arteries and arterioles NEC I77.8
- attention deficit F98
- – with hyperactivity F90.0
- autistic F84.0
- behaviour, behavioural
- – organic F07.9
- – – specified NEC F07.8
- – REM-sleep-related G47.800
- bipolar
- – affective F31.9
- – – current episode
- – – – hypomanic F31.0
- – – – manic F31.1

Disorder (of) — *continued*
- bipolar — *continued*
- – affective — *continued*
- – – current episode — *continued*
- – – – manic — *continued*
- – – – – with psychotic symptoms F31.2
- – – – mild or moderate depression F31.3
- – – – mixed F31.6
- – – – severe depression F31.4
- – – – – with psychotic symptoms
- – – in remission F31.7
- – – specified NEC F31.8
- – single manic episode F30.–
- – II F31.8
- body dysmorphic F45.2
- bone NEC M89.8
- brachial plexus G54.0
- brain G93.9
- – specified NEC G93.8
- breast NEC N64
- Briquet's F48.80
- carbohydrate
- – absorption, intestinal NEC E74.3
- – metabolism E74.–
- central nervous system G96.9
- – specified NEC G96.8
- cerebrovascular, sequelae I69.–
- cervical root NEC G54.2
- character F68.8
- childhood disintegrative NEC F84.3
- choroid H31.9
- – specified NEC H31.8
- circulatory system, postprocedural NEC I97
- cognitive, mild F06.7
- conduct, hyperkinetic F90.1
- conduction NEC I45.–
- conversion (*see also* Disorder, dissociative) F44.9
- delusional, organic F06.2
- depressive (*see also* Episode, depressive) F32.9
- – organic F06.32
- – recurrent F33.9
- – – current episode
- – – – mild F33.0
- – – – moderate F33.1
- – – – severe F33.2
- – – – – with psychotic symptoms F33.3
- – – in remission
- – – specified NEC F33.8
- – seasonal F33.–
- development, developmental
- – arithmetical (skills) F81.2
- – coordination F82
- – expressive writing F81.8
- – language F80.9
- – – specified NEC F80.8

Disorder (of) — *continued*
- metabolism, metabolic — *continued*
- - following abortion or ectopic or molar pregnancy O08.5
- - fructose E74.1
- - galactose E74.2
- - glutamic acid E72.81
- - γ-glutamyl cycle E72.81
- - glycine E72.5
- - glycogen E74.08
- - glycoprotein E77.9
- - - specified NEC E77.8
- - glycosaminoglycan E76.9
- - - specified NEC E76.8
- - histidine E70.80
- - hydroxylysine E72.3
- - iron E83.1
- - keto-acid, intermediary branched-chain E88.820
- - lipoprotein E78.9
- - - specified NEC E78.8
- - lysine E72.3
- - magnesium E83.4
- - - neonatal, transitory P71.2
- - mineral E83.9
- - - specified NEC E83.8
- - non-ketotic hyperglycinate E72.55
- - ornithine E72.4
- - parathyroid gland E21.9
- - - specified NEC E21.8
- - phosphorus E83.3
- - plasma-protein NEC E88.0
- - porphyrin E80.2
- - postprocedural NEC E89.8
- - purine E79.9
- - - specified NEC E79.8
- - pyrimidine E79.9
- - - specified NEC E79.8
- - pyruvate E74.40
- - specified NEC E88.8
- - sphingolipid E75.–
- - tryptophan E70.81
- - tyrosine E70.2
- - urea cycle E72.2
- - zinc E83.2
- mood F39
- - organic F06.3
- - persistent F34.9
- - - specified NEC F34.8
- - recurrent NEC F38.1
- - single NEC F38.0
- specified NEC F38.8
- motor
- - dissociative F44.4
- - function, developmental F82
- movement G25.9
- - binocular H51.9
- - - specified NEC G25.8

Disorder (of) — *continued*
- movement — *continued*
- - limb, paroxysmal nocturnal G25.80
- - specified NEC G25.8
- - stereotyped F98.4
- muscle
- - primary G71.9
- - - specified NEC G71.8
- - specified NEC M62.8
- - tone, newborn P94.9
- - - specified NEC P94.8
- myoneural G70.9
- - specified NEC G70.8
- - toxic G70.1
- myotonic G71.1
- nerve
- - accessory G52.81
- - acoustic H93.3
- - cranial G52
- - - eighth H93.3
- - - eleventh G52.81
- - - fifth NEC G50.8
- - - first G52.0
- - - multiple G52.7
- - - ninth G52.1
- - - second NEC H47.0
- - - seventh NEC G51.9
- - - specified NEC G52.8
- - - tenth G52.2
- - - twelfth G52.3
- - facial G51.9
- - - specified NEC G51.8
- - glossopharyngeal G52.1
- - hypoglossal G52.3
- - olfactory G52.0
- - optic NEC H47.0
- - plexus G54.9
- - - specified NEC G54.8
- - pneumogastric G52.2
- - root G54.9
- - - specified NEC G54.8
- - trigeminal G50.9
- - - specified NEC G50.8
- - vagus G52.2
- nervous system
- - autonomic G90.9
- - - specified NEC G90.8
- - central G96.9
- - - specified NEC G96.8
- - degenerative G31.9
- - - specified NEC G31.8
- - peripheral NEC G64
- - postprocedural G97.9
- - - specified NEC G97.8
- - specified NEC G98
- neurotic F48.9
- - specified NEC F48.8
- obsessive–compulsive F42

Dissociative — *continued*
- fugue F44.1
- motor disorders F44.4
- stupor F44.2
Disto-occlusion K07.2
Distress
- fetal P20.–
- intrauterine P20.–
- maternal, during labour and delivery O75.0
- respiratory of newborn P22.–
Disturbance — *see also* Disorder
- activity and attention F90.0
- cerebral status of newborn NEC P91.9
- - specified NEC P91.8
- electrolyte, neonatal, transitory P74.–
- endocrine E34.9
- gait, due to loss of postural reflexes R26.20
- hormone E34.9
- metabolic, neonatal, transitory P74.–
- potassium balance, newborn P74.3
- sensation, skin R20.8
- smell R43.8
- sodium balance, newborn P74.2
- - taste R43.8
- speech NEC R47.8
- visual H53.9
- - specified NEC H53.8
- voice R49.8
Diver's palsy or paralysis T70.3
Division of nerve, traumatic T14.4
Dizziness R42
Dolichocephaly Q67.2
Dorsalgia M54.9
- specified NEC M54.8
Dorsopathy M53.9
- deforming M43.9
- - specified NEC M43.8
- specified NEC M53.8
Double
- monster Q89.4
- vision H53.2
Down's syndrome Q90.–
Drop attack R26.22
Drowning T75.1
Drowsiness R40.0
Drug
- addiction — *code to* F10–F19 with fourth character .2
- adverse effect NEC, correct substance properly administered T88.7
- dependence — *code to* F10–F19 with fourth character .2
- harmful use — *code to* F10–F19 with fourth character .1
- overdose — *see* Table of drugs and chemicals, page 565
Drug — *continued*
- poisoning — *see* Table of drugs and chemicals, page 565
Drunkenness F10.0
Drusen (of)
- macula (degeneration) H35.3
- optic disc H47.30
Dry mouth R68.2
- due to sicca syndrome M35.0
Duane's syndrome H50.8
Dubin–Johnson syndrome E80.60
Dubowitz' syndrome Q87.13
Duchenne-type muscular dystrophy G71.07
Duodenitis K29.8
Duplication, chromosome NEC
- seen only at prometaphase Q92.4
- with complex rearrangements NEC Q92.5
Dwarfism
- Lorain–Levi E23.021
- pituitary E23.022
Dysaesthesia R20.3
Dysarthria R47.1
Dysautonomia, familial G90.1
Dysequilibrium syndrome, congenital G11.06
Dysfibrinogenaemia (congenital) D68.2
Dysfunction (of)
- autonomic
- - due to alcohol G31.23
- - somatoform F45.3
- bladder
- - neurogenic NEC N31.9
- - neuromuscular N31.9
- - - specified NEC N31.8
- hypothalamic NEC E23.3
- labyrinthine H83.2
- ovarian E28
- pineal gland E34.8
- polyglandular E31.–
- symbolic NEC R48.8
- testicular E29
Dysgenesis, pure gonadal Q99.1
Dysgeusia R43.21
Dyskinesia G24.9
Dyslalia F80.0
Dyslexia R48.0
- developmental F81.0
Dysmenorrhoea N94.6
- primary N94.4
- psychogenic F45.8
- secondary N94.5
Dysmorphism (due to)
- alcohol Q86.0
- warfarin Q86.2
Dysmorphophobia (nondelusional) F45.2
Dysostosis
- craniofacial Q75.1
- mandibulofacial Q75.4

Dysostosis — *continued*
- oculomandibular Q75.5
Dyspareunia N94.1
Dyspepsia K30
- psychogenic F45.3
Dysphagia R13
- psychogenic F45.8
Dysphasia R47.0
- developmental F80.2
Dysphonia R49.0
- isolated spasmodic G24.24
- psychogenic F44.4
Dysplasia (of)
- arterial, fibromuscular I77.3
- asphyxiating thoracic Q77.2
- diastrophic Q77.5
- eye Q11.2
- polyostotic fibrous Q78.1
- progressive diaphyseal Q78.3
- septo-optic Q04.4
- spinal cord Q06.1
Dyspnoea R06.0
Dyspraxia, developmental F82
Dyssynergia cerebellaris myoclonica, Hunt's G11.13
Dysthymia F34.1
Dystonia G24.9
- drug-induced G24.0
- idiopathic
- - familial G24.1
- - nonfamilial G24.2
- - orofacial G24.4
- nocturnal paroxysmal G47.813
- specified NEC G24.8
Dystrophy, dystrophia
- adiposogenital E23.61
- choroidal (central areolar) (generalized) (peripapillary) (hereditary) H31.2
- Landouzy–Déjerine G71.02
- muscular (*see also* muscular dystrophy) G71.0
- myotonica G71.12
- neuroaxonal G31.82
- reflex, sympathetic M89.0
- retinal (albipunctate) (pigmentary) (vitelliform) (hereditary) H35.5
- yellow liver K72
Dysuria R30.0

E

Eating strike R63.81
Eaton–Lambert syndrome C80† G73.1*
– unassociated with neoplasm G70.80
Ebola virus A98.4
Echinococcosis B67.–
Eclampsia O15.9
– during labour O15.1
– pregnancy O15.0
– puerperal O15.2
Edwards' syndrome Q91.3
Effusion (of)
– ear H92.–
– pleural NEC J90
Ehlers–Danlos syndrome Q79.6
Ekbom's syndrome G25.82
Elaboration of physical symptoms for psychological reasons F68.0
Electric current, effects T75.4
Electrocution T75.4
Electrolyte imbalance E87.8
Elevated, elevation
– blood glucose level R73.–
– erythrocyte sedimentation rate R70.0
– lactic acid dehydrogenase (LDH) level R74.0
– transaminase level R74.0
Embolism
– air
– – obstetric O88.0
– – postprocedural NEC T81.7
– – traumatic T79.0
– amniotic fluid O88.1
– aorta I74.1
– – abdominal I74.0
– artery, arterial I75.9
– – basilar I65.1
– – carotid I65.2
– – cerebellar I66.3
– – cerebral I66.9
– – – causing cerebral infarction I63.4
– – – specified NEC I66.8
– – extremity
– – – lower I74.3
– – – upper I74.4
– – iliac I75.5
– – peripheral I74.4
– – precerebral I65.9
– – – causing cerebral infarction I63.1
– – – specified NEC I65.8
– – specified NEC I75.8
– – vertebral I65.0
– blood-clot, obstetric O88.2

Embolism — *continued*
– fat
– – obstetric O88.8
– – traumatic T79.1
– following abortion and ectopic and molar pregnancy O08.2
– obstetric NEC O88.8
– pyaemic, obstetric O88.3
– septic
– – of intracranial and intraspinal venous sinuses and veins G08.–
– – obstetric O88.3
Emery–Dreifuss muscular dystrophy G71.01
Emphysema J43
– (subcutaneous) resulting from a procedure T81.8
Empyema of sinus (accessory) (nasal)
– acute J01.–
– chronic J32.–
Encephalitis G04.9
– acute disseminated G04.0
– adenoviral A85.1† G05.1*
– amoebic B60.2† G05.2*
– Australian A83.4
– California A83.5
– cytomegaloviral B25.8† G05.1*
– enteroviral A85.0† G05.1*
– equine
– – eastern A83.2
– – Venezuelan A92.2
– – Western A83.1
– herpesviral B00.4† G05.1*
– in (due to)
– – African trypanosomiasis B56.–† G05.2*
– – Chagas' disease B57.4† G05.2*
– – Lyme disease A69.2† G05.2*
– – naegleriasis B60.2† G05.2*
– – toxoplasmosis B58.2† G05.2*
– Japanese A83.0
– La Crosse A83.5
– lethargica A85.8
– listerial A32.1† G05.0*
– measles B05.0† G05.1*
– meningococcal A39.8† G05.0*
– mumps B26.2† G05.1*
– periaxial G37.0
– postchickenpox B01.1† G05.1*
– postimmunization G04.00
– postinfectious G04.80
– postmeasles B05.0† G05.1*
– rubella B06.00† G05.1*

Encephalitis — *continued*
- Russian spring–summer A84.0
- specified NEC G04.8
- St Louis A83.3
- syphilitic
- - congenital A50.4† G05.0*
- - late A52.1† G05.0*
- tuberculous A17.8† G05.0*
- varicella B01.1† G05.1*
- viral, virus A86
- - arthropod-borne NEC A85.2
- - herpes B00.4† G05.1*
- - mosquito-borne A83.–
- - sequelae B94.1
- - specified NEC A85.2
- - tick-borne
- - - central European A84.1
- - - Far Eastern A84.0
- zoster B02.0† G05.1*

Encephalocele Q01.9
- frontal Q01.0
- nasofrontal Q01.1
- nasopharyngeal Q01.81
- occipital Q01.2
- orbital Q01.83
- parietal Q01.80
- specified NEC Q01.8
- temporal Q01.82

Encephalomalacia, multi-cystic Q04.62

Encephalomyelitis G04.9
- adenoviral A85.1† G05.1*
- amoebic B60.2† G05.2*
- benign myalgic G93.3
- cytomegaloviral B25.8† G05.1*
- enteroviral A85.0† G05.1*
- equine, Venezuelan A92.2
- herpesviral B00.4† G05.1*
- in
- - African trypanosomiasis B56.–† G05.2*
- - Chagas' disease B57.4† G05.2*
- - Lyme disease A69.2† G05.2*
- - naegleriasis B60.2† G05.2*
- - toxoplasmosis B58.2† G05.2*
- listerial A32.1† G05.0*
- measles B05.0† G05.1*
- mumps B26.2† G05.1*
- postchickenpox B01.1† G05.1*
- zoster B02.0† G05.1*
- postimmunization G04.01
- postinfectious G04.81
- specified NEC G04.8
- syphilitic
- - congenital A50.4† G05.0*
- - late A52.1† G05.0*
- varicella B01.1† G05.1*

Encephalomyelocele Q01.*xx*0

Encephalopathy G93.4
- alcoholic G31.21

Encephalopathy — *continued*
- epileptic, early infantile G40.41
- hepatic K72.–
- HIV-associated B22.0
- hypertensive I67.4
- in (due to)
- - influenza J11.8
- - - influenza virus identified J10.8
- - vitamin B_{12} deficiency E53.80† G94.82*
- limbic, paraneoplastic G13.10
- myoclonic, early, symptomatic G40.45
- necrotizing, subacute G31.81
- postcontusional F07.2
- posthypoglycaemic (coma) E16.10
- postradiation G93.80
- spongiform, subacute A81.0
- toxic
- - early G92.–0
- - late G92.–1
- Wernicke's E51.2

Enchondromatosis Q78.4

Encopresis R15
- nonorganic origin F98.1

Endarteritis I77.6

Endocarditis (chronic) I38
- rheumatic
- - acute I01.1
- - chronic I09.1
- rheumatoid M05.3† I39.–*

Endophlebitis I80
- septic, of intracranial and intraspinal venous sinuses and veins G08.–

Enlargement, enlarged
- sulci R90.81
- ventricular R90.80

Enophthalmos H05.4

Enteritis
- campylobacter A04.5
- granulomatous K50
- regional K50

Enthesopathy, spinal M46.0

Enucleation, traumatic S05.7

Enuresis R32
- nonorganic origin F98.0
- sleep-related G47.811

Epiduritis G06.11

Epilepsy G40.9
- absence
- - childhood G40.33
- - juvenile G40.35
- generalized
- - idiopathic G40.3
- - specified NEC G40.4
- grand mal NEC G40.6
- Kozhevnikof's G40.50
- localization-related
- - idiopathic G40.0
- - symptomatic, with partial seizures

Epilepsy — *continued*
- localization-related — *continued*
- - symptomatic, with partial seizures — *continued*
- - - complex G40.2
- - - simple G40.1
- myoclonic
- - benign, in infancy G40.30
- - juvenile G40.36
- - severe, in infancy G40.890
- - with ragged red fibres G40.46
- petit mal
- - impulsive G40.36
- - specified NEC G40.7
- reflex G40.57
- specified NEC G40.8
- Unverricht–Lundborg G40.37
Epiloia Q85.1
Episode
- affective, mixed F38.0
- depressive F32.9
- - mild F32.0
- - moderate F32.1
- - recurrent brief F38.1
- - severe F32.2
- - - with psychotic symptoms F32.3
- - specified NEC F32.8
- manic F30.9
- - recurrent F31.8
- - specified NEC F30.8
Erb's
- disease G71.03
- paralysis due to birth injury P14.0
Erection
- non-painful, impaired REM sleep-related G47.801
- painful N48.3
- - REM-sleep-related G47.802
Erosion — *see also* Ulcer
- artery I77.2
Erythema
- chronicum migrans A69.2
- multiforme L51
- nodosum L52
Erythrocyanosis I73.8
Erythrocytosis, familial D75.0
Erythromelalgia I73.8
Esophoria H50.5
Esotropia, intermittent H50.3
Evaluation — *see* Observation
Evans' syndrome D69.3
Evasiveness R46.5
Eventration of diaphragm Q79.1
Examination (general) (routine) (for) (of)
- administrative purpose Z02.9
- - specified NEC Z02.8
- admission to
- - educational institution Z02.0

Examination (general) — *continued*
- admission to — *continued*
- - prison Z02.8
- - residential institution Z02.2
- - summer camp Z02.8
- adolescent development state Z00.3
- adoption Z02.8
- child
- - development Z00.1
- - health, routine Z00.1
- - rapid growth Z00.2
- driving licence Z02.3
- ears Z01.1
- eyes Z01.0
- follow-up, after
- - chemotherapy Z09.2
- - - for malignant neoplasm Z08.2
- - psychotherapy Z09.3
- - radiotherapy Z09.1
- - - for malignant neoplasm Z08.1
- - surgery Z09.0
- - - for malignant neoplasm Z08.0
- - treatment Z09.9
- - - fracture Z09.4
- - - malignant neoplasm Z08.9
- - - - specified NEC Z08.8
- - - specified NEC Z09.8
- growth in childhood Z00.3
- hearing Z01.1
- immigration Z02.8
- insurance purposes Z02.6
- medicolegal reason Z04
- naturalization Z02.8
- pre-employment Z02.1
- premarital Z02.8
- puberty development Z00.3
- recruitment, armed forces Z02.3
- special screening (for)
- - chromosomal abnormality Z13.7
- - congenital malformation and deformation Z13.7
- - developmental disorders in childhood Z13.4
- - disease and disorder NEC Z13.–
- specified NEC Z04
- sport, participation Z02.5
- vision Z01.0
Exanthem, Boston A88.0
Excessive
- crying of infant R68.1
- eating R63.2
- thirst R63.1
Exhaustion R53
- due to
- - exertion, excessive T73.3
- - exposure T73.2
- heat T67.5
- - anhydrotic T67.3

Exhaustion — *continued*
- heat — *continued*
- - due to salt depletion T67.4
Exomphalos Q79.2
Exophoria H50.5
Exophthalmos H05.–
- due to hypothyroidism E05.0
Exostosis, orbit H05.3
Exotropia H50.1
- intermittent H50.3
Exposure (to)
- air pressure, high, low and changes in W94
- cold, excessive, man-made W93
- deep-freeze unit, prolonged W93
- dry ice W93
- electric current W87
- - specified NEC W86
- - transmission line W85

Exposure (to) — *continued*
- environmental factor, man-made NEC W99
- heat, excessive, man-made W92
- liquid air, hydrogen or nitrogen W93
- radiation
- - infrared W90
- - ionizing W88
- - laser W90
- - nonionizing NEC W90
- - radiofrequency W90
- radioactive isotopes W88
- ultraviolet light W89
- visible light W89
- X-rays W88
Extrasystoles I49.4
Eye, eyeball — *see condition*

F

Fabry(–Anderson) disease E75.22
Fahr's disease G23.850
Failed, failure (of) (to)
– cardiac — *see also* Failure, heart
– – due to anaesthesia during labour and delivery O74.2
– – following caesarean or other obstetric procedures O75.4
– cardiorespiratory R09.2
– dosage during medical and surgical care Y63
– gain weight R62.8
– heart I50
– – due to hypertension I11
– – – with renal disease I13
– – rheumatic I09.9
– hepatic
– – alcoholic K70.4
– – due to drugs K71.1
– – specified NEC K72
– menstruation at puberty N91.0
– peripheral circulation NEC R57.9
– polyglandular, autoimmune E31.0
– renal N19
– – acute N17
– – chronic NEC N18.8
– – congenital P96.0
– – following abortion and ectopic and molar pregnancy 008
– – with hypertension I12
– sterile precautions during surgical and medical care Y62
– thrive R62.8
– – resulting from HIV disease B22.2
Fainting R55
Family history — *see* History, family
Fanconi(–de Toni)(–Debré) syndrome E72.04
Farber's syndrome E75.25
Fasciculation R25.3
Fasciitis, diffuse (eosinophilic) M35.4
Fatigue (*see also* Exhaustion) R53
– heat, transient T67.6
– syndrome F48.0
– – postviral G93.3
Fazio–Londe disease or syndrome G12.110
Feeble-mindedness F70.–
Feeding difficulties R63.3
Feigned
– illness, with obvious motivation Z76.5
– symptoms or disabilities F68.1
Feminization (syndrome), testicular E34.5
Fetus, fetal — *see also condition*
– alcohol syndrome (dysmorphic) Q86.0
– hydantoin syndrome Q86.1
Fever
– dengue A90
– – haemorrhagic A91
– enteroviral, exanthematous (A88)
– equine, Venezuelan A92.2
– haemorrhagic
– – arenaviral A96.–† G02.0*
– – dengue A91
– – viral, specified NEC A98.–
– Lassa A96.2
– Malta A23.–
– Mediterranean A23.–
– – familial E85.00
– recurrent A68
– relapsing A68
– rheumatic
– – with heart involvement I01
– – without heart involvement I00
– scarlet A38
– snail B65
– spotted A77
– typhoid A01.0
– typhus A75
– undulant A23.–
– viral
– – haemorrhagic, specified NEC A98.–
– – mosquito-borne, specified NEC A92.–
– yellow A95
Fibrillation
– atrial I48
– ventricular I49.0
Fibrodysplasia ossificans progressiva M61.1
Fibromyalgia M79.0
Fibroplasia, retrolental H35.1
Fibrosclerosis, multifocal M35.5
Fibrosis (of)
– cystic E84.9
– – with intestinal manifestations E84.1
– – with pulmonary manifestations E84.0
– liver, alcoholic K70.2
Fibrositis M79.0
Filariasis B74
Finding in blood (of) (substance not normally found in blood) R78.9
– abnormal level
– – heavy metal R78.7
– – lithium R78.8
– alcohol, excessive R78.0
– cocaine R78.2

Fredrickson's hyperlipoproteinaemia — *continued*
- type IV E78.11

Friedreich's
- ataxia G11.11
- paramyoclonus multiplex G25.32

Fructosuria, essential E74.1
Fucosidosis E77.11
Fugue
- dissociative F44.1
- postictal, in epilepsy G40.9

Fukuyama's muscular dystrophy G71.084
Fusion (of)
- ear ossicles Q16.3
- hemivertebra, with scoliosis Q76.30
- rib, congenital Q76.6
- skull, imperfect Q75.01
- spine
- – congenital, not associated with scoliosis Q76.42
- – specified NEC M43.2

G

Gait
- apraxia R26.23
- - frontal lobe R26.03
- ataxic R26.0
- cerebello-spastic R26.11
- disorder, from muscle weakness R26.12
- disturbance
- - due to loss of postural reflex R26.20
- - senile R26.21
- paralytic R26.1
- paretic R26.12
- spastic R26.10
- staggering R26.0

Galactorrhoea, not associated with childbirth N64.3
Galactosaemia E74.20
Gammaglobulin, increased levels in cerebrospinal fluid R83.40
Gamma heavy chain disease C88.2
Gammopathy
- monoclonal D47.2
- polyclonal D89.0

Ganglionitis, geniculate G51.1
- herpetic, acute B02.2† G53.04*
- postherpetic B02.2† G53.05*

Gangliosidosis E75.11
- GM_1 E75.10
- GM_2 E75.0
- GM_3 E75.12

Gangrene, Raynaud's I73.0
Ganser's syndrome F44.80
Gastritis, alcoholic K29.2
Gastroduodenitis K29.9
Gastroenteritis, influenzal J10.8
Gastroschisis Q79.3
Gaucher's disease E75.20
Gerstmann's syndrome, developmental F81.2
Gerstmann–Straussler–Scheinker disease or syndrome A81.81
Giddiness R42
Gigantism, pituitary E22.0
Gilbert's syndrome E80.4
Gilles de la Tourette's syndrome F95.2
Gillespie's ataxia G11.05
Glaucoma H40.9
- angle-closure, primary H40.2
- congenital Q15.0
- open-angle, primary H40.1
- secondary to
- - drugs H40.6
- - eye inflammation H40.4
- - eye trauma H40.3

Glaucoma — *continued*
- secondary to — *continued*
- - eye disorder NEC H40.5
- specified NEC H40.9

Glaucomatous flecks (subcapsular) H26.2
Glomerular disease N05
Glomerulonephritis N05
- diffuse sclerosing N18.–

Glucose, decreased levels in cerebrospinal fluid R83.81
Glue ear H65.3
Glycogen storage disease E74.0
Glycosuria, renal E74.0
Goitre
- congenital (nontoxic) E03.0
- endemic (iodine-deficiency) E01.2
- - diffuse E01.0
- - multinodular E01.1
- exophthalmic E05.0
- iodine-deficiency related (endemic) E01.2
- lymphadenoid E06.3
- nontoxic E04
- - congenital E03.0
- toxic E05.0

Goldblatt's kidney I70.1
Goldenhar's syndrome Q87.03
Goldstein's aphasia R47.0
Goodpasture's syndrome M31.0
Gout M10
Grand mal
- seizures G40.6
- status epilepticus G41.0

Granuloma
- eosinophilic D76.0
- epidural (extradural) G06.11
- foreign body (in soft tissue) NEC M60.2
- intracranial G06.0
- intraspinal G06.1
- midline, lethal M31.2
- orbit H05.1
- spinal cord G06.10
- subdural G06.12

Granulomatosis
- respiratory, necrotizing M31.3
- Wegener's M31.3

Graves' disease E05.0
- ophthalmic (euthyroid) H05.22

Growth, fetal, slow P05.9
Guillain–Barré syndrome G61.0
Gumma (syphilitic) of central nervous system A52.3
Guyon's canal syndrome G56.23

H

Haemangioma D18
Haemarthosis T14.3
Haematemesis K92.0
Haematoma T14.0
– arterial, traumatic T14.5
– extradural I62.1
– – traumatic S06.4
– postprocedural T81.0
– subdural I62.0
– – due to birth injury P10.0
– – traumatic S06.5
Haematomyelia G95.12
– traumatic T14.4
Haemochromatosis E83.10
Haemophilia
– A D66
– B D67
– C D68.1
– vascular D68.0
Haemorrhage
– adrenal E27.40
– brain stem I61.3
– cerebellar I61.4
– cerebral lobe I61.1
– choroidal H31.3
– epidural I62.1
– – traumatic S06.4
– extradural I62.1
– – traumatic S06.4
– fibrinolytic (acquired) D65
– gastric K92.2
– gastrointestinal K92.2
– hemisphere
– – cortical I61.1
– – subcortical I61.0
– – specified NEC I61.2
– intestinal K92.2
– intracerebral I61.9
– multiple localized I61.6
– – sequelae I69.1
– – specified NEC I61.8
– – traumatic S06.3
– intracranial I62.9
– – fetus or newborn P52.9
– – – due to
– – – – anoxia or hypoxia P52.–
– – – – birth injury P10.–
– – – – maternal injury P00.5
– – sequelae I69.2
– – traumatic S06.80
– intraventricular I61.5
– meningeal I60.8
Haemorrhage — *continued*
– optic nerve sheath H47.01
– orbit H05.20
– postprocedural T81.0
– retinal H35.6
– secondary and recurrent, traumatic T79.2
– subarachnoid I60.9
– – sequelae I69.0
– – specified NEC I60.8
– – traumatic S06.6
– subdural I62.0
– – traumatic S06.5
– unintentional, during surgical and medical care Y60
Hageman's disease D68.2
Hallervorden–Spatz disease G23.0
Hallucination R44.3
– auditory R44.0
– gustatory R44.21
– hypnagogic or hypnopompic G47.43
– olfactory R44.20
– specified NEC R44.2
– visual R44.1
Hallucinosis
– alcoholic F10.5
– organic F06.0
Hallux varus, congenital Q66.3
Haltia–Sanavouri neuronal ceroid lipofuscinosis E75.4
Hamartosis Q85.9
Hammer toe, congenital Q66.8
Hand–Schüller–Christian disease D76.0
Hansen's disease (*see also* Leprosy) A30.9
Harada's disease H30.8
Hartnup's disease E70.810
Hashimoto's thyroiditis E06.3
Hashitoxicosis (transient) E06.3
Hawkinsuria E70.10
Headache R51
– cluster G44.0
– – atypical G44.08
– – chronic G44.02
– – episodic G44.01
– cold stimulus G44.802
– cough, benign G44.803
– drug-induced NEC G44.4
– exertional, benign G44.804
– external compression G44.801
– icepick G44.800
– menopausal N95.1
– migraine (*see also* Migraine) G43.9
– post-lumbar-puncture G97.0

HIV — *see also* Human immunodeficiency virus disease
- asymptomatic, infectious status Z21
- laboratory evidence R75
Hoarseness R49.0
Hodgkin's disease C81
Hole of macula H35.3
Hollenhorst's plaque H34.2
Holmes–Adie syndrome G90.80
Holmes' ataxia G11.12
Holoprosencephaly Q04.2
Holt–Oram syndrome Q87.20
Homocystinuria E72.10
Horner's syndrome G90.2
Hospital hopper syndrome F68.1
Hostility R45.5
Human immunodeficiency virus disease B24
- asymptomatic status Z21
- laboratory evidence R75
- resulting in
- - acute HIV infection syndrome B23.0
- - bacterial infection NEC B20.1
- - Burkitt's lymphoma B21.1
- - candidiasis B20.4
- - cytomegaloviral disease B20.2
- - dementia B22.0† F02.4*
- - encephalopathy B22.0
- - failure to thrive B22.2
- - haematological abnormality NEC B23.2
- - immunological abnormality NEC B23.2
- - infection B20.9
- - - specified NEC B20.8
- - Kaposi's sarcoma B21.0
- - lymphadenopathy, generalized (persistent) B23.1
- - multiple infections B20.7
- - mycobacterial infection B20.0
- - mycosis NEC B20.5
- - neoplasm, malignant B21.9
- - - haematopoietic tissue B21.3
- - - lymphoid tissue B21.3
- - - multiple B21.7
- - - specified NEC B21.8
- - non-Hodgkin's lymphoma NEC B21.2
- - parasitic disease B20.9
- - *Pneumocystis carinii* (pneumonia) B20.6
- - pneumonitis, interstitial, lymphoid B22.1
- - specified NEC B20.8
- - tuberculosis B20.0
- - viral infection NEC B20.3
- - wasting syndrome B22.2
Hunger T73.0
Hunt's dyssynergia cerebellaris myoclonica G11.13
Hunter's syndrome E76.1
Huntington's chorea or disease G10.–
- dementia in G10.–† F02.2*
Hurler–Scheie syndrome E76.01
Hurler's disease or syndrome E76.00
Hurst's disease G36.1
Hyaline necrosis of aorta I71.9
Hydatidosis B67.–
Hydranencephaly Q00.07
Hydrocephalus
- congenital Q03.9
- - specified NEC Q03.8
- - with spina bifida Q05.4
- - - cervical Q05.0
- - - lumbar Q05.2
- - - sacral Q05.3
- - - thoracic Q05.1
- due to toxoplasmosis (congenital) P37.1
- newborn Q03.–
Hydroencephalocele Q01.*xx*1
Hydromeningocele
- cranial Q01.*xx*2
- spinal Q05.*x*0
Hydromicrocephaly Q02.–0
Hydromyelia Q06.4
- with syringomyelia and syringobulbia G95.0
Hydrops, labyrinthine H81.0
Hydrorachis Q06.4
Hydroxykynureninuria E70.812
Hydroxylysinaemia E72.31
Hygiene, personal, very low level R46.0
Hyperacusis H93.2
Hyperaesthesia R20.3
Hyperaldosteronism E26.9
- primary E26.0
- secondary E26.1
- specified NEC E26.8
Hyperalimentation R63.2
- specified NEC E67.–
Hyperammonaemia E72.26
Hyperbetalipoproteinaemia E78.02
Hypercalcaemia, hypocalciuric, familial E83.50
Hypercalciuria, idiopathic E83.5
Hypercarotinaemia E67.1
Hyperchloraemia E87.8
Hypercholesterolaemia
- familial E78.00
- pure E78.0
- with hyperglyceridaemia, endogenous E78.23
Hyperchylomicronaemia E78.3
Hyperemesis gravidarum
- mild O21.0
- with metabolic disturbance O21.1
Hyperfunction
- adrenomedullary E27.5
- pituitary gland E22.9
- - specified NEC E22.8
Hypergammaglobulinaemia D89.2
- polyclonal D89.0

Hyperglycaemia R73.9
- postpancreatectomy E89.10
Hyperglyceridaemia
- endogenous E78.10
- mixed E78.32
- pure E78.1
Hyperglycinaemia, nonketotic
- type I E72.53
- type II E72.55
Hyperheparinaemia D68.3
Hyperhydroxyprolinaemia E72.50
Hyperinsulinism (functional) E16.1
- with hypoglycaemic coma E15
Hyperkalaemia E87.5
Hyperkinetic syndrome F90.9
Hyperleucine-isoleucinaemia E71.10
Hyperlipidaemia E78.5
- combined, familial E78.4
- group
- - A E78.03
- - B E78.12
- - C E78.24
- - D E78.31
- mixed E78.2
- specified NEC E78.4
Hyperlipoproteinaemia E78.–
- Frederickson's
- - type I and V E78.30
- - type IIa E78.01
- - type IIb and III E78.21
- - type IV E78.11
- very-low-density-lipoprotein-type E78.14
Hyperlysinaemia E72.32
Hypermagnesaemia E83.40
Hypermetropia H52.0
Hypermobility syndrome M35.7
Hypernasality R49.2
Hypernatraemia E87.0
Hyperornithinaemia
- type I E72.42
- type II E72.43
Hyperosmolality E87.0
Hyperostosis
- ankylosing M48.1
- cortical, infantile M89.8
- skeletal, diffuse idiopathic M48.1
- skull M85.2
Hyperoxaluria
- type I E80.311
- type II E74.81
Hyperparathyroidism E21.3
- primary E21.0
- secondary NEC E21.1
- - renal origin N25.8
- specified NEC E21.2
Hyperphenylalaninaemia NEC E70.1
Hyperphoria, alternating H50.5
Hyperplasia
- mandibular K07.0
- maxillary K07.0
- pancreatic
- - endocrine cells, with glucagon excess E16.3
- - islet cells E16.9
- - - beta E16.1
- parathyroid E21.0
- pituitary growth hormone cell E22.00
- thymus, persistent E32.0
Hyperpnoea, central R06.32
Hyperprebetalipoproteinaemia E78.13
Hyperproconvertinaemia D68.2
Hyperprolactinaemia E22.1
Hyperprolinaemia
- type I E72.51
- type II E72.52
Hyperpyrexia, malignant G71.84
Hypersecretion
- ACTH E27.0
- - with pituitary hyperplasia E24.01
- antidiuretic hormone E22.2
- catecholamine E27.5
- corticotropin-releasing hormone E24.00
- follicle-stimulating hormone E22.81
- glucagon E16.3
- growth hormone E22.80
- growth hormone-releasing hormone E16.8
- intestinal hormones NEC E34.1
- luteinizing hormone E22.81
- thyroid-releasing hormone, causing thyrotoxicosis E05.80
- thyroid-stimulating hormone E05.8
- vasopressin, hypothalamic E22.20
Hypersensitivity T78.4
- drug T88.7
- labyrinth H83.2
Hypersomnia
- nonorganic F51.1
- organic G47.1
Hypersplenism D73.1
Hypertelorism Q75.2
Hypertension
- complicating pregnancy, childbirth and the pueperium O10
- essential (primary) I10
- gestational O13
- - with significant proteinuria O14
- intracranial, benign G93.2
- maternal, unspecified O16
- ocular H40.0
- secondary I15
- transient, of pregnancy O16
Hyperthermia, malignant T88.3
Hyperthyroidism E05.–
- neonatal, transitory P72.1
Hypertonia, congenital P94.1

Hypertropia H50.4
Hypertrophy
- hemifacial Q67.4
- lip, congenital Q18.6
- muscle M62.81
- thymus E32.0
Hypervalinaemia E71.14
Hyperventilation R06.4
- psychogenic F45.3
Hypervitaminosis A E67.0
Hypoaesthesia of skin R20.1
Hypoaldosteronism E27.4
Hypoalphalipoproteinaemia E78.61
Hypobaropathy T70.2
Hypobetalipoproteinaemia, familial E78.63
Hypocalcaemia, neonatal P71.1
- due to cow's milk P71.0
Hypochloraemia E87.8
Hypochondriasis F45.2
Hypochondrogenesis Q77.0
Hypochondroplasia Q77.4
Hypofunction
- labyrinth H83.2
- of pituitary gland E23.–
Hypoglycaemia E16.2
- drug-induced E16.0
- - with coma, nondiabetic E15
- functional, nonhyperinsulinaemic E16.1
- neonatal
- - due to maternal diabetes P70.1
- - iatrogenic P70.3
- - transitory P70.4
Hypoglycinaemia, leucine-induced E71.16
Hypoinsulinaemia, postprocedural E89.1
Hypokalaemia E87.6
Hypomagnesaemia E83.41
- neonatal P71.2
Hypomania F30.0
Hypomenorrhoea N91.5
Hyponasality R49.2
Hyponatraemia E87.1
Hypoparathyroidism E20.9
- idiopathic E20.0
- neonatal, transitory P71.4
- postprocedural E89.2
- specified NEC E20.8
Hypophosphataemia, familial E83.31
Hypophosphatasia E83.32
Hypoplasia, granular cell G11.04
Hypopituitarism E23.0
- drug-induced E23.1
- postprocedural E89.3
Hypoplasia
- brain Q04.34
- eye Q11.2
- mandibular K07.0
- maxillary K07.0
- spinal cord Q06.1
Hypoproconvertinaemia D68.2
Hypo-osmolality E87.1
Hypotelorism Q75.83
Hypotension I95.9
- chronic I95.8
- drug-induced I95.2
- idiopathic I95.0
- intracranial, following ventricular shunting G97.2
- orthostatic I95.1
- - neurogenic, isolated G90.30
- postural I95.1
- specified NEC I95.8
Hypothermia (accidental) T68
- not associated with low environmental temperature R68.0
Hypothyroidism E03.9
- congenital
- - iodine-deficiency E00.9
- - with goitre E03.0
- - without goitre E03.1
- due to medicaments and other exogenous substances E03.2
- iodine-deficiency
- - acquired E01.8
- - congenital E00.9
- - subclinical E02
- neonatal, transitory P72.2
- postinfectious E03.3
- postirradiation E89.00
- postsurgical E89.01
- specified NEC E03.8
Hypotonia, hypotony
- congenital P94.1
- eye H44.4
Hypotropia H50.4
Hypovolaemia, hypovolaemic E86
- shock R57.1
- - surgical T81.1
Hypoxia
- altitudinal W94
- birth P21.9
- intrauterine P20.–
Hysteria F44.–

I

Infection — *continued*
- paracoccidioidomycosis B41.–
- *Paragonismus* species B66
- *Parastrongylus cantonensis* B83.2
- perinatal period NEC P39
- *Rickettsia prowazekii* A75.0
- roundworm B77.–
- salmonella NEC A02.–
- sinus
- - acute J01.–
- - chronic J30.–
- spirochaetal NEC A69.–
- *Taenia solium* B69.–
- trichinellosis B75.–
- toxoplasmosis B58.–
- trypanosomiasis
- - African B56.–
- - American B57.–
- wound, post-traumatic NEC T79.3
- zygomycosis B46.–

Infertility
- female N97
- male N46

Inflammation
- chorioretinal H30.9
- - disseminated H30.1
- - focal H30.0
- - specified NEC H30.8
- orbit
- - acute H05.0
- - chronic H05.1
- sinus, acute J01.–
- vein I80

Influenza
- virus identified J10.8
- - with pneumonia J10.0
- virus not identified J11.8
- - with pneumonia J11.0

Inhalation
- dry ice W93
- liquid air, hydrogen or nitrogen W93
- liquid or vomitus T17
- stomach contents or secretions due to anaesthesia during labour and delivery O74

Injencephaly
- aperta Q00.21
- clausa Q00.20

Injection, jet, traumatic (industrial) T70.4

Injury T14.9
- amputation, traumatic T14.7
- blood vessel T14.5
- - carotid artery S15.0
- - jugular vein
- - - external S15.2
- - - internal S15.3
- - multiple, neck level S15.7
- - vertebral artery S15.1

Injury — *continued*
- birth — *see* Birth, injury
- brachial plexus S14.3
- - cord S14.32
- - division S14.31
- - trunk S14.30
- brain S06.9
- - diffuse S06.2
- - focal S06.3
- cauda equina S34.3
- conjunctiva S05.0
- cranial nerves — *see* Injury, nerve, cranial
- ear, superficial S00.4
- electric current W87
- eye S05.9
- - specified NEC S05.8
- face, crushing S07.0
- head S09.–
- - crushing S07.–
- - multiple S09.7
- - sequelae T90.9
- - specified NEC
- - superficial S00.–
- - with neck, crushing T04.0
- intracranial S06.9
- - sequelae T90.5
- - specified NEC S06.8
- - with prolonged coma S06.7
- lacrimal duct S05.8
- limb
- - lower T13.–
- - - sequelae T93.–
- - upper T11.–
- - - sequelae T92.–
- lip, superficial S00.5
- multiple body regions
- - crushing T04.–
- - specified NEC T06.–
- - sequelae T94
- muscle T14.6
- - at neck level S16
- neck S19.–
- - crushing S17
- - multiple S19.7
- - sequelae T91.–
- nerve T14.4
- - abdomen level S34.–
- - abducent S04.4
- - accessory S04.7
- - acoustic S04.6
- - ankle level S94.–
- - axillary S44.3
- - cranial
- - - eighth S04.6
- - - eleventh S04.7
- - - fifth S04.3
- - - first S04.80
- - - fourth S04.2

Injury — *continued*
- nerve — *continued*
- - vagus S04.82
- - visual cortex S04
- - whiplash S13
- - wrist level S64.–
- nose, superficial S00.3
- oral cavity, superficial S00.5
- orbit S05.–
- scalp, superficial S00.0
- sequelae NEC T94
- skull, crushing S07.1
- spinal cord T09.3
- - cervical S14.1
- - lumbar S34.1
- - sequelae T91.3
- - thoracic S24.1
- tendon T14.6
- - neck level S16
- thorax with abdomen, lower back and pelvis, crushing T04.1
- trunk T09.9
- - sequelae T91.–
- - sequelae T94
- vein, jugular
- - external S15.2
- - internal S15.3
- whiplash S13.43

Insect bite (nonvenomous) T14.0

Insomnia
- altitudinal T70.2
- nonorganic F51.0
- organic G47.0

Instability, spinal M53.2

Insufficiency
- adrenocortical E27.4
- - drug-induced E27.3
- - primary E27.0
- pituitary E23.0

Intolerance
- fructose, hereditary E74.11
- lactose E73.9
- - specified NEC E73.8
- lysinuric protein E72.01

Intoxication
- acute F1*x*.0
- - alcohol F10.0

Intoxication — *continued*
- acute — *continued*
- - caffeine F15.0
- - cannabinoids F12.0
- - cocaine F14.0
- - hallucinogens F16.0
- - hypnotics F13.0
- - multiple drug use F19.0
- - opioids F11.0
- - psychoactive substance NEC F19.0
- - sedatives F13.0
- - stimulants NEC F15.0
- - tobacco F17.0
- - volatile solvents F18.0
- bacterial, foodborne A05.–
- fetus or newborn, via placenta or breast milk P04.–
- pathological F1*x*.0

Intubation, failed or difficult, during labour and delivery O74.7

Inversion
- chromosome, normal individual Q95.1
- sleep–wake schedule, psychogenic F51.2

Iridocyclitis H20.9
- acute H20.0
- chronic H20.1
- lens-induced H20.2
- specified NEC H20.8
- subacute H20.0

Iritis H20.0

Irritable, irritability R45.4
- bowel syndrome K58.9
- infant R68.1
- neonatal cerebral P91.3

Isaac's neuromyotonia G71.1

Ischaemia, ischaemic
- cerebral
- - neonatal P91.0
- - transient G45.9
- - specified NEC G45.8
- contracture, Volkmann's T79.6
- muscle, traumatic T79.6

Issue of
- medical certificate (cause of death) (fitness) (incapacity) (invalidity) Z02.7
- repeat prescription Z76.0

J

K

Kahler's disease C90.0
Kanner's syndrome F84.0
Kaposi's sarcoma C46.–
Karyotype
– 45,X Q96.0
– 46,X
– – iso (Xq) Q96.1
– – with abnormality except iso (Xq) Q96.2
– 46,XX
– – hermaphrodite (true) Q99.1
– – male Q98.3
– – with streak gonads Q99.1
– 46,XY
– – with streak gonads Q99.1
– – female Q97.3
– 47,XXX Q97.0
– 47,XXY, with Klinefelter's syndrome Q98.0
– 47,XYY Q98.5
Kawasaki's syndrome M30.3
Kearns–Sayre syndrome H49.8
Kennedy's bulbospinal muscular atrophy G12.118
Keratitis H16
Kernicterus P57.9
– due to isoimmunization P57.0
– specified NEC P57.8
Kidney, Goldblatt's I70.1
Kleine–Levin syndrome G47.84
Klinefelter's syndrome
– karyotype 47,XXY Q98.0

Klinefelter's syndrome — *continued*
– male with
– – karyotype 46,XX Q98.2
– – more than two X chromosomes Q98.1
Klippel–Feil syndrome Q76.1
Klippel–Trénaunay–Weber syndrome Q87.21
Klumpke's paralysis due to birth injury P14.1
Korsakov's psychosis or syndrome
– alcoholic F10.6
– drug-induced F1*x*.6
– nonalcoholic F04
Kozhevnikof's epilepsy G40.50
Krabbe's disease E75.21
Kufs' disease E75.43
Kugelberg–Welander disease G12.101
Kuhnt–Junius degeneration H35.3
Kunjin virus disease A83.4
Kuru A81.80
Kussmaul breathing R06.31
Kwashiorkor E40
– marasmic E42
Kyasanur Forest disease A98.2
Kyphoscoliosis M41.–
Kyphosis M40.2
– congenital not associated with scoliosis Q76.42
– postural M40.0
– secondary NEC M40.1

L

Labyrinthitis H83.0
Laceration (*see also* Wound, open) T14.1
- accidental, complicating procedure T81.2
- blood vessel(s) T14.5
- cerebral S06.2
- eye S05.3
- – with prolapse or loss of intraocular tissue S05.2
- joint T14.3
- ligament T14.3
- muscle T14.6
- ocular S05.3
- – with prolapse or loss of intraocular tissue S05.2
- tendon T14.6
Lack of
- coordination specified NEC R27.8
- expected normal physiological development R62.8
- growth R62.8
- relaxation and leisure Z73.2
Lactose intolerance E73.9
- specified NEC E73.8
Lalling F80.0
Lance–Adams syndrome G25.38
Landau–Kleffner syndrome F80.3
Landouzy–Déjerine dystrophy G71.02
Langerhans' cell histiocytosis NEC D76.0
Language disorder, developmental F80.9
- expressive F80.1
- receptive F80.2
Laron type short stature E34.3
Laryngoplegia J38.0
Lassa fever A96.2
Laterocollis, spasmodic G24.33
Late
- talker R62.00
- walker R62.01
Launois–Bensaude adenolipomatosis E88.80
Laurence–Moon(–Bardet)–Biedl syndrome Q87.81
Laxity, ligamentous, familial M35.7
Leak, cerebrospinal fluid G96.0
- from spinal puncture G97.0
Leber's optic atrophy H47.21
Leigh's disease G31.81
Lennox–Gastaut syndrome G40.44
Leprosy A30.9
- borderline A30.3
- – lepromatous A30.4
- – tuberculoid A30.2
- indeterminate A30.0
Leprosy — *continued*
- lepromatous A30.5
- sequelae B92
- specified NEC A30.8
- tuberculoid A30.1
Leptomeningitis G03.–
- bacterial G00.9
- – specified NEC G00.8
Leptospirosis A27
Leriche's syndrome I74.0
Lermoyez' syndrome H81.30
Lesch–Nyhan syndrome E79.1
Lesion
- biomechanical M99.9
- – specified NEC M99.8
- brain, congenital Q04.9
- intracranial space-occupying R90.0
- nerve
- – axillary G58.83
- – femoral G57.2
- – genitofemoral G57.80
- – gluteal G57.00
- – ilioinguinal G57.81
- – long thoracic G58.84
- – median NEC G56.1
- – musculocutaneous G56.80
- – peroneal
- – – deep G57.31
- – – superficial G57.30
- – phrenic G58.80
- – plantar G57.6
- – popliteal
- – – lateral G57.3
- – – medial G57.4
- – pudendal G57.82
- – radial G56.3
- – saphenous G57.22
- – sciatic G57.0
- – suprascapular G58.82
- – sural G57.42
- – ulnar G56.2
- nervous system, congenital Q07.9
- – specified NEC Q07.8
Lethargy R53
Letterer–Siwe disease C96.0
Leucinosis E71.15
Leukaemia C95
- lymphoid C91
- monocytic C93
- myeloid C92
- plasma cell C90.1
- specified cell type C94

Leukoderma, syphylitic A51.3† L99.8*
Leukodystrophy, metachromatic E75.23
- juvenile E75.231
- late infantile E75.230
- late-onset E75.232
Leukoencephalitis, haemorrhagic (acute) (subacute) G36.1
Leukoencephalopathy
- HIV B22.0
- multifocal, progressive A81.2
- sclerosing, van Bogaert's A81.1
- vascular, progressive I67
Leukomalacia, cerebral, neonatal P91.2
Lewy body disease, diffuse G31.85
Libman–Sacks disease M32.1† I39*
Light
- effects of T67.–
- fetus or newborn, for gestational age P05.0
- headedness R42
Light-for-dates (infant) P05.0
Lightning, effects of T75.0
Lightwood–Albright syndrome N25.8
Limbic epilepsy personality syndrome F07.0
Limitation of activities due to disability Z73.6
Lipidaemia NEC E78.–
Lipofuscinosis, neuronal ceroid E75.4
- adult E75.43
- Haltia–Sanavouri E75.4
- infantile E75.40
- - late E75.41
- juvenile E75.42
Lipoma D17.7
- cauda equina D17.70
- corpus callosum D17.71
Lipomeningocele Q05.*x*1
Lisping F80.8
Lissencephaly Q04.31
Listeriosis NEC A32.8
- neonatal (disseminated) P37.2
Little's disease G80.–
Liver — *see condition*
Lobotomy syndrome F07.0
Lorain–Levi dwarfism (short stature) E23.021
Lordosis M40.5
- acquired M40.4
- congenital, not associated with scoliosis Q76.43
- - postural M40.4
- - specified NEC M40.4
Loss
- appetite R63.0
Loss — *continued*
- hearing H91.9
- - central H90.5
- - conductive H90.2
- - - unilateral H90.1
- - neural H90.5
- - noise-induced H83.3
- - ototoxic H91.0
- - perceptive H90.5
- - sensorineural H90.–
- - specified NEC H91.8
- - sudden (idiopathic) H91.2
- sensory, dissociative F44.6
- visual H54.7
- - both eyes H54.6
- - one eye H54.3
- - sudden H53.1
- voice R49.1
- weight, abnormal R63.4
Louis–Bar syndrome G11.3
Louping ill A84.8
Low's neuropathy G60.84
Lowe's syndrome E72.00
Lubag's dystonia–parkinsonism complex G24.16
Luft's disease G71.33
Lumbago M54.5
- due to intervertebral disc displacement M51.2
- with sciatica M54.4
Lung — *see also condition*
- abscess J85
- oedema, acute J81
- pressure collapse, due to anaesthesia during labour and delivery O74.1
Lupus erythematosus, systemic M32.9
- drug-induced M32.0
- specified NEC M32.8
Luria's dynamic aphasia R47.05
Lutz' disease B41.–
Lyme disease A69.2
Lymphangioma D18
Lymphocytes, increased levels in cerebrospinal fluid R83.61
Lymphohistiocytosis, haemophagocytic D76.1
Lymphoma
- cutaneous T-cell C84
- non-Hodgkin's C85.–
- - diffuse C83
- - follicular (nodular) C82
- peripheral T-cell C84
Lymphosarcoma C85.0

M

Malnutrition E46
- fetal P05.–
- maternal, affecting fetus or newborn P00.4
- protein–energy E46
- - mild E44
- - moderate E44
- - severe E43
- - - intermediate form E42
- severe
- - protein–energy E43
- - - intermediate form E42
- - with
- - - marasmus E41
- - - nutritional oedema E40
- sequelae E64.–

Malocclusion K07.4
Malta fever A23.–
Maltreatment syndrome T74.9
- - specified NEC T74.8

Management, procreative Z31.–
Mania F30.9
- with psychotic symptoms F30.2
- without psychotic symptoms F30.1

Manic–depressive illness F31.–
Mannosidosis E77.10
Maple-syrup-urine disease E71.00
Marasmus
- nutritional E41
- with kwashiorkor E42

Marburg virus disease A98.3
Marchiafava–Bignami syndrome or disease G37.1
Marcus Gunn's syndrome Q07.82
Marfan's syndrome Q87.4
Marinesco–Sjögren syndrome G11.15
Mastoiditis H70.9
- acute H70.0
- chronic H70.1
- specified NEC H70.8

McArdle's disease E74.04
Meadow's syndrome Q86.1
Measles B05.–
- German (*see also* Rubella) B06.–
- with
- - encephalitis B05.0† G05.1*
- - meningitis B05.1† G02.0*

Meconium in liquor P20.–
Mediterranean fever A23.–
- familial E85.00

Megalencephaly Q04.5
Megavitamin-B_6 syndrome E67.2
Meige's blepharospasm G24.5
Melaena K92.1
Melanoma, malignant, of skin C43
MELAS G71.36
Melkersson(–Rosenthal) syndrome G51.2
Mendelson's syndrome (due to anaesthesia during labour and delivery) O74.0
Ménière's disease, syndrome or vertigo H81.0
Meningioma D32.9
Meningismus R29.1
Meningitis G03.9
- adenoviral A87.1† G02.0*
- adhesive, chronic G96.1
- bacterial G00.9
- - specified NEC G00.8
- benign recurrent G03.2
- candidal B37.5† G02.1*
- carcinomatous C79.362
- chronic G03.1
- coxsackievirus A87.0† G02.0*
- cryptococcal B45.1† G02.1*
- echovirus A87.0† G02.0*
- enteroviral A87.0† G02.0*
- gonococcal A54.8† G01*
- Gram-negative G00.90
- Gram-positive G00.91
- *Haemophilus* (*influenzae*) G00.0
- herpesviral B00.3† G02.0*
- in (due to)
- - *Acinetobacter* G00.82
- - *Actinomyces* G00.805
- - African trypanosomiasis B56.–† G02.8*
- - anthrax A22.8† G01*
- - arenaviral haemorrhagic fever A96.–† G02.0*
- - *Bacteroides fragilis* G00.800
- - Chagas' disease B57.4† G02.8*
- - chickenpox B01.0† G02.0*
- - *Citrobacter* G00.811
- - *Clostridium* G00.804
- - coccidioidomycosis B38.4† G02.1*
- - cytomegaloviral disease B25.–† G02.0*
- - *Enterobacter* G00.812
- - *Escherichia coli* G00.83
- - Friedländer bacillus G00.840
- - *Fusobacterium* G00.801
- - HIV disease B20.–† G02.0*
- - infectious mononucleosis B27.–† G02.0*
- - *Klebsiella* G00.84
- - Kyasanur forest disease A98.2† G02.0*
- - Lyme disease A69.2† G01*
- - lymphocytic choriomeningitis A87.2† G02.0*
- - measles B05.1† G02.0*
- - mumps B26.1† G02.0*
- - neurosyphilis A52.1† G01*
- - *Nocardia* G00.85
- - *Pasteurella multocida* G00.86
- - *Peptococcus* G00.803
- - *Peptostreptococcus* G00.803
- - *Propionibacterium* G00.802
- - *Proteus* G00.87
- - *Pseudomonas* G00.88
- - rubella B06.0† G02.0*
- - salmonella infection A02.2† G01*

Mollaret's syndrome G03.2
Mönckeberg's (medial) sclerosis I70.2
Moniliasis B37.–
Monofixation syndrome H50.4
Mononeuritis multiplex G58.7
Mononeuropathy G58.9
– diabetic NEC (*see also* E10–E14 with fourth character .4) E14.4† G59.0*
– in (due to)
– – leprosy A30.–† G59.8*
– – radiation G97.80† G59.8*
– – vasculitis M30–M31† G59.8*
– – zoster B02.2† G59.8*
– limb
– – lower NEC G57.8
– – upper NEC G56.8
Mononucleosis, infectious B27.–
– cytomegaloviral B27.1
– Epstein–Barr virus B27.0
– gammaherpesviral B27.0
Monoplegia G83.3
– lower limb G83.1
– upper limb G83.2
Monosomy, whole chromosome
– meiotic nondisjunction Q93.0
– mitotic nondisjunction Q93.1
Monster Q89.7
– double Q89.4
Morbilli B05.–
Morel's laminar sclerosis G31.24
Morquio's syndrome E76.21
Mortality, unknown cause R99
Morton's metatarsalgia G57.62
Mosaicism
– sex chromosome
– – female, lines with various numbers of X chromosomes Q97.2
– – male Q98.7
– 45,X
– – cell lines NEC with abnormal sex chromosomes Q96.4
– – 46,XX Q96.3
– – 46,XY Q96.3
Motion sickness T75.3
Motor neuron disease G12.29
– Guamanian type G12.260
– in
– – Kii Peninsula G12.261
– – West New Guinea G12.262
– Madras type G12.27
– paraneoplastic G13.12
– Patrikios' G12.25
– segmental G12.28
– Western Pacific type G12.26
Mountain sickness T70.2
– due to prolonged visit at high altitude W94
Movement
– abnormal NEC R25.8
– – head R25.0
– disorder
– – limb, paroxysmal nocturnal G25.80
– – stereotyped F98.4
– eye, irregular NEC H55.–
Moyamoya disease
– primary I67.50
– secondary I67.51
Mucolipidosis
– type I E77.12
– type II E77.00
– type III E77.01
– type IV E75.13
Mucopolysaccharidosis E76.3
– type I E76.0
– type II E76.1
– type III E76.20
– type IV E76.21
– type VI E76.23
– type VII E76.24
Mucormycosis, rhinocerebral B46.1
Mucous patch, syphilitic A51.3
Multiple
– personality F44.81
– sclerosis G35.–
– – progressive
– – – primary G35.–1
– – – secondary G35.–2
– – relapsing/remitting G35.–0
Mumps B26.–
– encephalitis B26.2† G05.1*
– meningitis B26.1† G02.0*
– polyneuropathy B26.8† G63.0*
Münchhausen's syndrome F68.1
Muscular dystrophy G71.0
– autosomal recessive G71.080
– congenital G71.08
– distal G71.081
– dystrophin-deficient
– – benign (Becker-type) G71.00
– – severe (Duchenne-type) G71.07
– facioscapulohumeral G71.02
– humeroperoneal G71.082
– limb-girdle G71.03
– ocular G71.04
– oculopharyngeal G71.05
– scapuloperoneal G71.01
– specified NEC G71.08
Mutism
– akinetic G96.83
– deaf NEC H91.3
Myalgia M79.1
– epidemic B33.0
– exertional R25.21
Myasthenia
– congenital G70.2

Myasthenia — *continued*
- developmental G70.2
- gravis G70.0
- - acquired idiopathic autoimmune G70.00
- - penicillamine-induced G70.03
- - specified NEC G70.08
- - with
- - - autoimmune disease G70.02
- - - thymoma G70.01
- infantile, familial G70.24
- limb-girdle
- - familial G70.25
- - non-familial G70.26
Myelatelia Q06.1
Myelinolysis, central pontine G37.2
Myelitis G04.9
- acute transverse G37.3
- adenoviral A85.1† G05.1*
- amoebic B60.2† G05.2*
- cytomegaloviral B25.8† G05.1*
- enteroviral A85.0† G05.1*
- herpesviral B00.4† G05.1*
- in (due to)
- - African trypanosomiasis B56.-† G05.2*
- - Chagas' disease B57.4† G05.2*
- - HIV B23.8† G05.1*
- - influenza J11.8† G05.1*
- - - virus identified J10.8† G05.1*
- - Lyme disease A69.2† G05.2
- - measles B05.0† G05.1
- - mumps B26.2† G05.1*
- - naegleriasis B60.2† G05.2*
- - rubella B06.0† G05.1*
- - syphilis
- - - congenital A50.4† G05.0*
- - - late A52.1† G05.0*
- - toxoplasmosis B58.2† G05.2*
- - zoster B02.0† G05.1*
- listerial A32.1† G05.0*
- meningococcal A39.8† G05.0*
- mosquito-borne A83.-† G05.1*
- postchickenpox B01.1† G05.1*
- specified NEC G04.8
- subacute necrotizing G37.4
- tuberculous A17.8† G05.0*
Myelocele Q05.*x*3
Myelodysplasia of spinal cord Q06.1
Myeloma
- multiple C90.0
- solitary C90.2
Myelomatosis C90.0
Myelomeningocele Q05.*x*4
Myelopathy G95.9
- drug-induced G95.80
- in (due to)
- - artery compression syndromes M47.0† G99.2*
- - HIV disease B23.8† G99.2*

Myelopathy — *continued*
- in (due to) — *continued*
- - intervertebral disc disorders
- - - cervical, cervicothoracic M50.0† G99.2*
- - - lumbar M51.0† G99.2*
- - lathyrism G95.83
- - neoplastic disease C00-D48† G99.2*
- - spondylosis M47.-† G99.2*
- - vitamin B_{12} deficiency E53.80† G99.2*
- radiation-induced G95.82
- subacute necrotic G95.13
- toxin-induced G95.81
- vascular G95.1
Myocarditis
- in (due to)
- - bacterial disease I41.0
- - Chagas' disease B57.2† I41.2*
- - - acute B57.0† I41.2*
- - toxoplasmosis B58.8† I41.2*
- - viral disease I41.1
- influenzal J11.8
- - virus identified J10.8
- rheumatoid M05.3† I41.8*
Myoclonus G25.3
- Baltic G40.37
- cortical type
- - diffuse G25.30
- - focal or multifocal G25.31
- essential G25.32
- in (due to)
- - Alzheimer's disease G30.-† G26.-3*
- - brain tumour C71.-† C79.3† D33.-† G26.-3*
- - Creutzfeldt–Jakob disease A81.0† G26.-3*
- - cerebrovascular disease I60–I67† G26.-3*
- - dyssynergia cerebellaris myoclonica G11.13† G26.-3*
- - head injury S06.-† G26.-3*
- - olivopontocerebellar atrophy G11.22–G11.23† G26.-3*
- - (Ramsay–)Hunt syndrome G11.13† G26.-3*
- - toxic encephalopathy G29.-† G26.-3*
- oculopalatal G25.33
- peripheral G25.36
- post-anoxic action G25.38
- propriospinal G25.35
- segmental spinal G25.34
- sleep (hypnic) G25.37
- with ataxia G11.13
Myoglobinuria G72.80
Myokymia
- facial G51.4
- focal C64.-2
- generalized G64.-0
- syndrome G64.-1

Myopathy G72.9
- alcoholic G72.1
- - acute G72.10
- - chronic G72.11
- centronuclear G71.23
- congenital G71.2
- drug-induced G72.0
- familial granulovacuolar G71.805
- fingerprint body G71.26
- hereditary G71.9
- hypertrophic brachial G71.83
- in (due to)
- - acromegaly E22.0† G73.5*
- - amyloidosis E85.-† G73.7*
- - carcinoid syndrome E34.0† G73.7*
- - carnitine deficiency E71.31† G73.6*
- - Cushing's syndrome E24.-† G73.5*
- - disorder of fatty-acid metabolism E71.3† G73.6*
- - endocrine disease G73.5
- - glycogen storage disease E74.0† G73.6*
- - hydroxymethylglutaryl-CoA lyase deficiency E71.31† G73.6*
- - hyperparathyroidism E21.-† G73.5*
- - hyperthyroidism E05.-† G73.5*
- - hypoadrenalism E27.3-E27.4† G73.5*
- - hypoparathyroidism E20.-† G73.5*
- - hypothyroidism E00-E03† G73.5*
- - intrauterine exposure to toxins P04.-† G73.7*
- - isovaleryl-CoA-dehydrogenase deficiency E71.11† G73.6*
- - lactate dehydrogenase deficiency E74.86† G73.6*
- - lipid storage disorders E75.-† G73.6*
- - mannose-6-phosphate isomerase deficiency E74.83† G73.6*
- - metabolic disease G73.6
- - methylmalonyl-CoA mutase deficiency E71.12† G73.6*
- - multiple-chain acyl-CoA dehydrogenase deficiency E88.820† G73.6*
- - nutritional deficiencies E40-E64† G73.7*
- - osteomalacia M83.-† G73.7*
- - phophoglycerate kinase deficiency E74.85† G73.6*
- - phosphoglycerate mutase deficiency E74.84† G73.6*
- - polyarteritis nodosa M30.0† G73.7*
- - rheumatoid arthritis M05.3† G73.7*
- - sarcoidosis D86.88† G73.7*
- - scleroderma M34.8† G73.7*
- - sicca syndrome M35.0† G73.7*
- - syphilis A51.4† A52.7† G73.7*
- - systemic lupus erythematosus M32.1† G73.7*

Myopathy — *continued*
- in (due to) — *continued*
- - thalassaemia D56.-† D73.7*
- - toxic agents G72.2
- - trauma and ischaemia T79.6† G73.7*
- - vitamin D deficiency E55.-† G73.7*
- inflammatory NEC G72.4
- mitochondrial G71.3
- monomelic hypertrophic G71.82
- myotubular G71.23
- nemaline G71.24
- ocular G71.81
- - in hyperthyroidism E05.-† G73.50*
- - with mitochondrial abnormalities G71.35
- oculocraniosomatic G71.81
- quadriceps G71.86
- reducing body G71.281
- sarcotubular G71.280
- specified NEC G72.8
- with
- - cylindrical bodies G71.801
- - cytoplasmic bodies G71.800
- - rimmed vacuoles G71.803
- - spheromembranous bodies G71.804
- - tubular aggregates G71.25
- - zebra bodies G71.802

Myopia H52.1
- degenerative H44.2

Myosclerosis G71.806

Myositis M60.9
- eosinophilic, localized M60.83
- inclusion body M33.26
- infective M60.0
- interstitial M60.1
- nodular, focal M60.80
- ossificans
- - in (due to)
- - - burns M61.3
- - - quadriplegia or paraplegia M61.2
- - progressiva M61.1
- - traumatica M61.0
- proliferative, focal M60.80
- specified NEC M60.8
- syphilitic A51.4† M63.0*

Myotonia
- chondrodystrophic G71.10
- congenita
- - dominant G71.130
- - recessive G71.131
- drug-induced G71.11
- symptomatic G71.18

Myxoedema E03.9
- coma E03.5
- psychosis F06.8

N

Neoplasm — *continued*
- behaviour unknown or uncertain — *continued*
- - pharynx D37.0
- - pineal gland D44.5
- - pituitary gland D44.3
- - pluriglandular D44.8
- - pons D43.101
- - retroperitoneum D48.3
- - salivary glands, major D37.0
- - skin D48.5
- - specified site NEC D48.7
- - spinal cord
- - - cervical D43.40
- - - cervicothoracic D43.41
- - - lumbar D43.44
- - - lumbosacral D43.45
- - - overlapping lesion D43.48
- - - sacral D43.46
- - - thoracic D43.32
- - - thoracolumbar D43.43
- - thalamus D43.02
- - thymus D38.4
- benign
- - accessory sinuses D14.0
- - adrenal gland D35.0
- - aortic body D35.6
- - basal ganglia D33.02
- - bone
- - - face D16.4
- - - jaw, lower D16.5
- - - pelvic D16.8
- - - skull D16.4
- - brain D33.2
- - - basal ganglia D33.02
- - - corpus callosum D33.04
- - - hypothalamus D33.03
- - - infratentorial D33.1
- - - - overlapping D33.18
- - - lobe
- - - - frontal D33.000
- - - - occipital D33.003
- - - - parietal D33.002
- - - - temporal D33.001
- - - supratentorial D33.0
- - - - overlapping D33.08
- - - thalamus D33.02
- - - ventricle
- - - - lateral D33.010
- - - - third D33.011
- - brain stem D33.10
- - - fourth ventricle D33.103
- - - medulla D33.102
- - - midbrain D33.100
- - - overlapping D33.108
- - - pons D33.101
- - carotid body D35.5
- - cauda equina D33.7

Neoplasm — *continued*
- benign — *continued*
- - cerebellum D33.11
- - clavicle D16.7
- - coccyx D16.8
- - connective tissue D21.9
- - - abdomen D21.4
- - - face D21.0
- - - head D21.0
- - - hip D21.2
- - - limb
- - - - lower D21.2
- - - - upper D21.1
- - - neck D21.0
- - - pelvis D21.5
- - - shoulder D21.1
- - - thorax D21.3
- - - trunk NEC D21.6
- - corpus callosum D33.04
- - craniopharyngeal duct D35.3
- - endocrine gland D35.9
- - - specified NEC D35.7
- - eye D31.–
- - glomus jugulare D35.60
- - glomus tympanicum D35.61
- - heart D15.1
- - hypothalamus D33.03
- - larynx D14.1
- - lipomatous, specified site NEC D17.7
- - lymph nodes D36.0
- - mediastinum D15.2
- - meninges D32.9
- - - cerebral D32.0
- - - spinal D32.1
- - medulla D33.102
- - midbrain D33.100
- - middle ear D14.0
- - mouth D10
- - nasal cavity D14.0
- - nerve
- - - abducens D33.322
- - - accessory D33.37
- - - acoustic D33.35
- - - cervical D36.101
- - - cranial
- - - - eighth D33.35
- - - - eleventh D33.37
- - - - fifth D33.33
- - - - first D33.30
- - - - fourth D33.321
- - - - multiple D33.39
- - - - ninth D33.360
- - - - second D33.31
- - - - seventh D33.34
- - - - sixth D33.322
- - - - tenth D33.361
- - - - third D33.320
- - - - twelfth D33.38

Neoplasm — *continued*
- malignant — *continued*
- - bone — *continued*
- - - jaw, lower C41.1
- - - limbs C40
- - - orbital C41.0
- - - pelvic C41.4
- - - secondary C79.5
- - - skull C41.0
- - brain C71.9
- - - lobe
- - - - frontal C71.1
- - - - - secondary C79.300
- - - - occipital C71.4
- - - - - secondary C79.303
- - - - parietal C71.3
- - - - - secondary C79.302
- - - - temporal C71.2
- - - - - secondary C79.301
- - - overlapping lesion C71.8
- - - ventricle
- - - - lateral C71.50
- - - - - secondary C79.310
- - - - third C71.51
- - - - - secondary C79.311
- - brain stem
- - - fourth ventricle C71.73
- - - - secondary C79.353
- - - medulla C71.72
- - - - secondary C79.352
- - - midbrain C71.70
- - - - secondary C79.350
- - - multiple C71.78
- - - - secondary C79.358
- - - overlapping lesion C71.78
- - - pons C71.71
- - - - secondary C79.351
- - breast C50
- - bronchus C34
- - carotid body C75.4
- - cartilage
- - - articular C41.–
- - - - limbs C40
- - - laryngeal C32.3
- - cauda equina C72.1
- - - secondary C79.41
- - cerebellum C71.6
- - - secondary C79.36
- - cerebrum
- - - basal ganglia C71.01
- - - - secondary C79.32
- - - corpus callosum C71.00
- - - - secondary C79.34
- - - specified NEC C71.07
- - - thalamus C71.01
- - - - secondary C79.32
- - cervix uteri C53
- - cheek NEC C76.0

Neoplasm — *continued*
- malignant — *continued*
- - clavicle C41.3
- - coccyx C41.4
- - colon C18
- - - rectosigmoid C19
- - - with rectum C19
- - connective tissue C49.9
- - - abdomen C49.4
- - - face C49.0
- - - head C49.0
- - - hip C49.2
- - - limb
- - - - lower C49.2
- - - - upper C49.1
- - - neck C49.0
- - - orbit C69.6
- - - pelvis C49.5
- - - shoulder C49.1
- - - thorax C49.3
- - - trunk C49.6
- - corpus callosum C71.00
- - - secondary C79.34
- - corpus uteri C54
- - craniopharyngeal duct C75.2
- - digestive system NEC
- - - overlapping lesion C26.8
- - - secondary C78
- - endocrine gland NEC C75.9
- - eye C69.–
- - gallbladder C23
- - genital organs, overlapping
- - - female C57
- - - male C63.8
- - glomus jugulare C75.50
- - glomus tympanicum C75.51
- - glottis C32.0
- - haematopoietic tissue NEC C96.–
- - head NEC C76.0
- - hypothalamus C71.02
- - - secondary C79.33
- - independent (primary) multiple sites C97
- - kidney C64
- - larynx
- - - cartilage C32.3
- - - overlapping lesion C32.8
- - lip NEC C14.–
- - liver C22
- - - secondary C78
- - lung C34
- - lymph nodes, secondary C77
- - lymphoid tissue NEC C96.–
- - maxilla (superior) C41.0
- - mediastinum C38.3
- - - anterior C38.1
- - - posterior C38.2
- - medulla C71.72

Neoplasm — *continued*
- malignant — *continued*
- - medulla — *continued*
- - - secondary C79.352
- - meninges C70.9
- - - cerebral C70.0
- - - - secondary C79.37
- - - spinal C70.1
- - midbrain C71.70
- - - secondary C79.350
- - middle ear C30.1
- - muscle, extraocular C69.6
- - nasal cavity C30.0
- - nasopharynx C11
- - neck NEC C76.0
- - nerve
- - - abducens C72.502
- - - accessory C72.55
- - - acoustic C72.4
- - - cranial C72.5
- - - - eleventh C72.55
- - - - fifth C72.51
- - - - fourth C72.501
- - - - multiple C72.57
- - - - ninth C72.53
- - - - secondary C79.41
- - - - seventh C72.52
- - - - sixth C72.502
- - - - tenth C72.54
- - - - third C72.500
- - - - twelfth C72.56
- - - facial C72.52
- - - glossopharyngeal C72.53
- - - gluteal C47.21
- - - hypoglossal C72.56
- - - lumbar C47.41
- - - median C47.12
- - - obturator C47.53
- - - oculomotor C72.500
- - - olfactory C72.20
- - - - bulb C72.21
- - - optic
- - - - chiasm C72.31
- - - - retrobulbar C72.30
- - - peripheral C47.9
- - - - abdomen C47.47
- - - - face C47.07
- - - - head C47.07
- - - - hip C47.27
- - - - limb
- - - - - lower C47.27
- - - - - - secondary C79.45
- - - - - upper C47.17
- - - - - - secondary C79.46
- - - - neck C47.07
- - - - orbit C69.6
- - - - pelvis C47.57
- - - - shoulder C47.17

Neoplasm — *continued*
- malignant — *continued*
- - nerve — *continued*
- - - peripheral — *continued*
- - - - thorax C47.37
- - - - trunk C47.6
- - - peroneal C47.22
- - - pudendal C47.52
- - - radial C47.11
- - - roots
- - - - cervical C47.00
- - - - lumbar C47.40
- - - - sacral C47.50
- - - - secondary C79.41
- - - - thoracic C47.30
- - - sacral C47.51
- - - sciatic C47.20
- - - thoracic C47.31
- - - tibial C47.23
- - - trigeminal C72.51
- - - trochlear C72.501
- - - ulnar C47.13
- - - vagus C72.54
- - nervous system
- - - autonomic C47.9
- - - central C72.9
- - nose NEC C76.0
- - oesophagus C15
- - oral cavity NEC C14.–
- - orbit C69.6
- - oropharynx C10
- - ovary
- - overlapping lesion
- - - accessory sinuses C31.8
- - - biliary tract NEC C24.8
- - - bone and articular cartilage C41.8
- - - brain C71.8
- - - - with other parts of central nervous system C72.8
- - - brain stem C71.78
- - - connective and soft tissue C49.8
- - - digestive system NEC C26.8
- - - genital organs
- - - - female C57.8
- - - - male C63.8
- - - heart, mediastinum and pleura C38.8
- - - larynx C32.8
- - - lip, oral cavity and pharynx C14.8
- - - peripheral nerves and autonomic nervous system C47.8
- - - rectum, anus and anal canal C21.8
- - - respiratory and intrathoracic organs C39
- - - spinal cord C72.08
- - - urinary organs C68.8
- - pancreas C25
- - paraganglia NEC C75.57
- - parathyroid gland C75.0

Neoplasm — *continued*
- malignant — *continued*
- - parotid gland C07
- - pelviureteric junction C65
- - penis C60
- - peritoneum C48
- - pharynx NEC C14.0
- - pineal gland C75.3
- - pituitary gland C75.1
- - placenta C58
- - plasma cell NEC C90.2
- - plexus
- - - brachial C47.10
- - - - secondary C79.42
- - - cervical C47.02
- - - lumbar C47.42
- - - lumbosacral, secondary C79.43
- - - thoracic C47.32
- - pluriglandular C75.8
- - pons C71.71
- - - secondary C79.351
- - prostate C61
- - rectum C20
- - - with colon C19
- - renal pelvis C65
- - respiratory system NEC, secondary C78
- - retina C69.2
- - retrobulbar tissue C69.6
- - retro-ocular tissue C69.6
- - retroperitoneum C48
- - ribs C41.3
- - sacrum C41.4
- - sebaceous glands C44
- - sinus
- - - accessory, overlapping lesion C31.8
- - - ethmoidal C31.1
- - - frontal C31.2
- - - maxillary C31.0
- - - sphenoidal C31.3
- - skin NEC C44
- - small intestine C17
- - soft tissue NEC C49.9
- - - abdomen C49.4
- - - face C49.0
- - - head C49.0
- - - hip C49.2
- - - limb
- - - - lower C49.2
- - - - upper C49.1
- - - neck C49.0
- - - pelvis C49.5
- - - shoulder C49.1
- - - thorax C49.3
- - - trunk C49.6
- - spinal cord
- - - cervical C72.00
- - - cervicothoracic C72.01
- - - lumbar C72.04

Neoplasm — *continued*
- malignant — *continued*
- - spinal cord — *continued*
- - - lumbosacral C72.05
- - - overlapping lesion C72.08
- - - sacral C72.06
- - - secondary C79.40
- - - thoracic C72.02
- - - thoracolumbar C72.03
- - spine C41.2
- - sternum C41.3
- - stomach C16
- - subglottis C32.2
- - supraglottis C32.1
- - sweat glands C44
- - testis C62.–
- - thalamus C71.01
- - - secondary C79.32
- - thymus C37
- - thyroid gland C73
- - tongue, overlapping lesion C02.8
- - trachea C33
- - ureter C66
- - urinary organs, overlapping lesion C68.8
- - uterus C55
- - - cervix C53
- - - corpus C54
- - vagina C52
- - vertebral column C41.2
- - vulva C51
Neovascularization, retinal H35.0
Nephritis N05
- arteriosclerotic I12
Nephropathy N05
- hypertensive I12
- uraemic N18.8† G63.8*
Nephrosclerosis I12
Nephrosis, lipoid N04
Nervousness R45.0
Neuralgia M79.2
- glossopharyngeal G52.10
- - postzoster B02.2† G53.03*
- laryngeal, superior G52.20
- occipital G52.80
- postzoster B02.2† G53.0*
- - glossopharyngeal B02.2† G53.03*
- - trigeminal B02.2† G53.01*
- trigeminal G50.0
- - idiopathic G50.00
- - postherpetic B02.2† G53.00*
- - postzoster B02.2† G53.01*
- - secondary G50.09
Neurasthenia F48.0
Neurilemmoma, acoustic nerve H93.30
Neurinoma, acoustic nerve H93.30
Neuritis M79.2
- acoustic, in syphilis A52.1† H94.0*

Neuritis — *continued*
- brachial M54.1
- lumbar M54.1
- lumbosacral M54.1
- optic H46
- peripheral, pregnancy-related O26.8
- retrobulbar H46
- – in (due to)
- – – late syphilis A52.1† H48.1*
- – – meningococcal infection A39.8† H48.1*
- – – multiple sclerosis G53.–† H48.1*
- shoulder-girdle G54.5
- thoracic M54.1

Neuroacanthocytosis G25.53
Neurofibromatosis (nonmalignant) Q85.0
Neuroma
- interdigital
- – lower limb G57.83
- – upper limb G56.81
- traumatic G58.81

Neuromyelitis optica G36.0
Neuromyopathy
- alcoholic
- – acute G72.10
- – chronic G72.11
- paraneoplastic D48† G13.08*

Neuromyotonia G71.14
Neuropathy G62.9
- autonomic
- – diabetic (*see also* E10–E14 with fourth character .4) E14.4† G99.0*
- – peripheral, idiopathic G90.0
- congenital sensory G60.84
- Déjerine–Sottas G60.02
- diabetic (*see also* E10–E14 with fourth character .4) E14.4† G59.0*
- giant axonal, familial G60.85
- glossopharyngeal, herpes zoster, acute B02.2† G53.02*
- hereditary G60.9
- – motor and sensory
- – – type I G60.00
- – – type II G60.01
- – – type III G60.02
- – – type IV G60.1
- – – type V G60.03
- – – type VI G60.04
- – – type VII G60.05
- – pressure-sensitive G60.87
- – sensory and autonomic
- – – type I G60.80
- – – type II G60.81
- – – type III G60.82
- – – type IV G60.83
- – – type V G60.84
- – specified NEC G60.8
- hypoglossal, idiopathic G52.30

Neuropathy — *continued*
- idiopathic G60.9
- – progressive G60.3
- – specified NEC G60.8
- intercostal G58.0
- Low's G60.84
- optic H46
- – ischaemic H47.02
- – post-infection H47.03
- paraneoplastic, sensory D48.–† G13.01*
- serum G61.1
- small fibre G62.81
- tomaculous G60.87
- trigeminal
- – herpes zoster, acute B02.2† G53.00*
- – idiopathic G50.80
- – secondary G50.81
- with
- – hereditary ataxia G60.2
- – multiple endocrine neoplasia G60.86

Neurosis
- compensation F68.0
- depressive F34.1
- hypochondriacal F45.2
- occupational F48.82
- psychasthenic F48.83

Neurosyphilis A52.3
- asymptomatic A52.2
- juvenile A50.4
- – taboparetic A50.41
- late congenital A50.4
- symptomatic A52.1

Newborn — *see* Fetus
Niemann–Pick disease E75.26
Night
- blindness H53.6
- – vitamin A deficiency E50.5
- terrors F51.4

Nightmare F51.5
Nocardiosis A43
Nocturia R35
Noise, effects on inner ear H83.3
Noonan's syndrome Q87.14
Nose, congenital deformity Q67.4
Nosophobia F45.2
Nothnagel's vasomotor acroparaesthesia I73.8
Nyctohemeral rhythm inversion, psychogenic F51.2
Nystagmus H55.–
- central positional, idiopathic H81.40
- downbeat H55.–1
- lateral, phasic H55.–2
- retractorius H55.–5
- rotatory H55.–3
- see-saw H55.–4
- upbeat H55.–0

O

Oasthouse disease E72.03
Obesity E66.–
Observation (for)
– malignant neoplasm, suspected Z03.1
– nervous system disorder, suspected Z03.3
Obstruction
– aqueduct of Sylvius, congenital Q03.0
– due to foreign body accidentally left in operation wound or body cavity T81.5
– mechanical, due to electronic neurostimulator T85.1
– mitral (valve) (rheumatic) I05.0
Occlusion
– artery
– – basilar I65.1
– – carotid I65.2
– – cerebellar I66.3
– – cerebral I66.9
– – – anterior I66.1
– – – causing infarction I63.5
– – – middle I66.0
– – – multiple and bilateral I66.4
– – – posterior I66.2
– – – specified NEC I66.8
– – precerebral I65.9
– – – causing infarction I63.2
– – – multiple and bilateral I65.3
– – – specified NEC I65.8
– – retinal
– – – central H34.1
– – – specified NEC H34.2
– – – transient H34.0
– – vertebral I65.0
– retinal
– – vascular H34.9
– – – specified NEC H34.8
– – vein H34.8
Ochranosis (ochronosis), alkaptonuric E70.23
Oculopathy
– syphylitic
– – late congenital A50.3
– – secondary NEC A51.4† H58.8*
– toxoplasma B58.0
Oedema
– angioneurotic T78.3
– cerebral G93.6
– – due to birth injury P11.0
– – traumatic S06.1
– spinal cord
– – cervical S14.0
– – lumbar S34.0
Oedema — *continued*
– spinal cord — *continued*
– – thoracic S24.0
– Quincke's T78.3
Oesophagitis K20
Old age R54
Oligoclonal bands, increased, in cerebrospinal fluid R83.41
Oligomenorrhoea N91.5
– primary N91.3
– secondary N91.4
Oliguria R34
Ollier's disease Q78.4
Omphalitis of newborn P38
Omphalocele Q79.2
Onchocerciasis, onchocercosis B73
Ondine's curse G47.3
One-and-a-half syndrome H51.01
Opacity, vitreous, congenital Q14.0
Openbite K07.2
Ophthalmoplegia
– dysthyroid E05.0† G73.50*
– external H49.8
– – progressive H49.4
– internal (complete) (total) H52.50
– internuclear H51.2
– supranuclear, progressive G23.1
– total (external) H49.3
Orbitopathy, dysthyroid E05.0† G73.50*
Ornithine metabolism disorder E72.4
Orozco–Diaz syndrome G11.22
Orthopnoea R06.0
Ossification
– ligament, posterior longitudinal M48.8
– muscle M61.–
– – paralytic M61.2
– – specified NEC M61.5
– – with burns M61.3
– subperiosteal, post-traumatic M89.8
Osteitis
– condensans M85.3
– deformans M88.–
– fibrosa cystica generalisata E21.0
Osteoarthritis of spine M47.–
Osteochondrodysplasia NEC Q78.8
– with defects of growth of tubular bones and spine Q77.–
Osteochondrosis of spine M42.9
– adult M42.1
– juvenile M42.0
Osteodystrophy
– azotaemic N25.0

P

Pachygyria Q04.33
Pachymeningitis G03.–
– bacterial G00.–
Paget's disease of bone M88.9
– skull M88.0
Pain R52.9
– abdominal R10.9
– – lower R10.3
– – upper R10.1
– acute R52.0
– back, low M54.5
– chest R07.3
– – on breathing R07.1
– chronic R52.2
– – intractable R52.1
– disorder, somatoform F45.4
– face R51
– – atypical G50.1
– female genital organs N94.–
– generalized R52.9
– loin M54.5
– menstrual N94.–
– ocular H57.1
– pelvic R10.2
– perineal R10.2
– precordial R07.2
– psychogenic F45.4
– spine, thoracic M54.6
– thigh, in intervertebral disc disorder M51.1
– throat R07.0
Palsy
– Bell's G51.0
– bulbar, progressive G12.22
– – of childhood G12.110
– cerebral, infantile G80
– diver's T70.3
– gaze, conjugate H51.0
– – in brain stem syndromes G46.3
– facial G51.0
– – due to birth injury P11.3
– nerve
– – abducent H49.2
– – cranial
– – – fourth H49.1
– – – sixth H49.2
– – – third H49.0
– – facial G51.0
– – ocular, due to herpes zoster B02.2† G53.06*
– – oculomotor H49.0
– – peroneal G57.3
Palsy — *continued*
– nerve — *continued*
– – trochlear H49.1
– – ulnar, tardy G56.21
– pseudobulbar, progressive G12.23
Pancreas — *see condition*
Pancreatitis K85
– acute K85
– chronic K86.1
– – alcohol-induced K86.0
– haemorrhagic K85
– subacute K85
– suppurative K85
Pandysautonomia
– acute G90.00
– chronic G90.01
Panencephalitis, subacute
– rubella B06.03
– sclerosing A81.1
Panhypopituitarism E23.00
Panniculitis
– back and neck M54.3
– relapsing M35.6
Pansinusitis
– acute J01.4
– chronic J32.4
Papilloedema H47.1
Paracoccidioidomycosis B41.8
– disseminated B41.7
– generalized B41.7
Paraesthesia, skin R20.2
Parageusia R43.2
Paragonimiasis B66.4
Paralysis, paralytic
– agitans G20.–
– Benedikt's I67.9† G46.30*
– diaphragm J98.6
– diver's T70.3
– Erb's, due to birth injury P14.0
– gait R26.1
– gaze
– – downward H51.82
– – upward H51.81
– glottis J38.0
– Klumpke's, due to birth injury P14.1
– larynx J38.0
– limb
– – lower G83.1
– – – both G82.2
– – upper G83.2
– – – both G83.0
– Millard–Gubler I67.9† G46.31*

Pins and needles R20.2
Pituitary (gland)
– abscess E23.60
– apoplexy E23.63
– dwarfism E23.022
– gigantism E22.0
– hormone deficiency, multiple E23.00
– – anterior E23.07
– hyperfunction E22.–
– hypofunction E23.–
– insufficiency E23.0
– necrosis, postpartum E23.01
Plagiocephaly Q67.3
Plague
– meningitis A20.3
– septicaemic A20.7
Plasmacytoma C90.2
Platybasia Q75.82
Platyspondylisis Q76.47
Plexopathy, idiopathic brachial G54.5
Pneumonia J18
– aspiration J69.0
– – neonatal P24
– bacterial NEC J15
– congenital P23
– *Haemophilus influenzae* J14
– infective, acquired in utero or during birth P23
– neonatal
– – aspiration P24
– – congenital P23
– specified organism NEC J16
– *Streptococcus pneumoniae* J13
Pneumonitis
– aspiration (due to)
– – anaesthesia during labour and delivery O74.0
– – food and vomit J69.0
– rubella, congenital P35.0
Pneumothorax J93
Poisoning by drugs, medicaments and biological substances — *see* Table of drugs and chemicals, page 565
– sequelae T96
Poland's syndrome Q79.84
Poliomyelitis (acute) A80.9
– nonparalytic A80.4
– paralytic A80.3
– – vaccine-associated A80.0
– – wild virus
– – – imported A80.1
– – – indigenous
– sequelae B91.–
Polyangiitis overlap syndrome M30.8
Polyarteritis
– juvenile M30.2
– nodosa M30.0
– with lung involvement M30.1
Polycythaemia
– benign D75.0
– familial D75.0
– secondary D75.1
– vera D45
Polydipsia R63.1
Polydystrophy, pseudo-Hurler E77.01
Polymorphs, increased levels in cerebrospinal fluid R83.62
Polymyalgia rheumatica M35.3
– with giant cell arteritis M31.5
Polymyositis M33.2
Polyneuritis
– acute (post-)infective G61.0
– cranialis G52.7
Polyneuropathy G62.9
– alcoholic G62.1
– amyloid, familial E85.1
– – type I E85.10
– – type II E85.11
– – type III E85.12
– – type IV E85.13
– diabetic (*see also* E10–E14 with fourth character .4) E14.4† G63.2*
– drug-induced G62.0
– due to toxic agent NEC G62.2
– in
– – ciguatera fish poisoning T61.0† G63.8*
– – diphtheria A36.8† G63.0*
– – hepatic failure, chronic K72.–† G63.8*
– – hepatitis B infection
– – – acute B16.–† G63.0*
– – – chronic B18.–† G63.0*
– – HIV disease B23.8† G63.0*
– – infectious mononucleosis B27.–† G63.0*
– – leprosy A30.–† G63.0*
– – Lyme disease A69.2† G63.0*
– – mumps B26.8† G63.0*
– – shigellosis A03.–† G63.0*
– – rheumatoid arthritis M05.3† G63.6*
– – sarcoidosis D86.88† G63.8*
– – syphilis, late A52.1† G63.0*
– – – congenital A50.4† G63.0*
– – typhoid fever A17.8† G63.0*
– – uraemic nephropathy N18.8† G63.8*
– – vitamin B_{12} deficiency E53.80† G63.4*
– – xanthoma tuberosum E78.26† G63.3*
– – zoster B02.2† G63.0*
– inflammatory G1.9
– – demyelinating, chronic
– – – progressive G61.80
– – – relapsing–remitting G61.81
– – specified NEC G61.8
– postherpetic B02.2† G63.0*
– radiation-induced G62.80
– specified NEC G62.8
– tuberculous A17.8† G63.0*
Polyphagia R63.2

Pupil — *continued*
- Argyll Robertson, syphilitic A52.1† H58.0*
- myotonic H57.00
- - paraneoplastic H57.01
- springing H57.02

Purpura D69.–
- allergic D69.0
- fibrinolytic D65
- fulminans D65
- hypergammaglobulinaemic, benign D89.0
- nonthrombocytopenic NEC D69.2

Purpura — *continued*
- thrombocytopenic
- - idiopathic D69.3
- - thrombotic M31.1

Pygopagus Q89.4
Pyknolepsy G40.33
Pylorospasm NEC K31.3
Pyomyositis, tropical M60.0
Pyrexia
- during labour NEC O75.2
- heat T67.0

Q

R

Rabies A82.8
- sylvatic A82.0
- urban A82.1
Rachischisis Q05.*x*5
Radiations, optic S04.03
Radiculitis NEC M54.1
Radiculo-myelopathy G54.83
Radiculopathy NEC M54.1
- with
- - cervical disc disorder M50.1
- - lumbar and other intervertebral disc disorder M51.1
- - spondylosis M47.2
Radiculo-plexopathy G54.82
Radiotherapy session Z51.0
Raised
- antibody titre R76.0
- - acetylcholine receptor R76.80
- - anti-GM1 ganglioside R76.84
- - antineuronal R76.82
- - muscle antistriational R76.81
- - rheumatological R76.83
- immunoglobin level R76.87
Ramsay–Hunt ataxia G11.13
Rasmussen's syndrome G40.51
Raynaud's disease, gangrene, phenomenon or syndrome I73.0
Reaction
- abnormal, to surgical procedure Y83.–
- allergic, to correct drug or medicament properly administered T88.7
- anaphylactic T78.2
- - due to
- - - correct drug or medicament properly administered T88.6
- - - food T78.0
- - - serum T80.5
- drug T88.7
- inflammatory, due to internal prosthetic device, implant or graft T85.7
- toxic, to local anaesthesia
- - in labour and delivery O74.4
- - in puerperium O89.3
Reading disorder, specific F81.0
Rearrangement, chromosomal, balanced Q95
- in abnormal individual
- - non-sex chromosomes Q95.2
- - sex/non-sex chromosomes Q95.3
Reflex, abnormal R29.2
- pupillary H57.0
Rehabilitation Z50.9
- specified NEC Z50.8
- tobacco Z50.8
- vocational NEC Z50.7
Refsum's disease G60.1
- infantile E80.300
Relaxation, diaphragm J98.6
Renal failure — *see* Failure, renal
Rendu–Osler–Weber disease I78.0
Restless legs syndrome
- familial G25.83
- sporadic G25.82
Restlessness R45.1
Retardation
- fetal growth P05.9
- mental F79.–
- - mild F70.–
- - moderate F71.–
- - profound F73.–
- - severe F72.–
- - specified NEC F78.–
- physical R62.8
- - due to malnutrition E45
- reading, specific F81.0
- spelling, specific F81.1
Retention, urine R33
Reticuloendotheliosis, nonlipid C96.0
Reticulohistiocytoma (giant-cell) D76.3
Reticulosis
- haemophagocytic, familial D76.1
- histiocytic medullary C96.1
- nonlipid C96.0
Retinitis H30.9
- disseminated H30.1
- focal H30.0
- pigmentosa H35.5
Retinochoroiditis H30.9
- disseminated H30.1
- focal H30.0
Retinopathy H35.0
- atherosclerotic I70.80† H36.8*
- background H35.0
- Coats' H35.0
- diabetic (*see also* E10–E14 with fourth character .3) E14.3† H36.8*
- exudative H35.0
- hypertensive H35.0
- prematurity H35.1
- proliferative NEC H35.2
- - sickle-cell D57.–† H36.8*
- solar H31.0

S

Sacroiliitis NEC M46.1
Salaam attacks G40.40
Sandhoff's disease E75.03
Sandifer's syndrome G24.81
Sanfilippo's syndrome E76.20
Sanger–Brown ataxia G11.23
Sarcoidosis D86.8
Sarcoma, Kaposi's C46.–
Sarcosinaemia E72.54
Scar, chorioretinal H31.0
– postsurgical H59.8
Scarlatina, scarlet fever A38
Scheie's syndrome E76.02
Scheuermann's disease M42.0
Schilder's disease G37.0
Schistosomiasis B65
Schizencephaly Q04.61
Schmidt's syndrome E31.0
Schmorl's nodes M51.4
Schultze's simple acroparaesthesia I73.8
Schwannoma, acoustic nerve H93.30
Schwartz–Jampel syndrome G71.10
Sciatica M54.3
– due to intervertebral disc disorder M51.1
– with lumbago M54.4
Scleroderma M34.–
Sclerosis
– ALS G12.20
– amyotrophic lateral G12.20
– choroid H31.1
– concentric G37.5
– coronary (artery) I25.1
– diffuse G37.0
– laminar, Morel's G31.24
– liver, alcoholic K70.2
– Mönckeberg's (medial) I70.2
– multiple G35.–
– – progressive
– – – primary G35.–1
– – – secondary G35.–2
– – relapsing/remitting G35.–0
– systemic M34.9
– – drug-induced M34.2
– – progressive M34.0
– – with myelopathy M34.8
Scoliosis M41.9
– adolescent M41.1
– congenital Q67.5
– – due to bony malformation Q76.3
– – postural Q67.5
– idiopathic M41.2
– – infantile M41.0

Scoliosis — *continued*
– idiopathic — *continued*
– – juvenile M41.1
– neuromuscular M41.4
– secondary NEC M41.5
– specified NEC M41.8
– thoracogenic M41.3
– tuberous Q85.1
Scotoma H53.4
– scintillating H53.1
Screening (for)
– antenatal Z36.–
– chromosomal abnormalities Z13.7
– congenital malformation Z13.7
– developmental disorder in childhood Z13.4
Scurvy E54
Seckel's syndrome Q87.180
Secretion
– hormone
– – ectopic NEC E34.2
– – antidiuretic inappropriate E22.2
– increased — *see* Hypersecretion
Segawa's disease or syndrome G24.13
Seitelberger's syndrome G31.82
Seizure
– convulsive (*see also* Convulsions) R56.8
– epileptic G40.9
– isolated R56.8
Semicoma R40.1
Senescence (without mention of psychosis) R54
Senile, senility R54
– asthenia R54
– debility R54
– dementia F03
– psychosis F03
Sensation
– choking R06.82
– skin, disturbance R20.–
Separation, retinal layers H35.7
Sepsis, following infusion, injection or transfusion T80.2
Septicaemia A41.9
– anaerobic A41.4
– anthrax A22.7
– during labour O75.3
– following infusion, injection or transfusion T80.2
– Gram-negative organism A41.5
– *Haemophilus influenzae* A41.3
– herpesviral B00.7

Septicaemia — *continued*
- pneumococcal A40.3
- postprocedural T81.4
- specified organism NEC A41.8
- *Staphylococcus*, staphylococcal A41.2
- – *aureus* A41.0
- – coagulase-negative A41.1
- *Streptococcus*, streptococcal A40.9
- – group A A40.0
- – group B A40.1
- – group C A40.2
- – *pneumoniae* A40.3
- – specified NEC A40.8

Sequelae (of)
- burn T95
- complications (of)
- – early, of trauma T98.2
- – surgical and medical care NEC T98.3
- corrosion T95
- deficiency
- – nutritional E64.9
- – – specified NEC E64.8
- – vitamin
- – – A E64.1
- – – C E64.2
- effects of external causes NEC T98.1
- encephalitis, viral B94.1
- fracture
- – facial bones T90.2
- – pelvis T91.2
- – skull T90.2
- – spine T91.1
- – thorax T91.2
- frostbite T95
- infectious and parasitic diseases B94.9
- – specified NEC B94.8
- inflammatory disease of central nervous system G09
- injury
- – cranial nerves T90.3
- – head T90.9
- – – specified NEC T90.8
- – intracranial T90.5
- – limb
- – – lower T93.–
- – – upper T92.–
- – multiple body regions T94
- – neck T91.9
- – – specified NEC T91.8
- – nerve
- – – cranial
- – – limb
- – – – lower T93.4
- – – – upper T92.4
- – spinal cord T91.3
- – trunk T91
- – – specified NEC T91.8
- leprosy B92

Sequelae (of) — *continued*
- malnutrition E64.–
- – protein–energy E64.0
- poisoning due to
- – drug, medicament or biological substance T96
- – nonmedicinal substance T97
- poliomyelitis B91.–
- rickets E64.3
- trachoma B94.0
- tuberculosis, central nervous system B90.0

Serum neuropathy G61.1

Sheehan's syndrome E23.01

Shigellosis A03

Shock (due to) (during) (following) (from) R57.9
- abortion O08.3
- allergic T78.2
- anaesthesia T88.2
- anaphylactic (due to) T78.2
- – adverse food reaction T78.0
- – correct medicinal substance properly administered T88.6
- – serum T80.5
- cardiogenic R57.0
- ectopic or molar pregnancy O08.3
- electric W87
- – current T75.4
- endotoxic R57.8
- hypovolaemic R57.1
- – injury (immediate) (delayed) T79
- labour and delivery O75.1
- lightning T75.0
- obstetric O75.1
- postoperative NOS T81.1
- septic A41.9
- – following infusion, injection or transfusion T80.2
- specified NEC R57.8
- syndrome, toxic A48.3
- traumatic T79.4

Short, shortening, shortness (of)
- breath R06.0
- rib syndrome Q77.2
- stature E34.3
- – achondroplastic (Q77)
- – constitutional E34.3
- – Laron-type E34.3
- – pituitary E23.0
- – psychosocial E34.3
- – renal N25.0
- – thanatophoric Q77.1
- tendon and constricting band Q79.83

Shoulder-girdle neuritis G54.5

Shoulder–hand syndrome M89.0

Shuddering attacks, childhood G25.04

Shunt
- arteriovenous, for dialysis Z99.2
- CSF Z98.2

Shy–Drager syndrome G90.31
Sialidosis E77.12
Sicca syndrome M35.0
Sick sinus syndrome I49.5
Sickle-cell
– anaemia, with crisis D57.0
– beta thalassaemia D56
Sighing R06.83
Signs — *see* Symptoms
Simian B disease B00.4† G05.1*
Simmonds' disease E23.00
Simultanagnosia R48.104
Sinus
– branchial cleft Q18.0
– face and neck, medial Q18.8
– preauricular Q18.2
Sinusitis
– acute J01.9
– – ethmoidal J01.2
– – frontal J01.1
– – maxillary J01.0
– – specified NEC J01.8
– – sphenoidal J01.3
– chronic J32.9
– – ethmoidal J32.2
– – frontal J32.1
– – maxillary J32.0
– – specified NEC J32.8
– – sphenoidal J32.3
Siriasis T67.0
Sjögren's syndrome M35.0
Skew deviation H50.5
Sleep
– apnoea G47.3
– disorder G47.9
– drunkenness G47.82
– – emotional F51.9
– – nonorganic F51.9
– – – specified NEC F51.8
– – specified NEC G47.8
– paralysis G47.42
– rhythm inversion F51.2
– starts G47.831
– terrors F51.4
Sleeping sickness B56.9
– East African B56.1
– West African B56.0
Sleeplessness
– associated with menopause N95.1
– nonorganic F51.0
– organic G47.0
Sleep–wake
– schedule disorder G47.2
– – nonorganic F51.2
– transition disorder G47.83
Sleeptalking G47.832
Sleepwalking F51.3
Slim disease B22.2
Slowness, behavioural R46.4
Sly's syndrome E76.24
Small-for-dates (infant) P05.1
Smallpox B03
Smith–Lemli–Opitz syndrome Q87.181
Snapping jaw K07.6
Sneezing R06.7
Snoring R06.5
Social
– role conflict NEC Z73.5
– skills, inadequate NEC Z73.4
Sodium
– deficiency E87.10
– excess E87.0
– overload E87.0
Soemmerring's ring H26.4
Somnambulism F51.3
Somnolence R40.0
Sotos' syndrome Q87.31
Sparganosis B70.–
Spasm(s), spastic
– anal K59.4
– artery I73.9
– – cerebral G45.9
– carpopedal R29.0
– cerebral artery G45.9
– diplegia Q80.1
– dysarthria R47.10
– gait R26.10
– hemifacial, clonic G51.3
– infantile G40.40
– near reflex H52.5
– palsy, cerebral G80.0
– paralysis, congenital G80.0
– paraplegia, hereditary G11.4
– specified NEC R25.28
Speech
– disturbance NEC R47.8
– therapy Z50.5
Sphingolipidosis E75.3
– specified NEC E75.2
Spielmeyer–Vogt disease E75.42
Spina bifida Q05.9
– cervical Q05.5
– – with hydrocephalus Q05.0
– dorsal Q05.6
– – with hydrocephalus Q05.1
– lumbar Q05.7
– – with hydrocephalus Q05.2
– lumbosacral Q05.7
– – with hydrocephalus Q05.2
– occulta Q76.0
– sacral Q05.8
– – with hydrocephalus Q05.3
– thoracic Q05.6
– – with hydrocephalus Q05.1
– thoracolumbar Q05.6
– – with hydrocephalus Q05.1
– with hydrocephalus Q05.4

Spondylitis
- ankylosing M45
- brucella A23.–† M49.1*
- enterobacterial A04† M49.2*
Spondylolisthesis M43.1
- congenital Q76.2
Spondylolysis M43.0
- congenital Q76.2
Spondylopathy M48.9
- infective NEC M46.5
- inflammatory M46.9
- - specified NEC M46.8
- neuropathic, in
- - syringomyelia and syringobulbia G95.0† M49.4*
- - tabes dorsalis A52.1† M49.4*
- specified NEC M48.8
- traumatic M48.3
Spondylosis M47.9
- cervical M47.8
- lumbosacral M47.8
- specified NEC M47.8
- thoracic M47.8
- with
- - myelopathy NEC M47.1
- - radiculopathy NEC M47.2
Sprain, strain (joint) (ligament) T14.3
- atlantoaxial S13.41
- atlanto-occipital S13.42
- cervical S13.40
- cricoarytenoid S13.5
- cricothyroid S13.5
- head NEC S03.5
- - with neck T03.0
- jaw S03.4
- multiple body regions NEC T03.8
- neck NEC S13.6
- - with head T03.0
- pelvis NEC S33.7
- - with thorax and lower back T03.1
- sacroiliac S33.6
- spine
- - cervical S13.4
- - lumbar S33.5
- - - with thorax and pelvis T03.1
- - thoracic S23.3
- temporomandibular S03.4
- thorax, with pelvis and lower back T03.1
- thryoid cartilage S13.5
Staggering gait R26.0
Stammering
- organic origin R47.80
- psychogenic F98.5
Stargardt's disease H35.5
Starvation T73.0
- oedema E43
State
- climacteric, female N95.1

State — *continued*
- confusional, acute or subacute F05.–
- emotional shock and stress R45.7
- hallucinatory, organic (nonalcoholic) F06.0
- menopausal N95.1
- - artificial N95.3
- paranoid, organic F06.2
- postsurgical NEC Z98.–
- twilight, psychogenic F44.8
- vital exhaustion Z73.0
- withdrawal — *code to* F10–F19 with fourth character .3
- - alcohol F10.3
- - - with delirium F10.4
- - caffeine F15.3
- - - with delirium F15.4
- - cannabinoids F12.3
- - - with delirium F10.4
- - cocaine F14.3
- - - with delirium F14.4
- - hallucinogens F16.3
- - - with delirium F16.4
- - hypnotics F13.3
- - - with delirium F13.4
- - multiple drugs F19.3
- - - with delirium F19.4
- - opioids F11.3
- - - with delirium F11.4
- - psychoactive substances NEC F19.3
- - - with delirium F19.4
- - sedatives F13.3
- - - with delirium F13.4
- - stimulants NEC F15.3
- - - with delirium F15.4
- - tobacco F17.3
- - volatile solvents F18.3
- - - with delirium F18.4
- - with delirium — *code to* F10–F19 with fourth character .4
Stature, short — *see* Short, stature
Status
- asthmaticus J46
- epileptic absence G41.1
- epilepticus G41.9
- - complex partial G41.2
- - generalized convulsive G41.1
- - grand mal G41.0
- - petit mal G41.1
- - specified NEC G41.8
- - tonic–clonic G41.0
- human immunodeficiency virus infection, asymptomatic Z21
- migrainosus G43.2
- renal dialysis Z99.2
Steele–Richardson–Olszewski disease or syndrome G23.10
Steinert's disease G71.12

Stenosis
- aqueduct of Sylvius Q03.0
- artery
- - basilar I65.1
- - carotid I65.2
- - cerebellar I66.3
- - cerebral I66.9
- - - anterior I66.1
- - - causing infarction I63.5
- - - middle I66.0
- - - multiple and bilateral I66.4
- - - posterior I66.2
- - - specified NEC I66.8
- - precerebral I65.9
- - - causing infarction I63.2
- - - multiple and bilateral I65.3
- - - specified NEC I65.8
- - vertebral I65.0
- caudal M48.0
- intervertebral foramina
- - connective tissue M99.7
- - disc M99.5
- - osseous M99.6
- - subluxation M99.6
- mitral I05.2
- neural canal
- - connective tissue M99.4
- - intervertebral disc M99.5
- - osseous M99.3
- - subluxation M99.2
- spinal M48.0
- valvular I38
- - rheumatic I09.1
Stereotypies G25.87
- psychogenic F98.4
Sterility
- female N97
- male N46
Sternum bifidum Q76.7
Stiff man syndrome G25.8
Stokes–Adams syndrome I45.9
Stomatitis, aphthous K12.0
Storm, thyroid E05.5
Strabismus H50.9
- concomitant H50.4
- - convergent H50.0
- - divergent H50.1
- mechanical H50.6
- paralytic H49.9
- - specified NEC H49.8
- specified NEC H50.8
- vertical H50.2
Strain — *see also* Sprain
- low back M54.5
- mental NEC Z73.3
- muscle M62.6
- physical NEC 73.3
Strangury R30.0
Stress NEC Z73.3
Stricture
- artery I77.1
- auditory canal (external), congenital Q16.1
Stridor R06.1
Stroke I64
- sequelae I69.4
Struma lymphomatosa E06.3
Stuart–Prower disease D68.2
Stunting, nutritional E45
Stupor R40.1
- dissociative F44.2
- manic F30.2
Sturge–Weber(–Dimitri) syndrome Q85.81
Stuttering F98.5
- organic origin R47.80
Subluxation
- atlantoaxial, recurrent M43.4
- - with myelopathy M43.3
- complex (vertebral) M99.1
- joint, traumatic T14.3
- ligament, traumatic T14.3
- vertebral, recurrent NEC M43.5
Submersion, nonfatal T75.1
Subnormality, mental F79.–
- mild F70.–
- moderate F71.–
- profound F73.–
- severe F72.–
Sudeck's atrophy M89.0
Suffocation (by strangulation) T71
Sunstroke T67.0
Suppuration, sinus
- acute J01.–
- chronic J32.–
Surveillance, medical, following treatment Z09.–
- for neoplasm Z08.–
Suspiciousness R46.5
Sutures, wide cranial, of newborn P96.3
Swallowing, abnormal, non-REM-sleep-related syndrome G47.812
Sydenham's chorea I02.–
Symptoms
- elaboration, for psychological reasons F68.0
- feigning F68.1
- general NEC R68.–
- involving
- - appearance R46.–
- - awareness R41.–
- - behaviour R46.–
- - circulatory system R09.–
- - cognitive functions R41.–
- - emotional state R45.–
- - food and fluid intake R63.–

Symptoms — *continued*
- involving — *continued*
- - general sensations and perceptions R44.–
- - musculoskeletal system NEC R29.8
- - nervous system NEC R29.8
- - respiratory system R09.–
- nonspecific, in infancy R68.1
- physical
- - elaboration for psychological reasons F68.0
- - feigning F68.1
- psychological, feigning F68.1
Syncope R55
- carotid sinus G90.02
- heat T67.1
- psychogenic F48.84
Syndrome
- Aarskog's Q87.10
- aches, cramps and pains R25.21
- acquired immunodeficiency (AIDS) B24
- adrenal, meningococcic A39.1† E35.1*
- adrenogenital E25.–
- Albers–Schönberg Q78.2
- Albright(–McCune)(–Sternberg) Q78.1
- Alport's Q87.80
- alveolar hypoventilation G47.30
- amnesic
- - alcohol-induced F10.6
- - caffeine-induced F15.6
- - cannabinoid-induced F12.6
- - drug-induced — *code to* F11–F19 with fourth character .6
- - hallucinogen-induced F16.6
- - hypnotic-induced F14.6
- - multiple drug-induced F19.6
- - opioid-induced F11.6
- - organic (nonalcoholic) F04
- - psychoactive substance-induced NEC F19.6
- - sedative-induced F13.6
- - stimulant-induced NEC F15.6
- - volatile solvent-induced F18.6
- androgen resistance E34.5
- anterior spinal artery compression M47.0† G99.2*
- aortic
- - arch M31.4
- - bifurcation I74.0
- Apert's Q87.01
- Arnold–Chiari Q07.0
- Asperger's F84.5
- aspiration, neonatal P24
- Bartter's E26.8
- battered baby, child or spouse T74.1
- Beckwith–Wiedmann Q87.30
- Benedikt's I67.9† G46.30*
- benign fasciculation R25.30

Syndrome — *continued*
- Bernard(–Horner) G90.2
- blast injury T70.8
- Bouveret(–Hoffmann) I47.9
- brain (acute) (subacute) F05.–
- - post-traumatic, nonpsychotic F07.2
- brain stem stroke I67.9† G46.3*
- Brown's sheath H50.6
- Camurati–Engelmann Q78.3
- carcinoid E34.0
- carotid artery (hemispheric) G45.1
- carpal tunnel G56.0
- Carpenter's Q87.083
- cauda equina G83.4
- cerebellar G96.80
- - hereditary G11.9
- - stroke I67.9† G46.4*
- cervical
- - fusion Q76.1
- - sympathetic, posterior M53.0
- cervicobrachial M53.1
- cervicocranial M53.1
- Chediak(–Steinbrinck)–Higashi E70.32
- Churg–Strauss M30.1
- Claude's I67.9† G46.30*
- clumsy child F82
- Cockayne's Q87.11
- compartment T79.6
- compression, artery
- - anterior spinal or vertebral M47.0† G99.2*
- - coeliac I77.4
- Conn's E26.0
- Costen's K07.6
- CR(E)ST M34.1
- cri-du-chat Q93.4
- Crigler–Najjar E80.5
- Cross' E70.33
- cryptophthalmos Q87.082
- cubital tunnel, ulnar nerve G56.22
- Cushing's E24.9
- - alcohol-induced E24.4
- - drug-induced E24.2
- - pituitary-dependent E24.0
- - specified NEC E24.8
- dancing eyes, dancing feet G25.86
- Dandy–Walker Q03.1
- De Lange's Q87.12
- defibrination D65
- Denny-Brown D48.9† G13.01*
- dependence — *code to* F10–F19 with fourth character .2
- depersonalization–derealization F48
- Devic's G36.0
- dhat F48.81
- diencephalic E23.30
- Down's Q90.–

Syndrome — *continued*
- drug withdrawal, infant of dependent mother P96.1
- Duane's H50.8
- Dubin–Johnson E80.60
- Dubowitz' Q87.13
- dysarthria–clumsy hand I67.9† G46.71*
- dysequilibrium syndrome, congenital G11.06
- Eaton–Lambert G70.80
- – with neoplasm C80† G73.1*
- ectopic ACTH E24.3
- Edwards' Q91.3
- Ehlers–Danlos Q79.6
- Ekbom's G25.82
- epileptic (*see also* Epilepsy) G40.9
- – special G40.5
- Evans' D69.3
- facial pain
- – paroxysmal G50.0
- – specified NEC G44.85
- Fanconi(–de Toni)(–Debré) E72.04
- Farber's E75.25
- fatigue F48.0
- – postviral G93.3
- Fazio–Londe G12.110
- fetal
- – alcohol (dysmorphic) Q86.0
- – hydantoin Q86.1
- Fisher's G61.03
- flatback M40.3
- floppy baby, nonspecific P94.2
- Foville's
- – peduncular I67.9† G46.30*
- – pontine I67.9† G46.31*
- fragile X Q99.2
- frontal lobe F07.0
- Ganser's F44.80
- Gerstmann's, developmental F81.2
- Gerstmann–Straüssler–Scheinker A81.81
- Gilbert's E80.4
- Gilles de la Tourette's F95.2
- Goldenhar's Q87.03
- Goodpasture's M31.0
- Guillain–Barré G61.0
- Guyon's canal G56.23
- Goodpasture's M31.0
- headache NEC G44.8
- Heller's F84.3
- hemiparkinson–hemiatrophy G23.80
- Hermansky–Pudlak E70.34
- histiocytosis NEC D76.3
- HIV infection, acute B23.0
- Holmes–Adie G90.80
- Holt–Oram Q87.20
- Horner's G90.2
- hospital hopper F68.1
- Hunter's E76.1

Syndrome — *continued*
- Hurler–Scheie E76.01
- hydantoin, fetal Q86.1
- hyperkinetic F90.9
- hypermobility M35.7
- immobility (paraplegic) M62.3
- inappropriate secretion of antidiuretic hormone E22.2
- infant of diabetic mother P70.1
- – gestational P70.0
- iodine-deficiency, congenital (E00)
- irritable bowel K58.9
- – with diarrhoea K58.0
- jaw-winking Q07.82
- Joubert's G11.03
- Kanner's F84.0
- Kawasaki's M30.3
- Kearns–Sayre H49.8
- Kleine–Levin G47.84
- Klinefelter's Q98.4
- – karyotype 47,XXY Q98.0
- – male with
- – – karyotype 46,XX Q98.2
- – – more than two X chromosomes Q98.1
- Klippel–Feil Q76.1
- Klippel–Trénaunay–Weber Q87.21
- Korsakov's
- – alcohol- or drug-induced — *see* F10–F19 with fourth character .6
- – nonalcoholic F04
- lacunar I67.9† G46.7*
- – pseudobulbar I67.9† G46.73*
- – pure motor I67.9† G46.5*
- – pure sensory I67.9† G46.6*
- Lance–Adams G25.38
- Laudau–Kleffner F80.3
- Laurence–Moon(–Bardet)–Biedl Q87.81
- Lennox–Gastaut G40.44
- Leriche's I74.0
- Lermoyez' H81.30
- Lesch–Nyhan E79.1
- Lightwood–Albright N25.8
- limbic epilepsy personality F07.0
- lobotomy F07.0
- locked-in G96.82
- Louis–Bar G11.3
- Lowe's E72.00
- Maffucci's Q78.4
- malformation, congenital
- – due to exogenous cause NEC Q86.8
- – specified NEC, affecting multiple systems Q87.8
- malignant neuroleptic G21.0
- maltreatment T74.9
- – specified NEC T74.8
- Marchiafava-Bignami G37.1
- Marcus Gunn's Q07.82

Syndrome — *continued*
- swallowing, abnormal, non-REM-sleep-related G47.812
- tachycardia–bradycardia I49.5
- Takayasu's M31.4
- TAR Q87.25
- tarsal tunnel G57.5
- temperomandibular joint-pain-dysfunction K07.6
- testicular feminization E34.5
- thalamic I66.2† G46.21*
- thoracic outlet G54.0
- thrombocytopenia with absent radius Q87.25
- Tolosa–Hunt G44.850
- Tourette's F95.2
- toxic shock A48.3
- traumatic vasospastic T75.2
- Treacher Collins Q87.080
- Turner's Q96.–
- ulnar nerve cubital tunnel G56.22
- vasospastic, traumatic T75.2
- VATER Q87.26
- vertebro-basilar artery G45.0
- vertiginous H81.9
- vitreous, following cataract surgery H59.9
- von Hippel–Lindau Q85.82
- Wadia's G11.22
- Wallenberg I67.9† G46.32*
- Wardenburg–Klein E70.82
- wasting, resulting from HIV disease B22.2
- Waterhouse–Friderichsen A39.1† E35.1*
- Weaver's Q87.32
- Weber I67.9† G46.30*
- Werdnig–Hoffmann G12.0
- Wernicke's superior haemorrhagic polioencephalitis E51.2
- West's G40.40
- whistling face Q87.081
- withdrawal — *see* State, withdrawal
- Wolff–Hirschorn Q93.3
- Zellweger's Q87.82
- Zollinger–Ellison E16.8

Syphilis, syphilitic A53.9
- alopecia A51.3† L99.8*
- anal A51.1
- Argyll Robertson pupil A52.1† H58.0*
- asymptomatic A52.2

Syphilis, syphilitic — *continued*
- cardiovascular A52.0
- central nervous system A52.3
- congenital
- – early A50.2
- – – latent A50.1
- – – symptomatic A50.0
- – late A50.5
- – – encephalitis A50.4† G05.0*
- – – meningitis A50.4† G01*
- – – oculopathy A50.3
- – – polyneuropathy A50.4† G63.0*
- early A51.9
- – latent A51.5
- genital A51.0
- – gumma A52.3
- late
- – central nervous system A52.3
- – encephalitis A52.1† G05.0*
- – general paresis A52.1† G05.0*
- – latent A52.8
- – meningitis A52.1† G01*
- – optic atrophy A52.1† H48.0*
- – polyneuropathy A52.1† G63.0*
- – retrobulbar neuritis A52.1† H48.1*
- latent A53.0
- – early A51.5
- – late A52.8
- leukoderma A51.3† L99.8*
- mucous patch A51.3† L99.8*
- muscle A52.7† M63.0*
- parkinsonism A52.1† G22.–2*
- primary
- – anal A51.1
- – genital A51.1
- – specified site NEC
- secondary
- – meningitis A51.4† G01*
- – myositis A51.4† M63.0*
- – oculopathy NEC A51.4† H58.8*
- – skin and mucous membranes A51.3
- – specified site NEC A51.4
- symptomatic A52.1
- – late NEC A52.7

Syphiloma, central nervous system A52.3

Syringobulbia G95.0

Syringomyelia G95.0

Syringomyelocele Q05.*x*7

T

Thyroiditis — *continued*
- drug-induced E06.4
- Hashimoto's E06.3
- lymphocytic E06.3
Thyrotoxicosis E05.9
- factitia E05.4
- from ectopic thyroid tissue E05.3
- neonatal P72.1
- specified E05.8
- transient, with chronic thyroiditis E06.2
- with
- - diffuse goitre E05.0
- - multinodular goitre E05.2
- - single thyroid nodule E05.1
Tic (disorder) F95.9
- combined vocal and multiple motor F95.2
- douloureux G50.0
- drug-induced G25.60
- motor, chronic F95.1
- organic origin G25.61
- secondary G25.61
- specified NEC F95.8
- transient F95.0
- vocal, chronic F95.1
Tingling skin R20.2
Tinnitus H93.1
Tiredness R53
Titubation
- familial R25.00
- non-familial R25.01
Todd's paralysis (postepileptic) G83.80
Toe walking R26.24
Tolosa–Hunt syndrome G44.850
Torticollis M43.6
- congenital (sternomastoid) Q68.0
- psychogenic F45.8
- spasmodic G24.3
Tourette's syndrome F95.2
Toxic effect (*see also* Table of drugs and chemicals, page 565)
- reaction — *see* Reaction, toxic
- sequelae T97
Toxoplasmosis B58.–
- congenital P37.1
- pulmonary B58.3† J17.3*
Trachoma A71
- sequelae B94.0
Training (in)
- activities of daily living NEC Z50.8
- orthoptic Z50.6
Trait, personality, accentuation Z73.1
Trance F44.3
Translocation
- balanced Q95.–
- trisomy
- - 13 Q91.6
- - 18 Q91.2
- - 21 Q90.2
Trauma, acoustic H83.3
Travel sickness T75.3
Treacher Collins syndrome Q87.080
Tremor R25.1
- drug-induced G25.1
- dystonic G25.22
- essential G25.0
- hysterical F44.4
- intention G25.20
- isolated
- - facial G25.01
- - hand G25.03
- - head G25.00
- - rest G25.26
- - vocal G25.02
- kinetic G25.20
- midbrain G25.25
- multiple site G25.07
- orthostatic G25.23
- parkinsonian G20.–
- physiological G25.21
- specified NEC G25.2
- task-specific G25.24
Trichinellosis B75
Trichiniasis B75
Trigonocephaly Q75.03
Trimethylaminuria E88.81
Triploidy Q92.7
Trisomy
- autosomes Q92.9
- chromosome specified NEC Q92.8
- - partial
- - - major Q92.2
- - - minor Q92.3
- - whole
- - - meiotic nondisjunction Q92.0
- - - mitotic nondisjunction Q92.1
- - - mosaicism Q92.1
- 13
- - meiotic nondisjunction Q91.4
- - mitotic nondisjunction Q91.5
- - mosaicism Q91.5
- - translocation Q91.6
- 18
- - meiotic nondisjunction Q91.0
- - mitotic nondisjunction Q91.1
- - mosaicism Q91.1
- - translocation Q91.2
- 21 Q90.9
- - meiotic nondisjunction Q90.0
- - mitotic nondisjunction Q90.1
- - mosaicism Q90.1
- - translocation Q90.2
Tritanomaly H53.5
Tritanopia H53.5
Trypanosomiasis
- African B56.9
- American B57.2

U

Ulcer
- anastomotic K28.–
- aphthous, recurrent K12.0
- artery I77.2
- decubitus L89
- duodenal K26.–
- gastric K25.–
- gastrocolic K28.–
- gastroduodenal K27.–
- gastrointestinal K28.–
- gastrojejunal K28.–
- jejunal K28.–
- marginal K28.–
- oesophagus K22.1
- peptic K27.–
- plaster L89
- pressure L89
- postpyloric K26.–
- pylorus K25.–
- stomach K25.–
- stomal K28.–

Ulegyria Q04.81
Unconsciousness R40.2
Unhappiness R45.2
Unsteadiness on feet R26.8
Unverricht–Lundborg disease or epilepsy G40.37
Uraemia, uraemic N19
- chronic N18.–
- neuropathy N18.8
- newborn P96.0

Urticaria, giant T78.3
Use, harmful
- alcohol F10.1
- caffeine F15.1
- cannabinoids F12.1
- cocaine F14.1
- hallucinogens F16.1
- hypnotics F13.1
- multiple drugs F19.1
- opioids F11.1
- psychoactive substances NEC F19.1
- sedatives F13.1
- stimulants NEC F15.1
- tobacco F17.1
- volatile solvents F18.1

Uveitis, anterior H20.0

V

Vaginismus N94.2
Vaginitis, postmenopausal, atrophic N95.2
Valinaemia E71.14
Valvulitis
- chronic I38
- rheumatic
- - acute I01.1
- - chronic I09.1
Van Allen type amyloidosis E85.12
Van Bogaert–Scherer–Epstein disease E75.50
Van Bogaert's sclerosing leukoencephalopathy A81.1
Varicella B01.–
- congenital P35.8
- encephalitis B01.1† G05.1*
- encephalomyelitis B01.1† G05.1*
- meningitis B01.0† G02.0*
Varicose veins in pregnancy O22.0
Varix
- aneurysmal I77.0
- retinal H35.0
Vascular sheathing, retinal H35.0
Vasculitis
- allergic D69.0
- cryoglobulinaemic D89.10
- hypocomplementaemic M31.8
- retinal H35.0
Vasculopathy, necrotizing M31.9
- specified NEC M31.8
Vasovagal attack R55
VATER syndrome Q87.2
Venezuelan equine encephalitis virus disease A92.2
Ventriculitis (cerebral) G04.9
Verbosity, obscuring reason for contact R46.7
Vertebra, vertebral
- collapsed M48.5
- fracture — *see* Fracture, vertebra
- supernumerary, not associated with scoliosis (Q76)
Vertical talus Q66.8
Vertigo R42
- aural H81.31
- benign
Vertigo — *continued*
- benign — *continued*
- - paroxysmal H81.18
- - positional
- - - idiopathic H81.10
- - - post-traumatic H81.11
- central H81.48
- - drug-induced H81.41
- - positional, idiopathic H81.40
- childhood, benign paroxysmal G43
- drug-induced H81.90
- - central H81.41
- - peripheral H81.33
- epidemic A88.1
- infrasound T75.2
- Menière's H81.0
- otogenic H81.32
- peripheral H81.3
- - drug-induced H81.33
Vestige, branchial Q18.0
Vibration, effects T75.2
Violence, physical R45.6
Vision, visual
- colour, deficiency H53.5
- disturbance H53.9
- - specified NEC H53.8
- - subjective H53.1
- double H53.2
- field defect H53.4
- halos H53.1
- loss H54.7
- - both eyes H54.3
- - one eye H54.6
- low
- - both eyes H54.2
- - one eye H54.5
Volkmann's ischaemic contracture T79.6
Volume depletion E86
Vomiting R11
- in pregnancy, excessive O21.–
Von Economo–Cruchet disease A85.8
Von Gierke's disease E74.00
Von Hippel–Lindau syndrome Q85.82
Von Recklinghausen's disease Q85.0
- of bone E21.0
Von Willebrand's disease D68.0

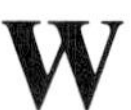

Wadia's syndrome G11.22
Waldenström's macroglobulinaemia C88.0
Wallenberg's syndrome I67.9† G46.32*
Wardenburg–Klein syndrome E70.82
Waterhouse–Friderichsen syndrome A39.1† E35.1*
Water
- deprivation T73.1
- pressure, effects T70.9
Weaver's syndrome Q87.32
Webbing of neck Q18.3
Weber–Christian disease M35.6
Weber's paralysis or syndrome I67.9† G46.30*
Wegener's granulomatosis M31.3
Weight
- gain, abnormal R63.5
- loss, abnormal R63.4
Weightlessness, effects T75.8
Wenckebach's block I44.1
Werdnig–Hoffmann disease or syndrome G12.0
Wernicke's
- developmental aphasia F80.2
- encephalopathy E51.2
- receptive aphasia R47.01
- superior haemorrhagic polioencephalitis syndrome E51.2
West's syndrome G40.40
Wheezing R06.2
Whiplash injury S13.43
Whipple's disease K90.8† M14.8*
Whistling face syndrome Q87.081
Whooping cough A37
Wilson's disease E83.01
Withdrawal
- state — *see* State, withdrawal
- symptoms, neonatal, from maternal use of drugs P96.1
Wolff–Hirschorn syndrome Q93.3
Wolman's disease E75.51
Word deafness F80.2
Worries R45.2
Wound, open T14.1
- cheek and temporomandibular area S01.4
- ear S01.3
- eyeball, penetrating S05.6
- - with foreign body S05.5
- eyelid and periocular area, open S01
- head S01.9
- - multiple S01.7
- - specified NEC S01.8
- lip S01.5
- neck S11
- - sequelae T91.0
- nose S01.2
- oral cavity S01.5
- scalp S01.0

X, Y, Z

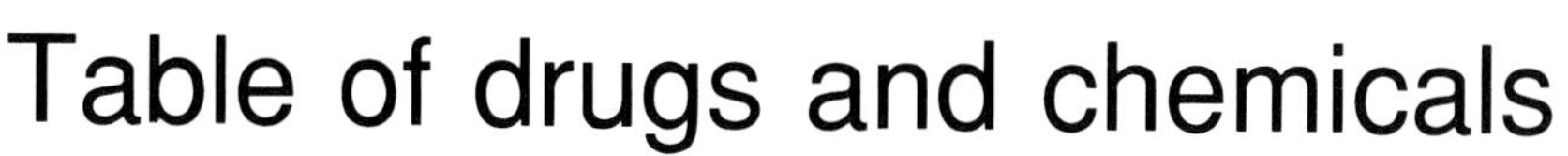

Table of drugs and chemicals

Substance	Poisoning		Adverse effect in therapeutic use
	Chapter XIX	Accidental	
Acetazolamide	T50.2	X44.–	Y54.2
Acid (corrosive) NEC	T54.2	X49.–	—
Acidifying agent NEC	T50.9	X44.–	Y43.5
Acrylamide	T65.81	X49.–	—
Adenohypophyseal hormone	T38.8	X44.–	Y42.8
Adhesive NEC	T52.8	X49.–	—
Adrenergic blocking agent NEC	T44.8	X43.–	Y51.8
α-Adrenoreceptor agonist NEC	T44.4	X43.–	Y51.4
α-Adrenoreceptor antagonist NEC	T44.6	X43.–	Y51.6
β-Adrenoreceptor agonist NEC	T44.5	X43.–	Y51.5
β-Adrenoreceptor antagonist NEC	T44.7	X43.–	Y51.7
Aerosol spray NEC	T59.–	X49.–	—
Aflatoxin	T64	X49.–	—
Alcohol			
– butyl	T51.3	X45.–	—
– deterrent NEC	T50.6	X44.–	Y57.3
– ethyl	T51.0	X45.–	—
– isopropyl	T51.2	X45.–	—
– methyl	T51.1	X45.–	—
– propyl	T51.3	X45.–	—
Aldosterone antagonist	T50.0	X44.–	Y54.1
Alkali (caustic)	T54.3	X49.–	—
Alkalizing agent NEC	T50.9	X44.–	Y43.5
Amantadine	T42.8	X41.–	Y46.7
Aminodarone	T45.30	X44.–	Y52.3
Aminoglycoside	T36.5	X44.–	Y40.5
4-Aminophenol derivatives	T39.1	X40.–	Y45.4
Aminophylline	T48.1	X44.–	Y55.6
Anabolic steroid (congener)	T38.7	X44.–	Y42.7
Anaesthetic, general	T41.2	X44.–	Y48.2
Anaesthetic, local	T41.3	X44.–	Y48.3
Analeptic NEC	T50.7	X44.–	Y48.4
Analgesic			
– nonopioid	T39.9	X40.–	Y43.3
– opioid	T40.2	X42.–	Y45.0
Androgen	T38.7	X44.–	Y42.7
Angiotensin converting enzyme inhibitor	T46.4	X44.–	Y52.4
Aniline (dye) (liquid)	T65.3	X49.–	—
Animals, venomous	T63.–	—	—
Anorexiant	T50.5	X44.–	Y57.0
Antacid NEC	T47.1	X44.–	Y53.1
Antagonist			
– aldosterone	T50.0	X44.–	Y54.1
– anticoagulant	T45.5	X44.–	Y44.3
– H_2 receptor	T47.0	X44.–	Y53.0
– mineralocorticoid	T50.0	X44.–	Y54.1
– opioid receptor	T50.7	X44.–	Y50.1
Anterior pituitary hormone NEC	T38.8	X44.–	Y42.8
Anthelminthic NEC	T37.4	X44.–	Y41.4
Antiadrenergic NEC	T44.9	X43.–	Y51.8
Antiallergic NEC	T45.0	X44.–	Y43.0
Anti-anaemia preparation NEC	T45.8	X44.–	Y44.0
Antiandrogen NEC	T38.6	X44.–	Y42.6

Substance	Poisoning		Adverse effect in therapeutic use
	Chapter XIX	Accidental	
Antianxiety drug NEC	T43.5	X41.–	Y47.9
Antiarteriosclerotic drug	T46.6	X44.–	Y52.6
Antiasthmatic drug NEC	T48.6	X44.–	Y55.6
Antibiotic	T36.9	X44.–	Y40.9
– antifungal, systemic	T36.7	X44.–	Y40.7
– antineoplastic	T45.1	X44.–	Y43.3
– local	T49.0	X44.–	Y56.0
Anticholinergic NEC	T44.3	X43.–	Y51.3
Anticholinesterase	T44.1	X43.–	Y51.0
Anticoagulant	T45.5	X44.–	Y44.2
Anticoagulant antagonist	T45.6	X44.–	Y44.3
Anti-common-cold drug NEC	T48.5	X44.–	Y55.3
Anticonvulsant NEC	T42.7	X41.–	Y46.6
Antidepressant	T43.2	X41.–	Y49.2
Antidiabetic NEC	T38.3	X44.–	Y42.3
Antidiarrhoeal drug NEC	T47.6	X44.–	Y53.6
Antidote NEC	T50.6	X44.–	Y57.2
– heavy metal	T45.8	X44.–	Y43.8
Antidysrhythmic NEC	T46.2	X44.–	Y52.2
Antiemetic	T45.0	X44.–	Y43.0
Antiepileptic	Y42.7	X41.–	Y46.6
Antiestrogen NEC	T38.6	X44.–	Y42.6
Antifungal			
– local NEC	T49.0	X44.–	Y56.0
– systemic	T36.7	X44.–	Y40.7
Anti-gastric-secretion drug NEC	T47.1	X44.–	Y53.1
Antigonadotrophin NEC	T38.6	X44.–	Y42.6
Antihyperlipidaemic	T46.6	X44.–	Y52.6
Antihypertensive drug NEC	T46.5	X44.–	Y52.5
Anti-infective			
– local	T49.0	X44.–	Y56.0
– systemic	T37.9	X44.–	Y41.9
Anti-inflammatory drug, nonsteroidal	T39.3	X40.–	Y45.3
– local NEC	T49.0	X44.–	Y56.0
Antimalarial	T37.2	X44.–	Y41.2
Antimuscarinic NEC	T44.3	X43.–	Y51.3
Antimycobacterial drug NEC	T37.1	X44.–	Y41.1
Antineoplastic NEC	T45.1	X44.–	Y43.3
Antiparasitic, systemic	T37.9	X44.–	Y41.9
Antiparkinsonism drug NEC	T42.8	X41.–	Y46.7
Antiprotozoal drug NEC	T37.3	X44.–	Y41.3
Antipruritic drug NEC	T49.1	X44.–	Y56.1
Antipsychotic drug NEC	T43.5	X41.–	Y49.3
Antipyretic NEC	T39.8	X40.–	Y45.9
Antirheumatic NEC	T39.4	X40.–	Y45.4
Antispasticity [antirigidity] drug NEC	T42.8	X41.–	Y46.8
Antithrombotic	T45.5	X44.–	Y44.4
Antithyroid drug NEC	T38.2	X44.–	Y42.2
Antitussive NEC	T48.3	X44.–	Y55.3
– codeine mixture (opiate)	T40.2	X42.–	Y45.0
Antivaricose drug	T46.8	X44.–	Y52.8
Antiviral drug NEC	T37.9	X44.–	Y41.5
Arsenic (compounds)	T57.0	X48.–	—
Astringent, local	T49.2	X44.–	Y56.2

Substance	Poisoning		Adverse effect in therapeutic use
	Chapter XIX	Accidental	
Barbiturate NEC	T42.3	X41.–	Y47.0
Benzenamine	T65.3	X49.–	—
Benzene (homologues)	T52.1	X46.–	—
– nitro- and amino-derivatives	T65.3	X49.–	—
Benzodiazepine NEC	T42.4	X44.–	Y47.1
Benzothiadiazine derivative	T50.2	X44.–	Y54.3
Beryllium (compounds)	T56.7	X49.–	—
Blood (product)	T45.8	X49.–	Y44.6
Bromine sedative	T42.6	X41.–	Y47.4
1-Butanol	T51.3	X45.–	—
Butyrophenone neuroleptic	T43.4	X41.–	Y49.4
Cadmium (compounds)	T56.3	X49.–	—
Caffeine	T43.6	X41.–	Y50.2
Calcium-channel blockers	T46.1	X44.–	Y52.1
Caloric agent	T50.7	X44.–	Y54.6
Cannabis (derivatives)	T40.7	X42.–	Y49.6
Carbamazepine	T42.1	X41.–	Y46.4
Carbon			
– dioxide	T59.7	X47.–	—
– monoxide	T58	X47.–	—
– tetrachloride	T53.0	X46.–	—
Carbonic anhydrase inhibitor NEC	T50.2	X47.–	Y54.2
Cardiac-stimulant glycoside	T46.0	X44.–	Y52.0
Cefalosporins	T36.1	X44.–	Y40.1
Chelating agent NEC	T50.6	X44.–	Y57.2
Chemical substance NEC	T65.8	X49.–	—
Chloral derivative	T42.6	X41.–	Y47.2
Chloramphenicol	T36.2	X44.–	Y40.2
Chlorofluorocarbons	T53.5	X46.–	—
Chloroquine	T37.2	X44.–	Y41.2
Cholinergic	T44.1	X43.–	Y51.1
Chromium (compounds)	T56.2	X49.–	—
Ciguatera fish [ciguatoxin]	T61.0	X49.–	—
Cinnarizine	T45.0	X44.–	Y43.0
Clioquinol	T37.81	X44.–	Y41.8
Clonidine	T46.5	X44.–	Y52.5
Cocaine	T40.5	X42.–	Y48.3
Codeine	T40.2	X42.–	Y45.0
Contraceptive (oral)	T38.4	X44.–	Y42.4
Contrast medium, X-ray	T50.8	X44.–	Y57.5
Copper (compounds)	T56.4	X49.–	—
Coronary vasodilators — *see* Vasodilator			
Corrosive substances	T54.9	X49.–	—
Cyanates	T65.00	X48.–	—
Cyanide	T65.0	X48.–	—
– hydrogen	T57.3	X48.–	—
Cyead	T62.201	X49.–	—
Cytarabine	T45.1	X44.–	Y43.1
Dapsone	T37.10	X44.–	Y41.1
Demulcent	T49.3	X44.–	Y56.3
Dental drug, topical application	T49.7	X44.–	Y56.7
Deoxybarbiturate	T42.3	X44.–	Y46.3

Substance	Poisoning		Adverse effect in therapeutic use
	Chapter XIX	Accidental	
Depressant, appetite [anorectic]	T50.5	X44.–	Y57.0
Detergent (local) (medicinal) NEC	T49.2	X44.–	Y56.2
– nonmedicinal	T55	X49.–	—
Diagnostic agent NEC	T50.8	X44.–	Y57.6
Digestant	T47.5	X44.–	Y53.5
Diltiazem	T46.1	X44.–	Y52.1
Dimethylaminopropionitrile	T65.821	X49.–	—
Dimethylbenzene	T52.2	X46.–	—
Dipyridamole	T46.31	X44.–	Y52.3
Diuretic	T50.2	X44.–	Y54.5
Dye NEC	T65.6	X49.–	—
Electrolytic agent	T50.3	X44.–	Y54.6
Emetic NEC	T47.7	X44.–	Y53.7
Emollient NEC	T49.3	X44.–	Y56.3
Enzyme NEC	T45.3	X44.–	Y43.6
Ergot alkaloid	T48.0	X44.–	Y55.0
Estrogen	T38.5	X44.–	Y42.5
Ethanol	T51.0	X45.–	—
Expectorant NEC	T48.4	X44.–	Y55.4
Fertilizer NEC	T65.8	X49.–	—
Fish	T61.2	X49.–	—
Flunarizine	T46.7	X44.–	Y52.7
Folic acid with ferrous salts	T45.2	X44.–	Y44.1
Foodstuffs	T62.9	X49.–	—
Fumes NEC	T59.9	X47.–	—
– metal — *see* specified metal			
Fungicide NEC	T60.3	X48.–	—
Fusel oil	T51.3	X45.–	—
Ganglionic blocking drug NEC	T44.2	X43.–	Y51.2
Garsava	T62.200	X49.–	—
Gas	T59.9	X47.–	—
– lacrimogenic [tear gas]	T59.3	X47.–	—
– motor (vehicle) exhaust	T58	X47.–	—
– therapeutic	T41.5	X44.–	Y48.5
– utility	T58	X47.–	—
Gasoline	T52.0	X46.–	—
Glucocorticosteroid NEC	T38.0	X44.–	Y42.0
– topically used	T49	X44.–	Y56
Glue NEC	T52.8	X49.–	—
Glycols	T52.3	X46.–	—
Glycoside, cardiac-stimulant	T46.0	X44.–	Y52.0
Guanethine	T46.5	X44.–	Y52.5
Hair treatment	T49.4	X44.–	Y56.4
Hallucinogen NEC	T40.9	X42.–	Y49.6
Herbicide NEC	T60.3	X48.–	—
Heroin	T40.1	X42.–	Y45.0
Hexacarbons NEC	T52.88	X46.–	—
N-Hexane	T52.80	X46.–	—
H_2 receptor antagonist	T47.0	X44.–	Y53.0

Substance	Poisoning		Adverse effect in therapeutic use
	Chapter XIX	Accidental	
Hormone and synthetic substitutes	T38.8	X44.–	Y42.8
– andronergic	T38.7	X44.–	Y42.7
– anterior pituitary	T38.8	X44.–	Y42.8
– antidiuretic	T38.8	X44.–	Y42.8
– cancer therapy	T45.1	X44.–	—
– glucocorticoids	T38.0	X44.–	Y42.0
– luteinizing	T38.8	X44.–	Y42.8
– ovarian	T38.5	X44.–	Y42.8
– oxytocic drugs	T48.0	X44.–	Y55.0
– parathyroid and derivative	T50.9	X44.–	Y54.7
– pituitary (posterior) NEC	T38.8	X44.–	Y42.8
– thyroid and substitute NEC	T38.1	X44.–	Y42.1
Hydantoin derivative	T42.0	X41.–	Y46.2
Hydrocarbon, halogenated	T53.9	X46.–	—
Hydrogen cyanide	T57.3	X49.–	—
Hydroxyquinoline derivative	T37.80	X44.–	Y41.8
Hypnotic NEC	T42.6	X41.–	Y47.9
Hypoglycaemic [antidiabetic]	T38.3	X44.–	Y42.3
β,β′-Iminodipropionitrile	T65.820	X49.–	—
Immunoglobulin	T50.9	X44.–	Y59.3
Immunosuppressive drug	T45.1	X44.–	Y43.4
Inhibitor			
– angiotensin-converting-enzyme	T46.4	X44.–	Y52.4
– carbonic-anhydrase	T50.2	X44.–	Y54.2
– monoamine-oxidase	T43.1	X41.–	Y49.1
– platelet-aggregation	T45.5	X44.–	Y44.4
Inorganic substances NEC	T57.8	X49.–	—
Insecticide	T60.2	X48.–	—
Insulin	T38.3	X44.–	Y42.3
Intestinal			
– atonia drug	T47.4	X44.–	Y53.4
– motility control drug	T47.6	X44.–	Y53.6
Iron preparation	T45.5	X44.–	Y44.0
Keratolytic drug NEC	T49.4	X44.–	Y56.4
Keratoplastic NEC	T49.4	X44.–	Y56.4
Kerosene	T52.0	X46.–	—
Ketone oils	T52.4	X46.–	—
Lacrimogenic gas	T59.3	X47.–	—
Lathyrus sativus	T62.210	X49.–	—
Laxative NEC	T47.4	X44.–	Y53.4
Lead (compounds)	T56.0	X49.–	—
Lipotropic drug NEC	T50.9	X44.–	Y57.1
Lithium salts (carbonate)	T43.5	X41.–	Y49.5
Lysergide [LSD]	T40.8	X42.–	Y49.6
Macrolide, antibiotic	T36.3	X44.–	Y40.3
Manganese (compounds)	T57.2	X49.–	—
– medicinal	T50.9	X44.–	Y54.9
Medicament NEC	T50.9	X44.–	Y57.9
Mercury (compounds)	T56.1	X49.–	—

Substance	Poisoning		Adverse effect in therapeutic use
	Chapter XIX	Accidental	
Mescaline	T40.90	X42.–	Y49.6
Metals	T56.9	X49.–	—
Metaraminol	T44.4	X43.–	Y51.4
Methadone	T40.3	X42.–	Y45.0
Methanol	T51.1	X45.–	—
Methaqualone (compound)	T42.6	X41.–	Y47.8
Methylbenzene	T52.2	X46.–	—
Methyl isobutyl ketone	T52.4	X46.–	—
Mineralocorticoids	T50.0	X44.–	Y54.0
Mineral salts NEC	T50.3	X44.–	Y54.9
Morphine	T40.2	X42.–	Y45.0
– antagonist	T50.7	X44.–	Y50.1
MPTP	T40.94	X42.–	Y49.8
Mycotoxins	T64	X49.–	—
Narcotic	T40.9	X42.–	Y49.9
Neuroleptic drug NEC	T43.5	X41.–	Y49.5
Neuromuscular blocking drug	T48.1	X44.–	Y55.1
Nicotine	T65.2	X49.–	—
Nicotinic acid (derivatives)	T46.7	X44.–	Y52.7
Nitrobenzene	T65.3	X49.–	—
Nitrogen oxide	T59.0	X47.–	—
Nitrous oxide	T41.00	X44.–	Y48.0
NSAID	T39.3	X40.–	Y45.3
Nuts	T62.20	X49.–	—
Ophthalmological (topical)	T49.5	X44.–	Y56.5
Opiate NEC	T40.6	X42.–	Y45.0
Opium (alkaloids)	T40.0	X42.–	Y45.0
Organophosphorus compound	T65.80	X49.–	—
Otorhinolaryngological	T49.6	X44.–	Y56.6
Oxytocic drugs	T48.0	X44.–	Y55.0
Paint NEC	T65.6	X49.–	—
Papaverine	T44.3	X43.–	Y51.3
Paraffin oil or wax	T52.0	X46.–	—
Paraldehyde	T42.6	X41.–	Y47.3
Parasympatholytic NEC	T44.3	X43.–	Y51.3
Parasympathomimetic	T44.1	X43.–	Y51.1
Parathyroid hormones (derivatives)	T50.9	X44.–	Y54.7
Penicillin	T36.0	X44.–	Y40.0
Perhexiline	T46.50	X44.–	Y52.3
Pesticide	T60.8	X48.–	—
Pethidine	T40.4	X42.–	Y45.0
Petroleum products NEC	T52.0	X46.–	—
Pharmaceutical excipient NEC	T50.9	X44.–	Y57.4
Phencyclidine	T40.93	X42.–	Y48.8
Phenothiazine antipsychotics and neuroleptics	T43.3	X41.–	Y49.3
Phosphorus (compounds)	T57.1	X49.–	—
Plant food	T62.2	X49.–	—
Plasma substitutes	T45.8	X44.–	Y44.7
Polyester fumes	T59.80	X47.–	—

Substance	Poisoning		Adverse effect in therapeutic use
	Chapter XIX	Accidental	
Preservative, wood	T60.–	X48.–	—
Progestogen NEC	T38.5	X44.–	Y42.5
1-Propanol	T51.3	X45.–	—
2-Propanol	T51.2	X45.–	—
Propionitrile	T65.82	X49.–	—
Protectant	T49.3	X44.–	Y56.3
Psilocin	T40.91	X42.–	Y49.6
Psilocybin	T40.92	X42.–	Y49.6
Psychodysleptic [hallucinogen] NEC	T40.9	X42.–	Y49.6
Psychostimulant (with abuse potential)	T43.6	X41.–	Y49.7
Psychotropic drug NEC	T43.9	X41.–	Y49.8
Pyrazolone derivative	T39.2	X40.–	Y45.8
Pyrethroids	T60.20	X48.–	—
Rauwolfia (alkaloids)	T46.5	X44.–	Y52.5
Rehydration salts (oral)	T50.3	X44.–	Y54.6
Relaxant, skeletal muscle [neuromuscular blocking agent]	T48.1	X44.–	Y55.1
Reserpine	T46.5	X44.–	Y52.5
Rifamycin	T36.6	X44.–	Y40.6
Rodenticide NEC	T60.4	X48.–	—
Salbutamol	T48.6	X44.–	Y55.6
Salicylate NEC	T39.0	X40.–	Y45.1
Salt, oral rehydration	T50.3	X44.–	Y54.6
Seafood, noxious	T61.9	X49.–	—
Sedative NEC	T42.7	X41.–	Y47.8
Seeds, poisonous	T62.8	X49.–	—
Sleeping draught, pill	T42.7	X41.–	Y47.9
Soap	T55	X49.–	—
Solvent, organic	T52.8	X46.–	—
Spasmolytic (autonomic nervous system)	T44.3	X43.–	Y51.3
Spermicide	T49.8	X44.–	Y56.8
Stimulant (central nervous system)	T50.9	X44.–	Y50.9
Streptomycin	T36.5	X44.–	Y40.5
Strychnine (salts)	T65.1	X48.–	—
Succinimide	T42.2	X41.–	Y46.0
Sulfonamide NEC	T37.0	X44.–	Y41.0
Sulfur dioxide	T59.1	X47.–	—
Sympatholytic NEC	T44.8	X43.–	Y51.8
Sympathomimetic NEC	T44.9	X43.–	Y51.9
Systemic drug	T45.9	X44.–	Y43.9
Tamoxifen	T38.6	X44.–	Y42.6
Tear gas	T59.3	X47.–	—
Tetrabenazine	T43.5	X41.–	Y49.5
Tetrachloromethane	T53.0	X46.–	—
Tetracycline	T36.4	X44.–	Y40.4
Theobromine	T48.6	X44.–	Y55.6
Theophylline	T48.6	X44.–	Y55.6
Thiobarbiturate anaesthetic	T41.1	X44.–	Y48.1
Thioxanthene neuroleptic	T43.4	X41.–	Y49.4
Thrombolytic	T45.5	X44.–	Y44.5

Substance	Poisoning		Adverse effect in therapeutic use
	Chapter XIX	Accidental	
Thylene oxide	T59.81	X47.–	—
Thyroid hormone (and substitutes)	T38.1	X44.–	Y42.1
Tin (compounds)	T56.6	X49.–	—
Tobacco NEC	T65.2	X49.–	—
Toluene	T52.2	X46.–	—
– diisocyanate	T65.00	X49.–	—
Topical agent NEC	T49.9	X44.–	Y56.9
Tranquillizer NEC	T42.4	X41.–	Y49.5
Trinitrotoluene	T65.3	X49.–	—
Uric acid metabolism drug NEC	T50.4	X44.–	Y54.8
Vaccine NEC	T50.9	X44.–	Y59.9
– bacterial	T50.9	X44.–	Y58.9
– – mixed	T50.9	X44.–	Y58.8
– BCG	T50.9	X44.–	Y58.0
– cholera	T50.9	X44.–	Y58.2
– diphtheria	T50.9	X44.–	Y58.5
– pertussis	T50.9	X44.–	Y58.6
– plague	T50.9	X44.–	Y58.3
– protozoal	T50.9	X44.–	Y59.2
– rickettsial NEC	T50.9	X44.–	Y59.1
– tetanus	T50.9	X44.–	Y58.4
– typhoid and paratyphoid	T50.9	X44.–	Y58.1
– viral NEC	T50.9	X44.–	Y59.9
– yellow fever	T50.9	X44.–	Y59.0
Valproic acid	T42.6	X41.–	Y46.5
Vapour NEC (*see also* Gas)	T59.9	X46.–	—
Vasodilator, peripheral	T46.3	X44.–	Y52.7
Vitamin NEC	T45.2	X44.–	Y57.7
– B_{12}	T45.2	X44.–	Y44.1
– D group	T45.2	X44.–	Y54.7
– K	T45.7	X44.–	Y44.3
Water balance drug	T50.3	X44.–	Y54.6
Wood preservative	T60.9	X47.–	—
Xylene	T52.2	X46.–	—
Zinc (compounds)	T56.5	X49.–	—